Advances in
Equine Upper Respiratory Surgery

Advances in
Equine Upper Respiratory Surgery

Edited by

Jan Hawkins, DVM, DACVS
Department of Veterinary Clinical Sciences
Purdue University
Indiana, USA

WILEY Blackwell

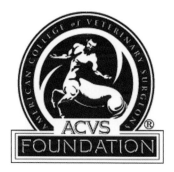

This work is a co-publication between the American College of Veterinary Surgeons Foundation and Wiley-Blackwell.

Library of Congress Cataloging-in-Publication Data

Advances in equine upper respiratory surgery / editor, Jan Hawkins.
      p.; cm.
   Includes index.
   Summary: Advances in equine upper Respiratory surgery is a comprehensive, up-to-date reference on surgical techniques in the upper respiratory tract in the horse, presenting theory and background as well as detailed procedures information.
   ISBN 978-0-470-95960-2 (cloth)
   I. Hawkins, Jan, editor.
   [DNLM: 1. Horse Diseases–surgery. 2. Respiratory Tract Diseases–veterinary. 3. Respiratory Tract Diseases–surgery. 4. Surgery, Veterinary–methods. 5. Surgical Procedures, Operative–veterinary. SF 959.R47]
   SF959.R47
   636.1'0897542–dc23
                                                                                      2014022277

A catalogue record for this book is available from the British Library.

Wiley also publishes its books in a variety of electronic formats. Some content that appears in print may not be available in electronic books.

Set in 9.5/11.5pt Palatino by Aptara Inc., New Delhi, India
Printed and bound in Singapore by Markono Print Media Pte Ltd

1 2015

Contents

Contributors

Benjamin J. Ahern, BVSc (Hons 1) MACVSc,
DACVSMR, DACVS
Surgeon, Randwick Equine Centre
Randwick, NSW, Australia

Warren Beard, DVM, MS, DACVS
Professor, Equine Surgery
Kansas State University
Manhattan, KS, USA

Heather Chalmers, DVM, PhD, DACVR
Assistant Professor, Radiology
Ontario Veterinary College, University of Guelph
Guelph, ON, Canada

Jonathan Cheetham, VetMB, PhD, DACVS
Principal Research Scientist and Equine Surgeon
Cornell College of Veterinary Medicine
Ithaca, NY, USA

Elizabeth Davidson, DVM, DACVS, DACVSMR
Associate Professor of Sports Medicine
New Bolton Center, University of Pennsylvania
Philadelphia, PA, USA

Thomas J. Divers, DVM, DACVIM, DACVEEC
Steffen Professor of Veterinary Medicine
Section Chief, Section of Large Animal Medicine
Cornell University
College of Veterinary Medicine
Ithaca, NY

Padraic M. Dixon, MVB, PhD, MRCVS, Dip EVDC
(Equine)
Professor, Equine Surgery
The Royal (Dick) School of Veterinary Studies
The University of Edinburgh
Midlothian, Scotland, UK

Norm G. Ducharme, DVM, MSc, DACVS
James Law Professor of Surgery
Section of Large Animal Surgery and Medical
    Director
Equine and Farm Animal Hospitals, Cornell
    University
Ithaca, NY, USA

David E. Freeman, MVB, MRCVS, PhD, DACVS
Professor
Large Animal Surgery Service Chief
Director, Island Whirl Equine Colic Research
    Laboratory
Large Animal Clinical Sciences
Gainesville, FL, USA

Katherine Garrett, DVM, DACVS
Associate, Diagnostic Imaging Director
Rood and Riddle Equine Hospital
Lexington, KY, USA

Catherine H. Hackett, DVM, PhD, DACVS-LA
Surgeon and Owner
Primus Equine Veterinary Surgery, PLLC
Ithaca, NY, USA

Jan Hawkins, DVM, DACVS
Section Head, Large Animal Surgery
Associate Professor of Large Animal
Surgery Department of Veterinary Clinical
  Sciences, Purdue University
West Lafayette, IN, USA

Daniel F. Hogan, DVM, DACVIM-Cardiology
Associate Professor, Cardiology
Chief, Comparative Cardiovascular Medicine and
  Interventional Cardiology
Department of Veterinary Clinical Sciences
Purdue University College of Veterinary Medicine
West Lafayette, IN, USA

Patricia Hogan, VMD, DACVS
Surgeon and Owner
Hogan Equine at Fair Winds Farm
Cream Ridge, NJ, USA

Nita Irby, DVM, DACVO
Senior Lecturer, Ophthalmology
Foundation Course Leader - Block V
Cornell University
College of Veterinary Medicine
Ithaca, NY

Eric J. Parente, DVM, DACVS
Professor of Surgery
New Bolton Center, University of Pennsylvania
Philadelphia, PA, USA

Justin Perkins, BVetMed, MS, CertES, DECVS,
MRCVS
Senior Lecturer
Department of Clinical Sciences and Services
The Royal Veterinary College

Hawkshead Lane
North Mymms
Hatfield
Hertfordshire
AL9 7TA
United Kingdom

Peter C. Rakestraw, MA, VMD, DACVS
Surgeon
Dayton, WY, USA

Michael W. Ross, DVM, DACVS
Professor of Surgery
Department of Clinical Studies, New Bolton
  Center
University of Pennsylvania
Philadelphia, PA, USA

Jim Schumacher, DVM, MS, DACVS
Professor
Department of Large Animal Clinical Sciences
University of Tennessee
Knoxville, TN, USA

Katie J. Smith, BVetMed, MSc, DACVS,
MRCVS
University Equine Surgeon
Cambridge Equine Hospital
Department of Veterinary Medicine
University of Cambridge
Cambridge, UK

Lloyd P. Tate, Jr., VMD, DACVS, ABLSM
Professor, Equine Surgery
College of Veterinary Medicine
North Carolina State University
Raleigh, NC, USA

Foreword

The American College of Veterinary Surgeons (ACVS) Foundation is excited to present *Advances in Equine Upper Respiratory Surgery* in the book series entitled *Advances in Veterinary Surgery*. The ACVS Foundation is an independently charted philanthropic organization devoted to advancing the charitable, educational, and scientific goals of the ACVS. Founded in 1965, the ACVS sets the standards for the specialty of veterinary surgery. The ACVS, which is approved by the American Veterinary Medical Association, administers the board certification process for diplomates in veterinary surgery and advances veterinary surgery and education. One of the principal goals of the ACVS Foundation is to foster the advancement of the art and science of veterinary surgery. The Foundation achieves these goals by supporting investigations in the diagnosis and treatment of surgical diseases; increasing educational opportunities for surgeons, surgical residents, and veterinary practitioners; improving surgical training of residents and veterinary students; and bettering animal patients' care, treatment, and welfare. This collaboration with Wiley-Blackwell will benefit all who are interested in veterinary surgery by presenting the latest evidence-based information on a particular surgical topic.

Advances in Equine Upper Respiratory Surgery is edited by Dr. Jan Hawkins, a diplomate of the ACVS and a prominent surgeon in the field of equine upper respiratory surgery. Dr. Hawkins has assembled many of the leaders in this field with state-of-the-art presentations on disorders and treatments of the larynx, soft palette, guttural pouch, and trachea. The ACVS Foundation is proud to partner with Wiley-Blackwell in this important series and is honored to present this book in the series.

—Mark D. Markel
Chair, Board of Trustees
ACVS Foundation

Section I

Recurrent Laryngeal Neuropathy

1 Recurrent Laryngeal Neuropathy: Grading of Recurrent Laryngeal Neuropathy

Katie J. Smith and Padraic M. Dixon

Introduction

Equine recurrent laryngeal neuropathy (RLN) has long been recognized in larger breeds of horses as a cause of laryngeal airway obstruction with production of abnormal respiratory noise during work and with variable levels of reduced athletic performance (Christley et al. 1997; Dixon et al. 2001; Marks et al. 1970; Morris and Seeherman 1990). The characterization and subjective evaluation of the degree of RLN present in affected horses has been the subject of much debate. Methods employed in the assessment of laryngeal function include listening to the horse's respiratory noise during exercise, palpation of the muscular process of the arytenoid cartilage to assess laryngeal muscle atrophy, and digital, endoscopic and electromyographic assessment of the laryngeal adductor reflex, laryngeal ultrasonography, and endoscopy, the latter of which has been the most commonly used technique for the past three decades.

Experienced clinicians can detect specific abnormal noise caused by RLN and subjectively assess the grade of RLN by noting the stage of exercise when the noise begins and by assessing the loudness and nature of any noise produced. In general, horses with milder degrees of RLN make more musical inspiratory "whistling" noises while more severely affected horses make harsher inspiratory and later biphasic noises, and do so after minimal work. However, there is no objective data on these correlations. Furthermore, fitter horses will make less noise than an unfit horse with a similar degree of RLN and some horses with endoscopically demonstrable low-grade RLN do not make any audible noise during exercise. Spectrum analysis of respiratory sounds recorded in exercising horses with a normal laryngeal endoscopic appearance and in horses with induced laryngeal hemiplegia has revealed unique patterns for RLN, characterized by specific frequency bands of inspiratory sounds (Cable et al. 2002; Derksen et al. 2001). However, the sensitivity and specificity of sound spectrograms (83% and 75%, respectively) indicate insufficient reliability to be used alone in dynamic investigation of upper airway abnormalities.

Palpation of the muscular process of the arytenoid can be used to detect cricoarytenoideus dorsalis muscle atrophy. The muscular process of the arytenoid on the affected side is discernibly more

Advances in Equine Upper Respiratory Surgery, First Edition. Edited by Jan Hawkins.
© 2015 ACVS Foundation. Published 2015 by John Wiley & Sons, Inc.

prominent than the unaffected contralateral cartilage in cases with notable muscle atrophy. This test may be of use in horses with severe RLN that have gross muscle wasting, but is less reliable in the earlier stages of disease as lower grades of atrophy are commonly palpable in many large, clinically normal horses that have subclinical RLN. Laryngeal palpation is also less accurate in heavily muscled horses such as draft horses and ponies.

The laryngeal adductor reflex ("thoracolaryngeal or slap test") has been used to assess laryngeal adductor function. The absence of a rapid arytenoid adduction movement following slapping the contralateral saddle area assessed endoscopically or via palpation of the larynx can be attributable in some cases to disruption of the adductory component of the recurrent laryngeal nerve. However, this test has fallen out of favor due to its lack of reliability (Newton-Clarke et al. 1994). An electromyographic technique to evaluate the duration of this reflex (comparing the left and right sides of the larynx) also held great promise (Cook and Thalhammer 1991), until it was shown that normal horses have a slower reflex on the left side, likely due the longer left recurrent laryngeal nerve (Hawe et al. 2001).

Ultrasonography has been used in laryngeal investigations (see Chapter 3) by assessing laryngeal adductor muscle atrophy and laryngeal dysplasia (Garrett et al. 2011). Although laryngeal adductor atrophy occurs ahead of abductor atrophy and this assessment has potential, there is little objective data on its value in grading the severity of RLN.

Resting endoscopic grading

Resting endoscopic assessment is currently the most common technique used to evaluate laryngeal function and indeed forms the mainstay of all upper airway assessments. Endoscopy to assess laryngeal function must be performed in unsedated horses (with the use of a twitch for restraint if necessary). There is a widespread consensus to use the right nasal passage when endoscopically assessing the larynx due to a purported reduction in artifactual changes in left cartilage movement and positioning, although this has not been substantiated scientifically. The endoscope is inserted via the right ventral meatus and positioned midline in the nasopharynx. Arytenoid symmetry and synchrony are observed during quiet breathing, following swallowing (induced by trans-endoscopic laryngeal flushing) and during transient nostril occlusion to induce maximal abduction.

Despite the common use of resting laryngeal endoscopy, limited agreement between authors resulted in the development of multiple different grading systems, including the widely used four-grade system of Hackett and Ducharme (Hackett et al. 1991), the five-grade system of Lane (Lane et al. 2006), and the six-grade system of Dixon et al. (Dixon et al. 2001). In 2003, an international panel of specialists reviewed the existing laryngeal grading systems and developed a consensus system of resting laryngeal grading known as the Havemeyer grading system comprising four main grades (Robinson 2004). The Havemeyer grading system essentially uses the four-grade system of Hackett and Ducharme (Hackett et al. 1991) but with grades 2 and 3 divided into subgrades (Table 1.1) (Robinson 2004). The three subgrades of grade 3 in the Havemeyer system are equivalent to grades 2, 3, and 4 of the system of Dixon et al. (Dixon et al. 2001).

An important disadvantage of all resting endoscopic grading systems is the use of a static system to characterize a dynamic process where an infinite range of movements is possible. Specifically, there has been controversy regarding the clinical significance of various forms of asynchrony and/or asymmetry, predominantly of the Havemeyer laryngeal function grades 2 and 3.1. However, a general consensus is that the inability to achieve full abduction of the affected arytenoid cartilage during resting examination is likely to be associated with compromised respiratory function during exercise. In addition, experienced clinicians anecdotally concur that laryngeal asymmetry at end exhalation and asynchronous arytenoid movement during inhalation are not causes for concern if horses can attain and *maintain* full bilateral arytenoid abduction after swallowing or nasal occlusion.

Incomplete laryngeal abduction at rest was once viewed as equivocal in terms of its ability to accurately predict dynamic laryngeal function (Hackett et al. 1991; Hammer et al. 1998; Lane et al. 2006). This is attributable to the fact that in the four-grade system of Hackett and Ducharme (Hackett et al.

Table 1.1   Havemeyer grading system of laryngeal function in the standing unsedated horse[a]

Grade character	Description	Sub-grade
1	All arytenoid cartilage movements are synchronous and symmetrical and full arytenoid cartilage abduction can be achieved and maintained.	
2	Arytenoid cartilage movements are asynchronous and/or larynx is asymmetric at times but full arytenoid cartilage abduction can be achieved and maintained.	2.1 Transient asynchrony, flutter, or delayed movements are seen. 2.2 There is asymmetry of the rima glottidis much of the time due to reduced mobility of the affected arytenoid and vocal fold but there are occasions, typically after swallowing or nasal occlusion when full symmetrical abduction is achieved and maintained.
3	Arytenoid cartilage movements are asynchronous and/or asymmetric. Full arytenoid cartilage abduction cannot be achieved and maintained.	3.1 There is asymmetry of the rima glottidis much of the time due to reduced mobility of the arytenoid and vocal fold but there are occasions, typically after swallowing or nasal occlusion, when full symmetrical abduction is achieved but not maintained. 3.2 Obvious arytenoid abductor deficit and arytenoid asymmetry. Full abduction is never achieved. 3.3 Marked but not total arytenoid abductor deficit and asymmetry with little arytenoid movement. Full abduction is never achieved
4	Complete immobility of the arytenoid cartilage and vocal fold.	

[a]Description generally refers to the left arytenoid cartilage in reference to the right. However, this grading system can apply to the right side.

1991) (where grade 3 was not subdivided), did not sufficiently differentiate between horses not able to attain and maintain full arytenoid abduction. Thus, horses with slight asymmetry but able to achieve full arytenoid abduction were in the same category as those with marked asymmetry and incapable of attaining even moderate arytenoid abduction. Therefore, the addition of subgrades to grade 3 was advantageous in differentiating horses with varying degrees of asymmetry in order to accurately predict dynamic laryngeal function. Importantly, research correlating resting and exercising laryngeal endoscopy (Barakzai and Dixon 2011) has documented a statistical correlation between grades of (resting) Havemeyer laryngeal function grades and laryngeal function during exercise. These authors showed a significant correlation between the four main Havemeyer grades of laryngeal function at rest and laryngeal function at exercise. Notably, there was also significant correlation between resting subgrades 3.1, 3.2, and 3.3 and exercising grades of laryngeal function, validating the Havemeyer system for endoscopically evaluating horses at rest. The Havemeyer grades have been correlated with

severity of histological abnormalities of the intrinsic laryngeal musculature (Collins et al. 2009). Correlations of the Havemeyer grades 2.1 and 2.2 with dynamic endoscopic grades have yet to be published.

One of the postulated disadvantages of using a more complex seven-grade/subgrade system as opposed to the previous four-grade system is the potential for variability during examinations. Significant inter- and intra-observer variability could introduce errors, which could have notable consequences in presale examinations or on decisions concerning laryngeal surgery. The observer variability and inter-horse repeatability using the Havemeyer grading system have been critically assessed (Perkins et al. 2009) and showed that reliability is high when experienced veterinarians conducted the endoscopic examinations. Importantly, there was moderate daily horse variability, which might suggest that results of endoscopy performed on a single day should be interpreted with caution. In addition, it has been recognized that there is a progressive deterioration of resting laryngeal function in approximately 12–15% of RLN-affected horses (Anderson et al. 1997; Davidson et al. 2007; Dixon et al. 2002).

Predictive value of resting laryngeal function

The sale of weanlings as training or resale prospects has prompted much evaluation of upper airway endoscopy in foals to determine if it can predict future racing performance. Major congenital abnormalities, including cleft soft palate, pharyngeal and subepiglottic cysts or laryngeal dysplasias, including branchial arch defects, will logically affect future athletic ability, unless they can be treated. Conversely, assessing laryngeal function in weanlings has been shown to be an unreliable predictor of laryngeal function as yearlings (Lane 2003).

In contrast to the unreliability of laryngeal endoscopic grading of foals, endoscopy in yearlings has shown more reliability as a predictive indicator of future performance (Garrett et al. 2010). In that study, a modified Havemeyer scale was employed, comprising grade 1, 2.1, 2.2, 3 (without subdividing grade 3), and 4. Analysis of the race records of horses at 2–4 years of age revealed that yearlings with grade 2.2 had fewer earnings than those with grade 1 or 2.1. A grade-3 laryngeal appearance was associated with fewer starts and less earnings at 3 and 4 years of age.

Dynamic grading

Laryngeal endoscopy during strenuous exercise (see Chapter 2) is the gold standard for assessing laryngeal function and is increasingly performed in the investigation of upper respiratory noise or poor performance using high-speed treadmill exercise at specialist referral centers and/or by overground endoscopy (Desmaizieres et al. 2009; Pollock et al. 2009). The subjective laryngeal function grading system used for dynamic laryngeal examinations is much simpler than that used for resting laryngeal evaluations (Table 1.2; Figure 1.1) (Robinson 2004) and has been altered little from the initial grading system suggested by Rakestraw (Rakestraw et al. 1991). Although studies have documented some variation between treadmill and field exercise, it remains unclear to what extent that incremental treadmill examination replicates racing conditions

Table 1.2   Grading system of laryngeal function as assessed in the horse during exercise[a]

Grade	Description
A	Full abduction of the arytenoid during inspiration
B	Partial abduction of the affected arytenoid cartilage (between resting position and full abduction)
C	Abduction less than resting position, including collapse into the contralateral half of the rima glottidis during inspiration

[a]Description generally refers to the left arytenoid cartilage in reference to the right. However, this grading system can apply to the right side.

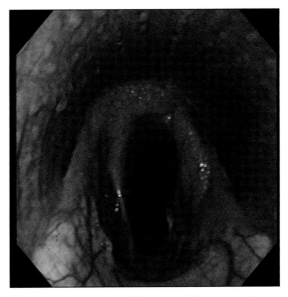

Figure 1.1   Collapse of the left arytenoid during exercise (Grade C).

in the Thoroughbred or Standardbred racehorse. An investigation into the comparison of overground versus high-speed treadmill endoscopy concluded that there was no difference in the prevalence of dynamic laryngeal disorders between the two techniques (Allen and Franklin 2010).

Post-laryngoplasty abduction grading

A grading system subjectively describing arytenoid positioning after laryngoplasty into five grades was

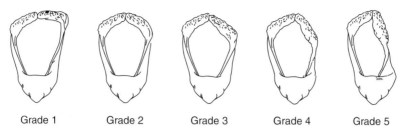

Grade 1   Grade 2   Grade 3   Grade 4   Grade 5

Figure 1.2   Grading of laryngoplasty abduction using five-grade system of Dixon et al. (2003).

Table 1.3   Postoperative grade of laryngeal position[a]

Grade	Description
1	Excessive abduction, that is, the affected arytenoid is close to or at maximal abduction (axial aspect of arytenoid at *circa* 80–90° to sagittal plane); hyperabducted with the apex of the corniculate process displaced beyond the midline, toward the normal side of the larynx
2	A high degree of arytenoid abduction (arytenoid at *circa* 50–80° to the sagittal plane), i.e., less than complete abduction
3	A moderate degree of arytenoid abduction (arytenoid at *circa* 45° to sagittal plane)
4	A slight degree of arytenoid abduction, that is, arytenoid is slightly more abducted than the normal resting position
5	No detectable arytenoid abduction

[a]Description generally refers to the left arytenoid cartilage in reference to the right. However, this grading system can apply to the right side.

described in 2003 (Table 1.3; Figure 1.2) (Dixon et al. 2003). Using this system, the degree of arytenoid abduction was assessed on day 1, day 7, and 6 weeks after surgery, showing significant loss of abduction in most horses in the 6 weeks following surgery. The presence of postoperative dysphagia and coughing correlated significantly with the degree of abduction, indicating that excessive (grade 1) abduction should be avoided.

In a further study, postoperative race performance was assessed in relation to the degree of surgical abduction obtained using the above five-grade laryngoplasty abduction system (Barakzai 2009). The findings indicated that horses with excessive abduction (grade 1) were significantly more likely to lose abduction by day 6 after surgery than horses with moderate (grade 3) abduction. Importantly, the postoperative grade of abduction

was not significantly correlated with markers of racing performance in National Hunt racehorses (Barakzai et al. 2009). However, there were very few cases with poor (grade 4 or 5) abduction included so conclusions regarding performance in such horses cannot be drawn.

References

Allen KJ, Franklin SH. 2010. Comparisons of overground endoscopy and treadmill endoscopy in UK Thoroughbred racehorses. *Equine Veterinary Journal* 42(3):186–191.

Anderson BH, Kannegieter NJ, Goulden BE. 1997. Endoscopic observations on laryngeal symmetry and movements in young racing horses. *New Zealand Veterinary Journal* 45(5):188–192.

Barakzai SZ. 2009. Variability of resting endoscopic grading for assessment of recurrent laryngeal neuropathy in horses. *Equine Veterinary Journal* 41(4):342–346.

Barakzai SZ, Dixon PM. 2011. Correlation of resting and exercising endoscopic findings for horses with dynamic laryngeal collapse and palatal dysfunction. *Equine Veterinary Journal* 43(1):18–23.

Barakzai SZ, Boden LA, Dixon PM. 2009. Postoperative race performance is not correlated with degree of surgical abduction after laryngoplasty in National Hunt Thoroughbred racehorses. *Veterinary Surgery* 38(8):934–940.

Cable CS, Ducharme NG, Hackett RP, Erb HN, Mitchell LM, Soderholm LV. 2002. Sound signature for identification and quantification of upper airway disease in horses. *American Journal of Veterinary Research* 63(12):1707–1713.

Christley RM, Hodgson DR, Evans DL, Rose RJ. 1997. Cardiorespiratory responses to exercise in horses with different grades of idiopathic laryngeal hemiplegia. *Equine Veterinary Journal* 29(1):6–10.

Collins N, Milne E, Hahn C, Dixon PM. 2009. Correlation of the Havemeyer endoscopic laryngeal grading system with histopathological changes in equine cricoarytenoideus dorsalis muscles. *Irish Veterinary Journal* 5:334–338.

Cook WR, Thalhammer G. 1991. Electrodiagnostic test for the objectve grading of recurrent laryngeal neuropathy in the horse. *Proceedings of the American Association of Equine Practitioners* 37:275–296.

Davidson EJ, Martin BB Jr, Parente EJ. 2007. Use of successive dynamic videoendoscopic evaluations to identify progression of recurrent laryngeal neuropathy in three horses. *Journal of the American Veterinary Medical Association* 230(4):555–558.

Derksen FJ, Holcombe SJ, Hartmann W, Robinson NE, Stick JA. 2001. Spectrum analysis of respiratory sounds in exercising horses with experimentally induced laryngeal hemiplegia or dorsal displacement of the soft palate. *American Journal of Veterinary Research* 62(5):659–664.

Desmaizieres LM, Serraud N, Plainfosse B, Michel A, Tamzali Y. 2009. Dynamic respiratory endoscopy without treadmill in 68 performance Standardbred, Thoroughbred and saddle horses under natural training conditions. *Equine Veterinary Journal* 41(4):347–352.

Dixon PM, McGorum BC, Railton DI, Hawe C, Tremaine WH, Pickles K, McCann J. 2001. Laryngeal paralysis: A study of 375 cases in a mixed-breed population of horses. *Equine Veterinary Journal* 33(5):452–458.

Dixon PM, McGorum BC, Railton DI, Hawe C, Tremaine WH, Pickles K, McCann J. 2002. Clinical and endoscopic evidence of progression in 152 cases of equine recurrent laryngeal neuropathy (RLN). *Equine Veterinary Journal* 34(1):29–34.

Dixon PM, McGorum BC, Railton DI, Hawe C, Tremaine WH, Dacre K, McCann J. 2003. Long-term survey of laryngoplasty and ventriculocordectomy in an older, mixed-breed population of 200 horses. Part 2: Owners' assessment of the value of surgery. *Equine Veterinary Journal* 35(4):397–401.

Garrett KS, Pierce SW, Embertson RM, Stromberg AJ. 2010. Endoscopic evaluation of arytenoid function and epiglottic structure in Thoroughbred yearlings and association with racing performance at two to four years of age: 2,954 cases (1998–2001). *Journal of American Veterinary Medical Association* 236(6):669–673.

Garrett KS, Woodie JB, Embertson RM. 2011. Association of treadmill upper airway endoscopic evaluation with results of ultrasonography and resting upper airway endoscopic evaluation. *Equine Veterinarian Journal* 43(3):365–371.

Hackett RP, Ducharme NG, Fubini SL, Erb HN. 1991. The reliability of endoscopic examination in assessment of arytenoid cartilage movement in horses. Part I:

Subjective and objective laryngeal evaluation. *Veterinary Surgery* 20(3):174–179.

Hammer EJ, Tulleners EP, Parente EJ, Martin BB Jr. 1998. Videoendoscopic assessment of dynamic laryngeal function during exercise in horses with grade-III left laryngeal hemiparesis at rest: 26 cases (1992–1995). *Journal of the American Veterinary Medical Association* 212(3):399–403.

Hawe C, Dixon PM, Mayhew IG. 2001. A study of an electrodiagnostic technique for the evaluation of equine recurrent laryngeal neuropathy. *Equine Veterinary Journal* 33(5):459–465.

Lane JG. 2003. Long-term longitudinal study of laryngeal function in 187 foals. In: Dixon PM, Robinson NE, Wad JF, (eds). *Proceedings of a Workshop on Equine Recurrent Laryngeal Neuropathy.* Havemeyer Foundation Monograph Series No (pp. 31–32). Newmarket, R&W Publications.

Lane JG, Bladon B, Little DR, Naylor JR, Franklin SH. 2006. Dynamic obstructions of the equine upper respiratory tract. Part 2: Comparison of endoscopic findings at rest and during high-speed treadmill exercise of 600 Thoroughbred racehorses. *Equine Veterinary Journal* 38(5):401–407.

Marks D, Mackay-Smith MP, Cushing LS, Leslie JA. 1970. Observations on laryngeal hemiplegia in the horse and treatment by abductor muscle prosthesis. *Equine Veterinary Journal* 2:159–166.

Morris EA, Seeherman HJ. 1990. Evaluation of upper respiratory tract function during strenuous exercise in racehorses. *Journal of American Veterinary Medical Association* 196(3):431–438.

Newton-Clarke MJ, Divers TJ, Valentine BA. 1994. Evaluation of the thoraco-laryngeal reflex ('slap test') as an indicator of laryngeal adductor myopathy in the horse. *Equine Veterinary Journal* 26(5):355–357.

Perkins JD, Salz RO, Schumacher J, Livesey L, Piercy RJ, Barakzai SZ. 2009. Variability of resting endoscopic grading for assessment of recurrent laryngeal neuropathy in horses. *Equine Veterinary Journal* 41(4):342–346.

Pollock PJ, Reardon RJ, Parkin TD, Johnston MS, Tate J, Love S. 2009. Dynamic respiratory endoscopy in 67 Thoroughbred racehorses training under normal ridden exercise conditions. *Equine Veterinary Journal* 41(4):354–360.

Rakestraw PC, Hackett RP, Ducharme NG, Nielan GJ, Erb HN. 1991. Arytenoid cartilage movement in resting and exercising horses. *Veterinary Surgery* 20(2):122–127.

Robinson NE. 2004. Consensus statements on equine recurrent laryngeal neuropathy: conclusions of the Havemeyer workshop. Stratford-Upon-Avon. *Equine Veterinary Education* 16:333–336.

2 Recurrent Laryngeal Neuropathy: Diagnosis, Dynamic Endoscopy

Elizabeth Davidson

Introduction

For years, resting endoscopic evaluation of the upper airway has been used for assessment of laryngeal function. Horses with endoscopic evidence of complete paralysis of the laryngeal cartilage(s) at rest are easy to diagnose and their impact on performance is clear. Affected horses have upper airway obstruction and abnormal respiratory noise during strenuous exercise because of dynamic collapse of the affected arytenoid cartilage. However, the clinical significance of asynchronous or asymmetric laryngeal cartilage movement has been controversial. Endoscopic evaluation at rest may make the clinician suspect the possibility of laryngeal dysfunction during exercise but resting endoscopy does not replicate the function of the larynx during exercise. Therefore, dynamic exercising upper airway endoscopy is the gold standard for accurate identification of laryngeal dysfunction.

The use of exercising upper airway endoscopy to evaluate horses with exercise intolerance, respiratory noise, or poor performance is well documented (Dart et al. 2001; Kannegieter and Dore 1995; Lane et al. 2006; Martin et al. 2000; Tan et al.

2005) and dynamic upper airway observations from these treadmill studies have shaped our current knowledge of laryngeal function during exercise and remain the foundation of our understanding. One of the recent advances in the equine respiratory medicine is the advent of overground endoscopy which enables the clinician to instrument and evaluate the upper airway while the horse is exercising in its natural environment. Initial studies have validated its use as a viable alternative to treadmill endoscopy. Whether performed on the treadmill or overground, exercising endoscopy remains the best way to assess upper airway dynamics.

Treadmill endoscopy

Treadmill endoscopy is performed with the horse exercising on a high-speed treadmill. Equine treadmills are uniquely designed to exercise horses at racing speeds and are widely available at referral institutions. Although treadmill protocols vary among individual institutions, the basic process is similar, with the goal to mimic racing or show conditions. In general, horses are first acclimated to the treadmill. Horses are walked, trotted, and cantered

Advances in Equine Upper Respiratory Surgery, First Edition. Edited by Jan Hawkins.
© 2015 ACVS Foundation. Published 2015 by John Wiley & Sons, Inc.

during the training session. Since most horses are not accustomed to treadmill exercise, the treadmill often evokes excitement and apprehension and a competent and patient horse-handling team is critical for familiarization and testing to proceed safely.

After acclimation, the treadmill exercise stress test is performed. Simulating race day conditions, horses undergo a warm-up phase of walking, trotting, and moderate cantering (trotting/pacing in Standardbreds) at approximately 7 m/s for 1600 m, analogous to the gallop to the starting gate. Following the warm up the treadmill is stopped, and the endoscope is secured to the halter and the tip of the endoscope is positioned so that continuous visualization of the larynx is obtained. The high-speed test immediately follows with the horse exercising as fast as they are capable of. Ideally the horse should be capable of sustaining maximal speed for 1600–2400 m. Most referral centers with a high-speed treadmill employ an incremental speed (stepwise) treadmill test whereby the speed is increased over constant time intervals. For some horses, uphill exercise (1–3° incline) may be appropriate; this is especially true for horses used in competitions that include jumping (i.e., steeple chasing, eventing). Racehorses are exercised until target maximal heart rates (>200 beats per minute) are achieved or until the horse is fatigued to the point of not being able to keep up with the speed of the treadmill. The exact intensity is dictated by the fitness and temperament of the individual horse, but in many cases will approach 12–14 m/s. Depending on the institutions' protocol and the horse's temperament, the entire procedure from acclimation to testing takes 1–3 days to complete.

Standardbreds are routinely outfitted with the same equipment used in training or racing (bridle, head-check, and harness). Racing Thoroughbreds are equipped with a halter only. Non-racing performance horses (show horses) are also equipped with a halter. If the respiratory noise is associated with head and neck flexion, horses should be equipped with bridle, long reins, or side reins to achieve enforced poll flexion. With long reins, an additional person is in charge of the horse's reins and stands next to the treadmill and behind the horse to keep it "on the bit." The entire exercising endoscopic evaluation is video recorded and reviewed on slow-motion playback at the end of the exercise session.

Overground endoscopy

Traditionally exercising endoscopy was performed on the high-speed treadmill. However, treadmill testing does not fully duplicate training or racing conditions. Factors such as the weight of the rider, excitement of race day, footing conditions, and the rapid changes of pace cannot be reproduced during treadmill testing. Therefore, exercising endoscopic examination in the field has advantages over treadmill endoscopy because the exercise test can be performed in the environment typically used for competition and horses can be examined in a manner appropriate for their discipline. For example, dressage horses can be examined in a collected frame and racehorses in company with other horses. In addition, the effect of track and rider can be accounted for and training sessions to acclimate horses to treadmills are not required. Disadvantages are minor and are related to inability to flush the endoscope on demand. Mucous accumulation on the camera or foggy image due to nasopharyngeal air temperature changes may occur because flushing on command is not possible.

Several commercially available overground endoscopic systems are available. The Dynamic Respiratory Scope (DRS®) system utilizes a backpack for electronics and lavage system which is secured to the rider's saddle pad or sulky harness. The semi-rigid endoscope is secured in position via a specialized bridle. This system also includes a handheld viewer for remote real time visualization of the upper airway within a range of 500 m. The telemetric system records the entire examination and is battery operated for portability.

Key practical points to minimize difficulties when using the equipment include the following. Preparation of the horse and securing the endoscope in the correct position should be optimal because it is difficult to reposition the endoscope during exercise; only small adjustments are possible. Mounted endoscopy should be performed with an experienced rider; the newest DRS® models are fitted to saddle pads, not on rider. As with treadmill endoscopy, the DRS® does not negate resting endoscopic evaluation as gross anatomically abnormalities may preclude exercising examination. Resting endoscopy will also assess the horse's compliance and cooperation.

Using the DRS®, exercising endoscopic observations in horses with recurrent laryngeal neuropathy (RLN) is comparable to those reported in treadmill endoscopy studies (Desmaizieres et al. 2009; Pollock et al. 2009). The ability to assess the effect of head and neck position, the rider, and other overground conditions are the main advantages of overground endoscopy.

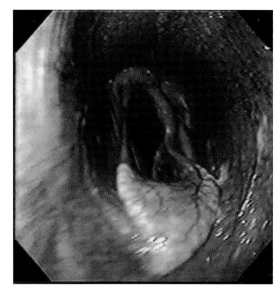

Figure 2.3   Exercising videoendoscopic appearance of the larynx of a horse with exercising laryngeal grade C. Note the severe collapse of the arytenoid and vocal fold.

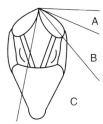

Figure 2.1   Diagram illustrating grades of exercising laryngeal function: grade A, full abduction; grade B, incomplete abduction; grade C, severe collapse of arytenoid and vocal fold.

Exercising laryngeal function

Whether the upper airway examination is performed on the treadmill or in the field, the goal of the examination in horses with RLN is to assess dynamic laryngeal function. During exercise, laryngeal function is categorized as grade A, B, or C (Figure 2.1) (Rakestraw et al. 1991). Horses with exercising laryngeal grade A are able to obtain and maintain full abduction of the arytenoid cartilages during inspiration. Horses with exercising laryngeal grade B are able to maintain the affected arytenoid in a relative fixed but incompletely abducted position; a position between full abduction and resting position (Figure 2.2). Horses with exercising laryngeal grade C have severe dynamic collapse of the affected arytenoid cartilage and vocal fold during exercise with abduction being less than a resting position (Figure 2.3).

Resting versus exercising laryngeal grading systems

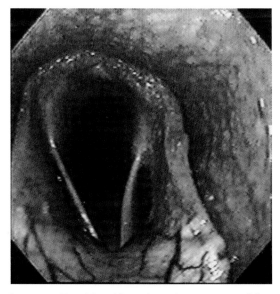

Figure 2.2   Exercising videoendoscopic appearance of the larynx of a horse with exercising laryngeal grade B. Note the concurrent collapse of the left vocal fold.

The vast majority of laryngeal endoscopic assessment is done in the resting, standing horse and RLN grading systems have been developed to characterize and categorize resting laryngeal movements. The three most commonly used resting laryngeal function grading systems are the four-grade system (Hackett et al. 1991), the five-grade system (Kannegieter and Dore 1995; Lane et al. 2006), and the six-grade system (Dixon et al. 2001). Of the three systems, the four-grade system is most widely used. A seven-grade "Havemeyer" system (Robinson 2004) was developed by a panel of respiratory experts in hope that clearly defined criteria would help minimize variability and therefore result in a reliable and consistent system. It is an amalgamation of the four, five, and six grading systems and represents a consensual agreement of respiratory clinicians worldwide.

The real value of any resting grading system is its correlation with laryngeal function during exercise. The combined results of numerous treadmill studies (Barakzai and Dixon 2011; Davidson et al. 2011; Franklin et al. 2006; Lane et al. 2006; Martin et al. 2000) indicate there is good correlation between resting laryngeal grades and exercising laryngeal function. The majority of horses that are able to fully abduct their arytenoid cartilages at rest will have normal laryngeal function during exercise (exercising laryngeal grade A). On the contrary, horses with complete immobility of the arytenoid cartilage at rest will have axial collapse of the affected arytenoid and vocal cord during exercise (exercising laryngeal grade C). However, between 1% and 7% (Barakzai and Dixon 2011; Garrett et al. 2011; Lane et al. 2006; Martin et al. 2000) of horses with "normal" resting laryngeal grades will experience dynamic arytenoid cartilage collapse during exercise. Presumptive assumption of exercising laryngeal function based on resting endoscopy is not correct in all horses.

Horses with asynchronous and/or asymmetric arytenoid cartilage movements that cannot achieve or maintain full arytenoid abduction (Havemeyer laryngeal grade 3) deserve special consideration. Previous reports vary regarding the proportion of horses with this "equivocal" resting laryngeal grade that are able to maintain arytenoid abduction versus those that experience arytenoid cartilage collapse during exercise. The initial treadmill study (Rakestraw et al. 1991) indicated that only 16% of grade 3 (using the four-grade system) horses experience dynamic collapse of the arytenoid cartilage. Subsequent studies (Dart et al. 2001; Hammer et al. 1998; Martin et al. 2000) refuted those results citing that the majority, 77–88%, of grade 3 horses will have axial collapse of affected arytenoid cartilage during exercise. Another treadmill study (Lane et al. 2006) using the five-grade system found only 40% of horses with grades 3 or 4 were unable to maintain arytenoid cartilage abduction at speed. In another study using the Havemeyer seven-grade system (Barakzai and Dixon 2011), 66% of grade 3 horses had dynamic arytenoid cartilage collapse and the likelihood of collapse increased with increasing Havemeyer subgrades 3.1, 3.2, 3.3. While it appears that the majority of grade 3 horses are unable to maintain laryngeal abduction during exercise, exercising endoscopy is clearly indicated for affected horses, especially subgrades 3.1 and 3.2.

The combined results of numerous treadmill studies indicate that failure to obtain and maintain arytenoid cartilage abduction at rest is the major criterion to determine the probability of abnormal laryngeal function during exercise. However, these studies also confirm that decisions about laryngeal function of horses that rely solely on resting endoscopy and do not include an exercise test are inadequate. While recognized associations between resting and exercising laryngeal function may provide general guidelines about the likelihood of dynamic laryngeal function, or dysfunction, not all horses should receive predetermined exercising assessments based on resting laryngeal grades. Clinicians should make individual patient assessments, not assessments based on groups of horses, and whenever possible perform exercising endoscopic evaluation of the larynx. Resting endoscopic examination should not be used as the only diagnostic method, especially in horses with questionable laryngeal function.

Bilateral laryngeal collapse

Bilateral laryngeal dynamic collapse is an abnormality that has been primarily reported in Norwegian Coldblooded Trotters (Strand et al. 2009). This disorder is characterized by marked bilateral collapse of the vocal folds and concurrent bilateral loss of arytenoid cartilage abduction during exercise (Figure 2.4). Diagnosis can only be made by

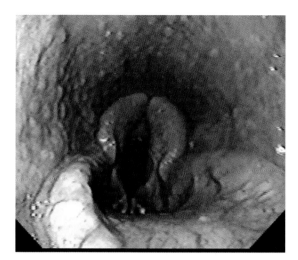

Figure 2.4   Exercising videoendoscopic appearance of the larynx of a horse with bilateral laryngeal collapse induced by rein tension.

exercising endoscopy. Upper airway obstruction is observed when the affected horse is driven into the bit and tension is applied to the long reins. An uncommon manifestation of RLN has been suggested as the etiology of this disorder. Affected horses are able to obtain and maintain full arytenoid abduction during resting endoscopic evaluation and during treadmill endoscopy without rein tension, it is unclear if RLN is the primary cause of this condition; neuromuscular histopathology has not been performed. Another proposed cause is that the disorder is secondary to conformation changes in the throat region associated with head and neck flexion and the small airway diameter of certain breeds. Bilateral laryngeal collapse has also been infrequently identified in other breeds/disciplines (Davidson et al. 2011) exercised with flexed neck and rein tension.

Dynamic collapse of the apex of corniculate process

Dynamic collapse of the apex of the corniculate process of the arytenoid cartilage is an uncommon laryngeal obstructive disorder. It has been reported in 4–6% of horses undergoing treadmill endoscopy (Barakzai et al. 2007; Dart et al. 2001, 2005; Tan et al. 2005). It is characterized by the apex of one cornic-

ulate process, usually the left, luxating to a position that is ventral and axial to the other corniculate process. The corniculate cartilage maintains abduction and does not axially collapse into the airway; it just slides ventral to the other. Concurrent dynamic collapse of other upper airway structures such as the aryepiglottic fold is common as the horse becomes fatigued. Although the underlying etiology of axial collapse of the corniculate process is unknown, it has been speculated that this disorder may be an atypical form of RLN.

The adductor branch of the recurrent laryngeal nerve and the adductor muscles, including the arytenoideus transversus muscle, are more severely affected (Duncan et al. 1991) in horses with RLN. Severe atrophy of the transverse arytenoid muscle may result in insufficient function and loss of the dorsal articulation between the right and left arytenoid cartilages. Without dorsal support, the apex of one corniculate process may be predisposed to collapsing under the other corniculate as airway pressure increase during exercise. Another proposed etiology is that the disorder may not be attributed to RLN but to an aberrant transverse arytenoid ligament. Histological findings of one horse revealed an enlarged wide transverse arytenoid ligament resulting in gap formation between the dorsal margins of the corniculate processes (Barakzai et al. 2007)

Vocal fold collapse

Axial collapse of the vocal fold is considered to occur passively as a result of arytenoid cartilage collapse (Figures 2.2 and 2.3). When there is loss of cricoarytenoideus dorsalis muscle function, there is decreased tension on the vocal fold predisposing it to collapse during exercise (Holcombe et al. 2006). Dynamic collapse of the vocal fold occurs with increased frequency as the resting laryngeal grade increases from 1 to 4 and with increasing subgrades of grade 3 (Barakzai et al. 2011). However, vocal fold collapse has also been reported in horses which are capable of maintaining adequate arytenoid abduction during exercise (Dart et al. 2001; Franklin et al. 2006; Kannegieter and Dore 1995; Lane et al. 2006; Martin et al. 2000). In these horses, solitary collapse of the vocal fold without concurrent arytenoid cartilage collapse likely reflects the pathology of the cricothyroid muscle and is not unusual endoscopic evidence of RLN.

Enforced poll flexion

Flexion of the poll has been shown to increase upper airway impedance in normal horses (Petsche et al. 1994). This is particularly important in horses which are required to exercise with a flexed head and neck, for example, show (combined driving, gaited, or show jumping) or dressage horses. In some horses with RLN, dynamic arytenoid cartilage collapse is only evident or markedly exacerbated when horses are exercised with enforced poll flexion (Davidson et al. 2011; Franklin et al. 2006; Van Erck 2011). Since this position is a contributing factor for the development of laryngeal collapse, exercising endoscopic evaluation with and without head and neck flexion should be performed in horses in suspected laryngeal dysfunction, especially those which are ridden with poll flexion.

Progression of RLN

Although it is commonly believed that complete arytenoid cartilage paralysis is preceded by progressive deterioration, few reports validate this statement (Anderson et al. 1997; Davidson et al. 2007; Dixon et al. 2002; Garrett et al. 2011). The reported incidence of RLN progression is low 5–15% (Anderson et al. 1997; Dixon et al. 2002) and slows with a median period of 12 months (Dixon et al. 2002). Progression of the disease is most commonly identified by deterioration of laryngeal function at rest combined with the onset of abnormal-exercise-related respiratory noise (Anderson et al. 1997; Dixon et al. 2002). Progressive loss of laryngeal function has also been identified during repeated treadmill endoscopic evaluation of horses (Davidson et al. 2007; Garrett et al. 2011).

Implications of RLN in show horses

Compared to racehorses, RLN does not always impede the performance of the show horse; they are able to compete despite laryngeal dysfunction. Research studies have demonstrated that at

exercise intensities less than VO_{2peak}, RLN does not have significant physiological consequences (Ehrlich et al. 1995) which may explain why some show horses can compete successfully despite the disease. Treadmill reports indicate that resting laryngeal grade 3 horses are less likely to have dynamic arytenoid cartilage collapse when exercised at submaximal intensities (Davidson et al. 2011; Rakestraw et al. 1991) compared to maximally exercised racehorses (Dart et al. 2001; Hammer et al. 1998; Martin et al. 2000). Brakenhoff observed RLN (resting laryngeal grade 3 or 4) in 35% of adequately performing competitive draft horses. In fact, some of the highest placed horses had untreated laryngeal dysfunction (Brakenhoff et al. 2006). At lower than maximal exercise intensities, the aerobic capacity of a horse affected with RLN seems to be adequate for many nonracing endeavors. However, since RLN can be progressive, declines in performance or abnormal respiratory noise are impetuses for additional endoscopic evaluation.

References

Anderson BH, Kannegieter NJ, Goulden BE. 1997. Endoscopic observations on laryngeal symmetry and movements in young racing horses. *New Zealand Veterinary Journal* 45(5):188–192.

Barakzai SZ, Es C, Milne EM, Dixon PM. 2007. Ventroaxial luxation of the apex of the corniculate process of the arytenoid cartilage in resting horses during induced swallowing or nasal occlusion. *Veterinary Surgery* 36(3):210–213.

Barakzai SZ, Dixon PM. 2011. Correlation of resting and exercising endoscopic findings for horses with dynamic laryngeal collapse and palatal dysfunction. *Equine Veterinary Journal* 43(1):18–23.

Brakenhoff JE, Holcombe SJ, Hauptman JG, Smith HK, Nickels FA, Caron JP. 2006. The prevalence of laryngeal disease in a large population of competition draft horses. *Veterinary Surgery* 35(6):579–583.

Dart AJ, Dowling BA, Hodgson DR, Rose RJ. 2001. Evaluation of high-speed treadmill videoendoscopy for diagnosis of upper respiratory tract dysfunction in horses. *Australian Veterinary Journal* 79(2):109–112.

Dart AJ, Dowling BA, Smith CL. 2005. Upper airway dysfunction associated with collapse of the apex of the corniculate process of the left arytenoid cartilage during exercise in 15 horses. *Veterinary Surgery* 34(6):543–547.

Davidson EJ, Martin BB, Jr, Parente EJ. 2007. Use of successive dynamic videoendoscopic evaluations to identify progression of recurrent laryngeal neuropathy in three horses. *Journal of the American Veterinary Medical Association* 230(4):555–558.

Davidson EJ, Martin BB, Boston RC, Parente EJ. 2011. Exercising upper respiratory videoendoscopic evaluation of 100 nonracing performance horses with abnormal respiratory noise and/or poor performance. *Equine Veterinary Journal* 43(1):3–8.

Desmaizieres LM, Serraud N, Plainfosse B, Michel A, Tamzali Y. 2009. Dynamic respiratory endoscopy without treadmill in 68 performance Standardbred, Thoroughbred and saddle horses under natural training conditions. *Equine Veterinary Journal* 41(4):347–352.

Dixon PM, McGorum BC, Railton DI, Hawe C, Tremaine WH, Pickles K, McCann J. 2001. Laryngeal paralysis: A study of 375 cases in a mixed-breed population of horses. *Equine Veterinary Journal* 33(5):452–458.

Dixon PM, McGorum BC, Railton DI, Hawe C, Tremaine WH, Pickles K, McCann J. 2002. Clinical and endoscopic evidence of progression in 152 cases of equine recurrent laryngeal neuropathy (RLN). *Equine Veterinary Journal* 34(1):29–34.

Duncan ID, Reifenrath P, Jackson KF, Clayton M. 1991. Preferential denervation of the adductor muscles of the equine larynx. II: Nerve pathology. *Equine Veterinary Journal* 23(2):99–103.

Ehrlich PJ, Seeherman HJ, Morris E, Kolias C, Cook WR. 1995. The effect of reversible left recurrent laryngeal neuropathy on the metabolic cost of locomotion and peak aerobic power in Thoroughbred racehorses. *Veterinary Surgery* 24(1):36–48.

Franklin SH, Naylor JR, Lane JG. 2006. Videoendoscopic evaluation of the upper respiratory tract in 93 sport horses during exercise testing on a high-speed treadmill. *Equine Veterinary Journal Supplement* Aug(36): 540–545.

Garrett KS, Woodie JB, Embertson RM. 2011. Association of treadmill upper airway endoscopic evaluation with results of ultrasonography and resting upper airway endoscopic evaluation. *Equine Veterinary Journal* 43(3):365–371.

Hackett RP, Ducharme NG, Fubini SL, Erb HN. 1991. The reliability of endoscopic examination in assessment of arytenoid cartilage movement in horses. Part I: Subjective and objective laryngeal evaluation. *Veterinary Surgery* 20(3):174–179.

Hammer EJ, Tulleners EP, Parente EJ, Martin BB, Jr. 1998. Videoendoscopic assessment of dynamic laryngeal function during exercise in horses with grade-III

left laryngeal hemiparesis at rest: 26 cases (1992–1995). *Journal of the American Veterinary Medical Association* 212(3):399–403.

Holcombe SJ, Rodriquez K, Lane J, Caron JP. 2006. Cricothyroid muscle function and vocal fold stability in exercising horses. *Veterinary Surgery* 35(6):495–500.

Kannegieter NJ, Dore ML. 1995. Endoscopy of the upper respiratory tract during treadmill exercise: A clinical study of 100 horses. *Australian Veterinary Journal* 72(3):101–107.

Lane JG, Bladon B, Little DR, Naylor JR, Franklin SH. 2006. Dynamic obstructions of the equine upper respiratory tract. Part 1: Observations during high-speed treadmill endoscopy of 600 Thoroughbred racehorses. *Equine Veterinary Journal* 28(5):393–399.

Martin BB Jr, Reef VB, Parente EJ, Sage AD. 2000. Causes of poor performance of horses during training, racing, or showing: 348 cases (1992–1996). *Journal of the American Veterinary Medical Association* 216(4):554–558.

Petsche VM, Derksen FJ, Robinson NE. 1994. Tidal breathing flow-volume loops in horses with recurrent airway obstruction (heaves). *American Journal of Veterinary Research* 55(7):885–891.

Pollock PJ, Reardon RJ, Parkin TD, Johnston MS, Tate J, Love S. 2009. Dynamic respiratory endoscopy in 67 Thoroughbred racehorses training under normal ridden exercise conditions. *Equine Veterinary Journal* 41(4):354–360.

Rakestraw PC, Hackett RP, Ducharme NG, Nielan GJ, Erb HN. 1991. Arytenoid cartilage movement in resting and exercising horses. *Veterinary Surgery* 20(2):122–127.

Robinson NE. 2004. Consensus statements on equine recurrent laryngeal neuropathy: Conclusions of the Havemeyer workshop. September 2003, Stratford-Upon-Avon, Warwickshire, UK. *Equine Veterinary Education* 16(6):333–336.

Strand E, Fjordbakk CT, Holcombe SJ, Risberg A, Chalmers HJ. 2009. Effect of poll flexion and dynamic laryngeal collapse on tracheal pressure in Norwegian Coldblood Trotter racehorses. *Equine Veterinary Journal* 41(1):59–64.

Tan RH, Dowling BA, Dart AJ. 2005. High-speed treadmill videoendoscopic examination of the upper respiratory tract in the horse: The results of 291 clinical cases. *Veterinary Journal* 170(2):243–248.

Van Erck E. 2011. Dynamic respiratory videoendoscopy in ridden sport horses: Effect of head flexion, riding and airway inflammation in 129 cases. *Equine Veterinary Journal Supplement* Nov(40):18–24.

3 Ultrasonography of the Larynx for the Diagnosis of Recurrent Laryngeal Neuropathy

Heather Chalmers

Introduction to laryngeal ultrasound

One of the more recent additions to the spectrum of diagnostic tests available for the evaluation of upper airway disease in horses is laryngeal ultrasound (Chalmers et al. 2006a). The general advantages of ultrasound in equine practice are that ultrasound is noninvasive, widely available, cost-effective, portable, and is generally well tolerated by horses. While endoscopy continues to be an essential technique to evaluate the upper airway, some of the limitations of endoscopy are addressed with the concurrent use of ultrasound. Endoscopy allows evaluation of the superficial morphology of luminal structures of the upper airway and focuses on the laryngeal function in the resting and exercising states. Ultrasonography is complementary to this, and is useful for imaging of non-luminal structures and can facilitate assessment of deeper tissues that are not readily seen or palpated.

Patient preparation and equipment

Laryngeal ultrasound can be performed in the standing, unsedated horse and is generally well tol-erated. Clipping of hair is usually not necessary, but is recommended. If hair is not clipped alcohol should be applied to the hair and skin as dirt, organic debris, or grooming products will attenuate the ultrasound beam and should be avoided or removed prior to the study. A range of ultrasound probes can be suitable for laryngeal ultrasound, but factors to consider in choosing a probe include probe frequency and footprint size. The frequency of the probe will affect image resolution and depth of penetration, with higher frequency probes having superior resolution with lower penetration. For laryngeal ultrasound, a probe with at least 8 MHz or higher is recommended because the depth of penetration required does not typically exceed 4–5 cm. Most practitioners using ultrasound will have at least one probe suitable for imaging of tendons, which would typically be a linear style probe in the 12–15 MHz range. These probes can be ideal for the larynx, especially in lean race horses in which the larynx is usually well imaged despite the larger footprint associated with these probes. For older horses, heavier horses, and draft breeds, linear probes may be too bulky to achieve satisfactory image quality. The larger size of many linear probes can be prohibitive especially when

Advances in Equine Upper Respiratory Surgery, First Edition. Edited by Jan Hawkins.
© 2015 ACVS Foundation. Published 2015 by John Wiley & Sons, Inc.

attempting to image the larynx from the lateral acoustic window. This is particularly problematic in horses with a rostral location of the larynx relative to the ramus of the mandible and horses with a narrow inter-mandibular space. A more specialized probe option is a "hockey stick"-style transducer, which is shaped like a hockey stick and offers the advantages of a small footprint and a fine handle that is affixed at an angle to the probe face. This probe provides versatility in maneuvering around the larynx without compromising image resolution and can be situated between the ramus of the mandible and the lateral aspect of the larynx, allowing a more extensive examination from the lateral acoustic window. Where multiple probe options are available, the highest frequency probe that has a footprint that can be easily manipulated in the throat region should be chosen.

How to perform a laryngeal ultrasound examination

A precise understanding of the normal function and anatomy of the upper airway is essential for both performing and interpreting the laryngeal ultrasound. The basic laryngeal ultrasound examination has been described using five acoustic windows (Chalmers et al. 2006a). Where indicated, the examination should be extended to include other structures of interest such as mandibular lymph nodes, salivary and thyroid glands, and jugular bifurcation. Occasionally, a complete evaluation of the larynx will not be possible with ultrasound due to mineralization of the laryngeal cartilages, intra luminal and intra ventricular air, and/or rostral location of the larynx relative to the mandibular rami. Turning the horse's head away from the side being imaged will help to move the mandible away from the lateral aspect of the larynx and should facilitate imaging of the larynx from the lateral acoustic window when this is problematic in a neutral head position. The dorsal midline position of the *cricoarytenoideus dorsalis* (CAD) muscles makes ultrasonography difficult; however, with some technical expertise the rostral portions of the CAD can be observed using percutaneous ultrasound (Garrett et al. 2011). To facilitate CAD imaging, concurrent laryngeal palpation is often useful.

By placing one hand on the opposite side of the larynx and gently pushing the larynx toward the side being imaged, the muscular process of the arytenoid cartilage of interest is positioned more laterally and imaging of the insertion of the CAD is facilitated. An advanced acoustic window for imaging of the CAD is the transesophageal approach. A specialized transesophageal ultrasound probe, originated for human applications and resembling a flexible 1-m endoscope, can be inserted via the nostril and passed into the cranial esophagus. This offers superior images of the CAD, but due to the specialized nature of the equipment this is of limited availability.

Use in recurrent laryngeal neuropathy

Recurrent laryngeal neuropathy (RLN) is the recognized cause of laryngeal hemiplegia and has been characterized as a distal axonopathy affecting the left recurrent laryngeal nerve (Duncan et al. 1974). RLN results in neurogenic atrophy of the intrinsic laryngeal muscles save the cricothyroid muscle which is innervated by the external branch of the cranial laryngeal nerve (Duncan et al. 1974). The ultrasonographic criteria used to diagnose RLN hinge on the ability of ultrasound to detect an altered appearance of the intrinsic laryngeal muscles in affected horses (Chalmers et al. 2006b; Garrett et al. 2011). The technique focuses on the cricoartyenoideus lateralis (CAL) muscle which is the primary adductor of the arytenoid cartilage. As an adductor, the CAL muscle has generally received less attention than the CAD muscle because the restoration of abductor function has been a major focus of RLN therapies (Derksen et al. 1986; Goulden and Anderson 1982). The CAL muscle is an ideal candidate for diagnostic purposes because it is affected earlier and more severely than the CAD (Cahill and Goulden 1986a, 1986b; Duncan et al. 1974). The CAL is imaged from the lateral acoustic window, while imaging of the CAD is more challenging (Chalmers et al. 2006a; Garrett et al. 2011). Since the CAL of affected horses undergoes histological changes associated with neurogenic atrophy, the ultrasound technique focuses on the detection of characteristic alterations in CAL muscle echogenicity and echotexture. Echogenicity

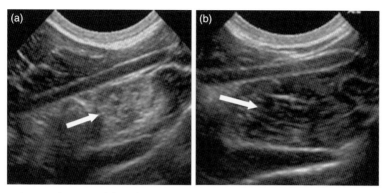

Figure 3.1   Composite ultrasound images of the left (a) and right (b) lateral acoustic windows from a 3-year-old Standardbred filly presenting for poor performance. The CAL muscles are depicted with white arrows. In (a), the left CAL muscle is observed to have increased echogenicity relative to the extrinsic laryngeal muscles in the near field and relative to the contralateral CAL (b). In (b), the normal right CAL is observed to have hypoechoic appearance, and is isoechoic to the extrinsic laryngeal muscles. These findings strongly suggest the presence of neurogenic atrophy in the left CAL muscle and support a diagnosis of recurrent laryngeal neuropathy. In both images, the thyroid and arytenoid cartilages are seen on either side of the CAL muscle as hypoechoic linear structures with slightly echoic margins.

refs to the level of brightness of a tissue, while echotexture refers to the characteristic patterns of echos generated by tissues. Both echogenicity and echotexture relate to subtle differences in acoustic impedance among tissue types, which in turn determines the fundamental ability of different tissues to reflect sound waves and create echoes that return to the ultrasound probe and are depicted on the resulting image.

When using ultrasound in horses suspected of having RLN, the operator should pay particular notice of the appearance of the CAL and CAD muscles. Both subjective and objective criteria have been described, but the subjective assessment of CAL echogenicity has been the most diagnostically useful (Chalmers et al. 2006a; Garrett et al. 2011). Most commonly, increased echogenicity of the left CAL muscle will be identified in horses with RLN (Figure 3.1) (Chalmers et al. 2006a; Garrett et al. 2011). Increased echogenicity can be established through visual inspection and experience, and should be confirmed by comparison to the ipsilateral extrinsic laryngeal muscles, the ipsilateral cricothyroid muscle, and/or the contralateral CAL muscle. These comparisons are made without altering the ultrasound machine settings for depth, overall gain, or time gain compensation as changing these parameters will change the absolute echogenicity and the perception of muscle bright-

ness. The exact relationship between histological changes, the increased echogenicity seen with ultrasound, and the timing of onset of the ultrasound changes relative to the course of disease in RLN has not yet been determined.

The use of laryngeal ultrasound should be considered to substantially augment and in some cases supersede the resting endoscopic findings in horses affected with RLN (Chalmers et al. 2006a; Garrett et al. 2011). The ultrasound and endoscopic examinations can be performed in series or in parallel depending on the intention of the clinician and the specifics of the patient in question. When the clinician chooses to utilize laryngeal ultrasound in combination with resting endoscopy, the specificity in the diagnosis of RLN is increased by requiring a positive diagnosis with both modalities to consider a horse positive for RLN. This is especially relevant for the evaluation of resting grade 2 and 3 horses, to increase the sensitivity of diagnosis one should use the tests in parallel, meaning that a positive result from either test should warrant additional evaluation using exercising endoscopy. Where exercising upper airway endoscopy is routinely performed, either on a treadmill or using over-ground endoscopy, laryngeal ultrasound is recommended to provide the clinician with additional structural information about laryngeal tissues.

Use in other laryngeal abnormalities

In addition to the application of laryngeal ultrasound in the evaluation of RLN, there are several reports outlining the use of laryngeal ultrasound in the diagnosis and characterization of laryngeal infections, masses, and deformities (Chalmers et al. 2006a, 2009; Garrett et al. 2009, 2010; Koenig 2012) For these various conditions, laryngeal ultrasound has been described as a complementary diagnostic test that allows the clinician to further establish the extent and location of diseased tissue.

Summary

While upper airway endoscopy is an essential and invaluable tool in the assessment for RLN, the concurrent use of laryngeal ultrasound greatly expands the diagnostic accuracy and capabilities in the resting horse. Laryngeal ultrasound is especially useful in horses with resting laryngeal grades 2 and 3, in which the exercising status of the larynx may be accurately predicted with ultrasound than with resting endoscopy (Chalmers et al. 2006b; Garrett et al. 2011). The ultrasonographic findings can serve to further emphasize the need for exercising examination, can confirm a diagnosis made with resting endoscopy, and may provide key information regarding the status of relevant non-luminal tissues in patients with laryngeal infection, masses, and deformity.

References

Cahill JI, Goulden BE. 1986a. Equine laryngeal hemiplegia. Part I. A light microscopic study of peripheral nerves. New Zealand Veterinary Journal 34(10):161–169.

Cahill JI, Goulden BE. 1986b. Equine laryngeal hemiplegia. Part IV. Muscle pathology. New Zealand Veterinary Journal 34(11):186–190.

Chalmers HJ, Cheetham J, Yeager AE, Ducharme NG. 2006a. Ultrasonography of the equine larynx. Veterinary Radiology and Ultrasound 47(5):476–481.

Chalmers HJ, Cheetham J, Mohammed HO, Yeager AE, Ducharme NG. 2006b. Ultrasonography as an aid in the diagnosis of recurrent laryngeal neuropathy in horses. In: Proceedings of the 2006 ACVS Veterinary Symposium, pp. 3–4.

Chalmers HJ, Yeager AE, Viel L, Caswell J, Ducharme NG. 2009. Ultrasonography in horses with arytenoid chondritis. In: Proceedings of 4th World Equine Airways Symposium, Berne, Switzerland.

Derksen FJ, Stick JA, Scott EA, Robinson NE, Slocombe RF. 1986. Effects of laryngeal hemiplegia and laryngoplasty on airway flow mechanics in exercising horses. American Journal of Veterinary Research 47:16–26.

Duncan ID, Griffiths IR, McQueen A, Baker GO. 1974. The pathology of equine laryngeal hemiplegia. Acta Neuropathologica (Berlin) 27:337–348.

Garrett KS, Woodie JB, Embertson RM, Pease AP. 2009. Diagnosis of laryngeal dysplasia in five horses using magnetic resonance imaging and ultrasonography. Equine Veterinary Journal 41(8):766–771.

Garrett KS, Woodie JB, Cook JL, Williams NM. 2010. Imaging diagnosis – nasal septal and laryngeal cyst like malformations in a Thoroughbred weanling colt diagnosed using ultrasonography and magnetic resonance imaging. Veterinary Radiology and Ultrasound 51(5):504–507.

Garrett KS, Woodie JB, Embertson RM. 2011. Association of treadmill upper airway endoscopic evaluation with results of ultrasonography and resting upper airway endoscopic evaluation. Equine Veterinary Journal 43(3):365–371.

Goulden BE, Anderson LG. 1982. Equine laryngeal hemiplegia. Part III. Treatment by laryngoplasty. New Zealand Veterinary Journal 30:1–5.

Koenig JB, Silveira A, Chalmers H, Buenviaje G, Lillie B. 2012. Laryngeal neuroendocrine tumour in a horse. Equine Veterinary Education 24(1):12–16.

4   **Laser Ventriculocordectomy**

Jan Hawkins

Introduction

Ventriculectomy (VE) or ventriculocordectomy (VCE) is a surgical procedure utilized to manage recurrent laryngeal neuropathy (RLN) in horses, with VCE being preferred over VE (Brown et al. 2003; Robinson et al. 2006). Surgical removal of the vocal cord and laryngeal saccule is believed to stabilize the paralyzed arytenoid cartilage, widen the ventral aspect of the rima glottidis, and decrease respiratory noise associated with RLN. The traditional surgical approach for VCE is ventral laryngotomy in combination with a roaring burr to remove the laryngeal ventricle and excision of the vocal cord with scissors.

In the 1980s the Nd:YAG laser was introduced to equine surgery. The Nd:YAG laser had the advantage of being used endoscopically. Some surgeons then began to shift from laryngotomy to laser surgical techniques. Tate described standing, noncontact ablation of the laryngeal ventricle (Bristol 1995) and later Tulleners (Tulleners 1996) described a technique for VE and VCE with the horse being recumbent prior to prosthetic laryngoplasty. Standing laser surgical techniques have the primary advan-

tage of avoiding general anesthesia but the disadvantages of patient movement and the reluctance of some horses to cooperate with manipulation of the endoscope and/or surgical instrumentation inserted via the nasal passages. Currently, with the widespread availability of surgical lasers at referral centers laser VCE is performed by most surgeons and VCE via laryngotomy is less frequently performed. Owner satisfaction with laser VCE is high as most owners prefer not to manage an open laryngotomy incision.

There are multiple variations/techniques for laser VCE. The techniques described include standing and recumbent contact and noncontact laser surgical techniques and the use of specific, dedicated surgical instruments.

Instrumentation

Either the 980-nm diode or 1064-nm Nd:YAG laser can be used for VCE. The most commonly used laser is the 980-nm diode. Several different models are available with the primary difference being the amount of wattage each laser unit can

Advances in Equine Upper Respiratory Surgery, First Edition. Edited by Jan Hawkins.
© 2015 ACVS Foundation. Published 2015 by John Wiley & Sons, Inc.

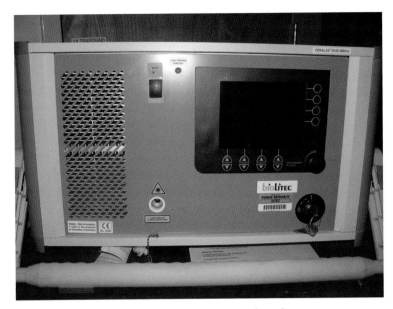

Figure 4.1   A 120-watt diode laser used for contact and noncontact ventriculocordectomy.

generate. Most commercially available units being marketed to equine surgeons have a maximum wattage of 25 watts. Lasers with maximum wattage of 25 watts, limits the surgeon to contact surgical techniques and makes noncontact techniques not effective for photoablation. For those surgeons who want the flexibility of taking advantage of all of the capabilities of the diode laser, a unit capable of greater than 25 watts should be considered. The unit we currently use at our institution is capable of 120 watts (Figure 4.1).

A standard, sculpted 600-μm laser fiber is used for the procedure. This fiber is reusable and can be used multiple times. A dedicated laser fiber cleaving device is needed to trim the end of the fiber between uses. Bronchoesophageal forceps (Richard Wolf or Sontec Instruments, Colorado, USA; model No. 1404–881) are needed for eversion of the laryngeal ventricle or grasping of the vocal cord and a custom designed transnasal or oral roaring burr is also available for eversion of the laryngeal ventricle (Sontec Instruments, Colorado, USA; Virgina Roaring Burr, model No. 1271–284 left) (Figure 4.2). Finally, stocks and a head support are useful for standing laser surgical procedures. For recumbent VCE, a mouth speculum is useful to aid access of the larynx via the oral cavity.

Laser VCE techniques

The major consideration for laser VCE is whether or not to perform the procedure standing or under general anesthesia. For horses, when VCE is to be performed as a standalone procedure standing is obviously preferred. Likewise, some surgeons prefer to perform standing VCE prior to

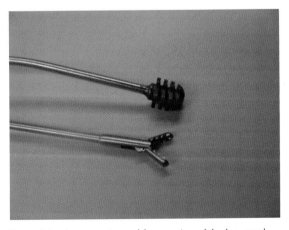

Figure 4.2   Instruments used for eversion of the laryngeal ventricle. These include bronchoesophageal grasping forceps and a transnasal/oral roaring burr.

prosthetic laryngoplasty rather than prolonged general anesthesia surgical times or the day following prosthetic laryngoplasty. It is the author's preference to perform VCE with the horse in right lateral recumbency prior to prosthetic laryngoplasty. I have found that VCE under general anesthesia has the following advantages: no patient movement, decreased hemorrhage, and shorter surgical times mainly because the horse does not move or resent the insertion of the endoscope or instruments into the nasal passages. For the majority of cases, VCE under general anesthesia adds 10–15 minutes to the total anesthesia time. During the time the horse is having VCE performed, it can be prepped for prosthetic laryngoplasty.

General surgical considerations for laser VCE

Any technique selected to complete laser VCE should follow these principles. Iatrogenic damage to the vocal process of the arytenoid cartilage should be avoided. Laser incision/contact too close to the vocal process can result in arytenoid chondritis. To avoid this approximately 2–3 mm of vocal cord should remain attached to the vocal process (Figure 4.3). Therefore, all laser fiber contact should begin just ventral to the vocal process. Likewise, the most ventral aspect of the vocal cord should not be damaged with the laser. This is to prevent cicatrix formation at the ventral aspect of the rima glottidis between the two vocal folds (Figures 4.4a and 4.4b), especially when performed bilaterally. Hemorrhage is always a concern regardless of the technique used for VCE. Hemorrhage always occurs to some degree but in some horses excessive hemorrhage can develop which makes visualization challenging (Figure 4.5). Some surgeons favor local injection with vasoconstrictors, such as epinephrine, but the author has not had much success with these agents. If hemorrhage obscures visualization, options for control include: time to allow a clot to form followed by endoscopic lavage, dropping of the head, direct pressure with a gauze sponge held with bronchoesophageal forceps, or increasing the wattage delivered to the area of hemorrhage to aid in coagulation. None of these techniques work 100% of the time and in some instances

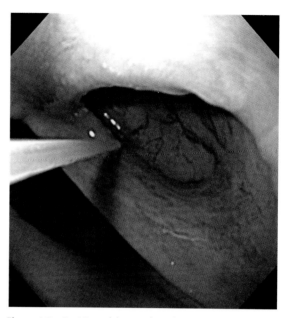

Figure 4.3   Incision of the vocal cord 2–3-mm ventral to the vocal process of the arytenoid cartilage.

hemorrhage is persistent enough that the procedure must be abandoned. Fortunately in most instances, if the surgeon is patient enough hemorrhage will abate and the procedure can be completed.

Standing laser VCE

The horse is restrained in stocks with the head secured in cross ties or supported with head support and held by an assistant (Hawkins and Andrews-Jones 2001). The horse is sedated with detomidine hydrochloride (5–10 mg, IV) and butorphanol tartrate (5–10 mg, IV). The right and left rostral nasal passage is desensitized with topical application of mepivacaine or cetacaine (Cetylite Industries, Inc., Pennsauken, NJ, USA) spray. The endoscope is inserted into the right nasal passage and the vocal cord and laryngeal ventricle are visualized. The mucous membrane of the vocal cord, laryngeal ventricle, and dorsal surface of the epiglottis is desensitized with topical anesthetic delivered via an endoscopic sprayer.

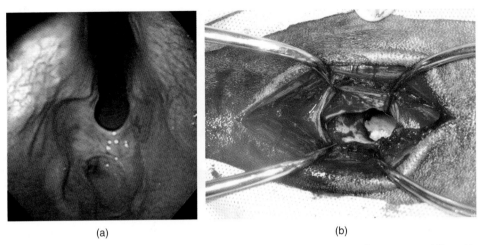

(a)   (b)

Figure 4.4   (a) An endoscopic photograph of a Quarter Horse, gelding with ventral cicatrix formation post bilateral laser ventriculocordectomy. (b) An intraoperative photograph of the ventral cicatrix as seen via laryngotomy. Rostral is to the left and caudal is to the right.

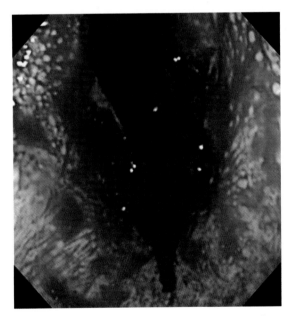

Figure 4.5   Endoscopic photograph of excessive hemorrhage obscuring visualization of the remaining portions of the vocal cord and laryngeal ventricle.

Recumbent laser VCE

The horse is anesthetized routinely and positioned in right lateral recumbency (Tulleners 1996). The horse can either be nasotracheally intubated or left unintubated. The horse cannot be maintained under inhalation anesthesia because of the risk for airway fire when the diode laser is used. While the laser is activated anesthesia is maintained with a continuous infusion of xylazine hydrochloride, ketamine hydrochloride, and guaifenesin (triple drip). Once the laser procedure is completed, the horse is intubated (if not already) and inhalation anesthesia is commenced.

A mouth speculum is used to open the mouth. A hand is inserted into the oral cavity to manually displace the epiglottis from the soft palate. The endoscope is inserted into the oral cavity to visualize the larynx. Suction is required for smoke evacuation during the procedure to improve visualization (Figure 4.6). Once the laryngeal ventricle and vocal cord are identified, the laser procedure is completed with one of the following options.

Noncontact/contact laser photoablation of the vocal cord and ventricle

Noncontact/contact laser photoablation of the vocal cord and ventricle is preferred by some surgeons because it is easy and straightforward to perform. It requires no specialized equipment besides the laser and laser fiber. However, to be effective it is best performed at higher laser wattages of 25–75 watts and some surgeons even prefer wattages approaching 100 watts. I prefer to use 30–45 watts

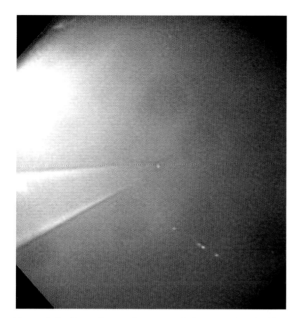

Figure 4.6   Excessive smoke accumulation associated with intraoral laser ventriculocordectomy.

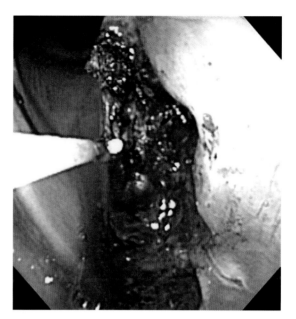

Figure 4.7   Contact photoablation of the vocal cord and laryngeal ventricle with a 600-µm sculpted laser fiber.

in a contact fashion, continuous wave, with laser energy delivered in a pattern of 3 seconds on and 1 second off. A 600-µm sculpted laser fiber is used to ablate the vocal cord first. Under endoscopic guidance, the vocal cord is ablated just ventral to the vocal process and the laser fiber is "paintbrushed" over the cord until the cord is level with the laryngeal lumen (Figure 4.7). Following vocal cord ablation the laryngeal ventricle is ablated in a contact fashion. In general, for photoablation of the vocal cord and laryngeal ventricle approximately 7000–10 000 joules of laser energy is needed. Iatrogenic injury to the arytenoid cartilage should be avoided to decrease the risk for arytenoid chondritis.

Contact laser VCE with instrumentation

Contact laser VCE with instrumentation can be performed with the aid of either bronchoesophageal grasping forceps (Hawkins and Andrews-Jones 2001; Tulleners 1996) or a custom-designed roaring burr (Henderson et al. 2007; Robinson et al. 2006; Sullins 2005). Bronchoesophageal grasping forceps are used to evert the laryngeal ventricle (Figure 4.8). Once everted the laryngeal ventricle is excised using a sculpted diode laser fiber. The

laser is set to 15–25 watts, continuous wave, and deployed at an interval of 3 seconds on and 1 second off. Starting dorsally the ventricle is incised until transected. Once the laryngeal ventricle has been excised, the vocal cord is photoablated as previously described.

An alternative to the use of bronchoesophageal forceps is to use the roaring burr to evert the laryngeal ventricle (Figure 4.9). There are two variations of the roaring burr. One is used to remove the right (turns counter clockwise) laryngeal ventricle and the other is used to remove the left (turns clockwise) laryngeal ventricle. When using the roaring burr for laser VCE the dorsal, ventral, and caudal ligaments of the vocal cord are incised with the laser. The roaring burr is then inserted into the left nasal passage if standing or via the oral cavity if recumbent. The burr is inserted into the laryngeal ventricle as far as possible. The burr is rotated clockwise and gentle traction is placed on the burr to evert the laryngeal ventricle. The laser fiber is then used to incise the everted laryngeal ventricle starting from the ventral to dorsal as needed to completely excise the ventricle. Continual tension with the burr and clockwise rotation greatly aid the dissection process. It has been the authors' experience that the use of the roaring burr results in a larger amount of

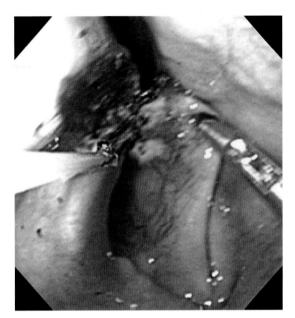

Figure 4.8   Eversion of the right laryngeal ventricle with bronchoesophageal grasping forceps.

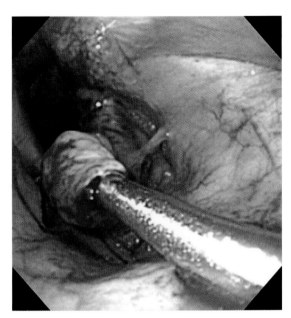

Figure 4.9   Intraoperative endoscopic photograph of eversion of the laryngeal ventricle using an intraoral roaring burr.

ventricle removal when compared to eversion with bronchoesophageal grasping forceps. However, I have found the use of the roaring burr to be more difficult than using bronchoesophageal grasping forceps. It can be challenging to rotate the roaring burr through a complete revolution with the tip of the burr being bent to aid insertion into the laryngeal ventricle. With the tip of the roaring burr bent to aid insertion into the ventricle makes rotation through a complete revolution difficult. Obviously the use of the roaring burr has a steeper learning curve and requires more practice than when using bronchoesophageal grasping forceps.

Aftercare

All horses following laser VCE are treated with oral or IV phenylbutazone (2.2–4.4 mg/kg, q12h) and dexamethasone (20–40 mg, IV). Antimicrobials are optional for VCE performed as a solitary procedure. When VCE is combined with prosthetic laryngoplasty, all horses will be treated with antimicrobials. Healing post laser VCE is generally complete within 30–45 days postoperatively (Figure 4.10). It is recommended that horses receive a minimum of 30 days off from exercise following laser VCE.

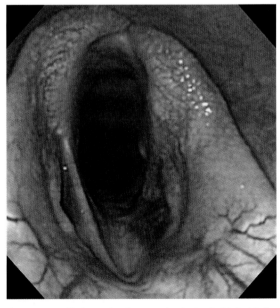

Figure 4.10   Endoscopic photograph of a healed left-sided laser ventriculocordectomy.

References

Bristol DG, Palmer SE, Tate LP, Bowman KF. 1995. Complications of Nd:YAG laser ventriculectomy in the horse, a review of 106 consecutive cases. *Journal of Clinical Laser Medicine and Surgery* 13: 377–381.

Brown JA, Derksen FJ, Stick JA, Hartmann WM, Robinson NE. 2003. Ventriculocordectomy reduces respiratory noise in horses with laryngeal hemiplegia. *Equine Veterinary Journal* 35(6):570–574.

Hawkins JF, Andrews-Jones L. 2001. Neodymium: yttrium aluminum garnet laser ventriculocordectomy in standing horses. *American Journal of Veterinary Research* 62(4):531–537.

Henderson CE, Sullins KE, Brown JA. 2007. Transendoscopic, laser-assisted ventriculocordectomy for treatment of left laryngeal hemiplegia in horses: 22 cases (1999–2005). *Journal of American Veterinary Medical Association* 231(12):1868–1872.

Robinson P, Dersken FJ, Stick JA, Sullins KE, DeTolve PG, Robinson NE. 2006. Effects of unilateral laser-assisted ventriculocordectomy in horses with laryngeal hemiplegia. *Equine Veterinary Journal* 38(6):491–496.

Sullins KE. 2005. Videoendoscopic laser ventriculocordectomy in the standing horse using a transnasal sacculectomy burr. *Proceedings of the American Association of Equine Practitioners*, Vol. 51.

Tulleners EP. 1996. Instrumentation and techniques in transendoscopic upper respiratory tract laser surgery. In: Baxter GM, ed. *The Veterinary Clinics of North America: Equine Practice.* (pp. 373–395). Philadelphia, PA: W.B. Saunders Company.

5 Prosthetic Laryngoplasty

Eric J. Parente and Jan Hawkins

Introduction

The objective of prosthetic laryngoplasty (PL) is to maintain a stable glottis that will provide enough airflow for the horse to perform its intended use without complications. This objective is accomplished by placing a loop(s) of suture from the caudal border of the cricoid through the muscular process of the arytenoid. While performing, PL may seem simple but there are many variables that will impact the success of the procedure.

Preoperative evaluation to definitively diagnose recurrent laryngeal neuropathy (RLN) cannot be underestimated. Laryngeal dysplasia (branchial arch defect), chondropathy, or failed laryngoplasty can all appear endoscopically similar to RLN, yet they would all likely warrant different treatments. Any question on the part of the examiner about the presence of RLN should prompt further diagnostic evaluation. High-speed treadmill or overground endoscopy would be the best choice to confirm the diagnosis of RLN.

Prior to surgery, horses are treated with prophylactic antimicrobials and anti-inflammatories that proceed through the perioperative period. Horses are clipped of all hair centered at the ventral aspect of the linguofacial vein. Once anesthetized, an orotracheal endotracheal tube or nasotracheal endotracheal tube can be used. Nasotracheal intubation with a 20-mm tube is preferred, since it will allow easier assessment of intraoperative arytenoid abduction and can allow adequate room for laser ventriculocordectomy prior to the laryngoplasty, if so chosen (see Chapter 4).

Surgical techniques for prosthetic laryngoplasty

The horse is positioned in right lateral recumbency with the horse's head extended as much as possible. One of the authors (Hawkins) maintains an extended head position with the aid of a board placed against the poll. The board is then stabilized with two short poles positioned in the surgery table. It is beneficial to have the nose tipped down slightly which will in turn elevate the caudal aspect of the mandible up and away from the larynx (Figure 5.1). In addition, a 3-liter fluid bag should be placed under the larynx to prevent the larynx from sinking away from the surgeon during the procedure. The skin

Advances in Equine Upper Respiratory Surgery, First Edition. Edited by Jan Hawkins.
© 2015 ACVS Foundation. Published 2015 by John Wiley & Sons, Inc.

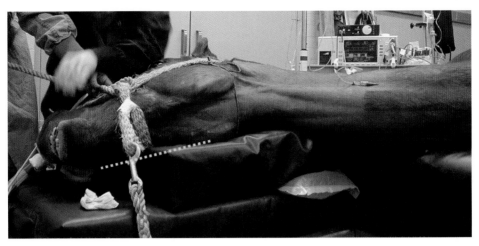

Figure 5.1   Horse in right lateral recumbency with dotted line demonstrating the slight tipped down position of the nose to provide better access to the lateral side of the larynx.

incision is centered at the intersection of the caudal aspect of the cricoid and linguofacial vein. The incision is made 6–10-cm long and parallels the ventral border of the vein, slightly curved ventrally. Sharp dissection is required to separate the vein from the omohyoideus muscle. Dissection through the omohyoideus muscle should be avoided. Once through the fascia, blunt dissection is performed to create space on the dorsolateral side of the larynx. The muscular process and the caudal border of the cricoid cartilage should be easily palpated. The caudal laryngeal artery should be palpated along the caudal border of the cricoid and bluntly dissected to a more ventral position to allow suture placement dorsally, minimizing the risk of puncture. The muscular process should be clearly exposed either by separation of the cricopharyngeus and thyropharyngeus muscles or caudal to the cricopharyngeus muscle (modified procedure). The latter is preferred since it obviates the need to later pass the suture under the cricopharyngeus, and minimizes soft tissue interference (Figure 5.2).

Once the muscular process is exposed, sutures can be placed or the cricoarytenoideus (CAD) muscle/tendon can be transected to access the cricoarytenoid joint and allow better visual assessment of the eventual needle placement through the muscular process (Parente et al. 2011). To transect the CAD muscle and tendon, a curved hemostat is passed from the thyroid cartilage dorsally under the CAD. The muscle is then clamped to minimize any hem-

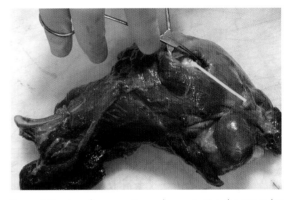

Figure 5.2   A cadaver specimen demonstrating the muscular process exposed caudal to the cricopharyngeus muscle. The yellow line demonstrates the eventual position of the sutures.

orrhage and then transected 2–3-mm caudal to the muscular process. This leaves a small section of tendon attached to the muscular process that can then be used to retract the muscular process rostrally to access the CAD joint. Facilitated ankylosis of the joint can then be performed (see Chapter 7).

Once the exposure of the muscular process of the arytenoid cartilage and cricoid cartilage is complete, sutures can be placed. There are multiple opinions for suture material and suture placement. Previous studies indicate that the maximal load on the suture is under 50 N (Witte et al. 2010) and the type of needle impacts the stability of the construct (Ahern and Parente 2010). For these reasons No. 5 Ethibond on the V37 needle (Ethicon Inc.,

Somerville, NJ, USA) is preferred by this author (Parente). There is also some disagreement about the number of sutures placed and their relative position. Regardless of the type of suture material and the number of sutures, the goal is to create a stable construct that will maintain the desired arytenoid abduction. The suture is first placed through the cricoid. The specific position of the needle is determined at the time of surgery based on the individual cricoid conformation. Since the tail end of the suture will eventually wrap over the caudal edge of the cricoid cartilage, the variability of the caudal edge of the cricoid may impact long-term suture position. If the tail end of the suture were to slide ventrally on the cricoid cartilage postoperatively, this would result in relative loosening and loss of abduction.

The first suture is placed in the most dorsal position possible. If there is a midline notch that can be accessed, the tail end of the first suture can be placed within that notch. Thus it is important to find a "notch" the tail end of the suture can slide into or make sure the suture is as ventral as it can be when the suture is tied so that no further loosening can take place over time postoperatively. The tip of the needle is placed just deep to the cricoid edge and slid forward parallel to the plane of the cartilage and then the tip is rotated up through the cricoid cartilage. Again care should be exercised not to lose control of the needle at any time to ensure there is no penetration into the laryngeal lumen. Intraoperative endoscopy is invaluable in ensuring that the laryngeal mucosa is not penetrated during needle insertion through the cricoid.

After the needle is passed through the cricoid it is passed through the muscular process, if the cricopharyngeus muscle was reflected rostrally. If the cricopharyngeus and thyropharyngeus muscles were separated to expose the muscular process, the suture is placed under the cricopharyngeus muscle before passing it through the muscular process. The needle is passed from a caudal medial to rostral lateral direction and an attempt is made to have the needle exit just dorsal to the sagittal ridge of the muscular process. The second suture is placed similarly just lateral to the first through both the cricoid and then muscular process. The needle is then passed through the muscular process parallel to the first, with the needle passing through the sagittal ridge of the muscular process.

When tying the suture ends together to create abduction, it is important to ensure that the suture ends slide freely. If the sutures do not slide freely through the cartilage, the more lateral side of the suture loop can be under greater tension than the medial side of the loop. This will result in equilibration over time and thus an overall loosening and potential loss of abduction. For this reason the suture placed second (more lateral) is used to create the abduction desired and then the first suture is slid through both cartilages and then tied. The second suture which initially was maintaining the position of the arytenoid is then slid through both cartilages before it is tied.

Inability to slide the first suture can be because of soft tissue interference or that the second suture passes through the first suture. If the latter occurs, it can be corrected by freeing the sutures from each other and pulling the "pierced" suture through even further so it becomes a discarded portion once the knot is tied.

Once both sutures are well placed, the videoendoscope is passed down the left nostril to the level of the larynx. First, the laryngeal lumen is assessed to make sure there is no suture penetration through the mucosa at the caudal margin of the cricoid. If that were to occur, that suture should be cut and removed without dragging the contaminated suture through the lumen. The endoscope is then focused on the front of the larynx to judge abduction of the arytenoid (Figure 5.3). While the amount of abduction is very subjective, aiming for approximately 90% of full abduction is desired (Rakesh et al. 2008).

Alternative laryngoplasty technique

An alternative to the two-suture laryngoplasty technique described by Parente is to substitute No. 5 Fiberwire™ (Arthrex, Naples, FL, USA) for the first suture and a Securos (Securos, Fiskdale, MA) tieback suture for the second suture. The sutures are placed as previously described; however, they are tied in a different sequence. The Securos tie back system consists of a tension device, crimp clamps, and a crimper to secure the crimps (Scherzer and Hainisch 2005). Once the Fiberwire suture and the Securos suture have been positioned, the Fiberwire suture is tied once (one throw of a square knot) and the suture ends are clamped with Carmalt

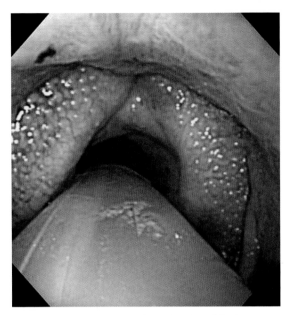

Figure 5.3   Intraoperative endoscopic view of the larynx while creating abduction. The nasotracheal tube is 20-mm inner diameter.

hemostats (Figure 5.4). The Fiberwire is resistant to damage with the Carmalts. The Securos tension device is then used to tighten the suture. The suture is tightened under endoscopic guidance. The purpose of this suture is to abduct the arytenoid, just sort of "ideal" abduction. Final arytenoid abduction is achieved when the Securos suture is ten-

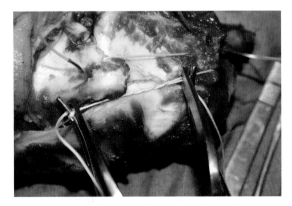

Figure 5.4   Gross dissection of an equine larynx depicting tensioning of the Fiberwire suture with the Securos tension device. The tension device is tightened against Carmalt hemostats clamped to the Securos suture.

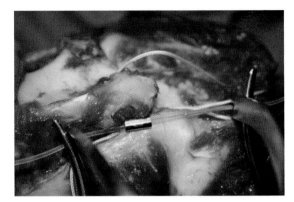

Figure 5.5   Gross postmortem photograph depicting tightening of the Securos suture with the tension device. Note the presence of a single crimp and the Carmalts securing the suture against the tension device. Finally note that once the Securos suture has been tightened the Fiberwire suture loosens.

sioned. Once the Fiberwire suture is tensioned, the first throw of the knot is clamped with a needle holder and the tension device is removed and the knot is completed. Next, a single crimp is positioned over the ends of the Securos suture and the suture is tensioned manually to tighten the suture. Once the suture has been hand tightened, the suture is clamped with Carmalts approximately 2 cm from the crimp and the tension device is used to tighten the suture (Figure 5.5). Arytenoid abduction is assessed with intraoperative endoscopy and once satisfactory abduction is achieved, the crimp is clamped twice with the crimping device (Figure 5.6). The advantages of this technique are that

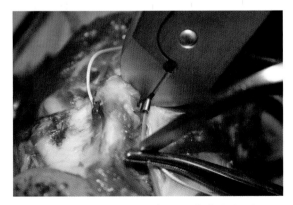

Figure 5.6   Gross postmortem photograph depicting the crimping of the clamp with the Securos crimping device.

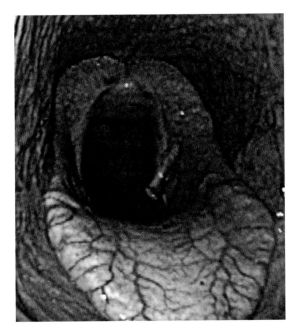

Figure 5.7 Endoscopic view of the larynx the morning after laryngoplasty.

the first suture is used to position the arytenoid just short of ideal abduction and the second suture positions the arytenoid in the ideal location. In addition, dissection of laryngeal cadavers has revealed that the first suture frequently loosens when the Securos suture is tightened and crimped (Figure 5.5).

Once the sutures are tied the subcutaneous tissues and skin are closed routinely. An adherent drape/bandage with a few 4 × 4 gauze sponges are placed over the incision to protect it during recovery but can be removed immediately thereafter.

Postoperative course and aftercare

Postoperatively another endoscopic examination is performed the morning after surgery (Figure 5.7). The position of the left arytenoid should be assessed relative to the right during maximal abduction following the induction of swallowing. There should be minimal evidence of inflammation and no evidence of feed material within the airway (Figure 5.6). The horse is maintained in a stall with hand walking for 1 month before returning to exercise and fed hay from the ground. Antimicrobials and anti-inflammatories are generally continued for 1 week. Skin suture removal is recommended at 2 weeks.

References

Ahern BJ, Parente EJ. 2010. Mechanical evaluation of the equine laryngoplasty. *Veterinary Surgery* 39(6):661–666.

Parente EJ, Birks EK, Habecker P. 2011. A modified laryngoplasty approach promoting ankylosis of the cricoarytenoid joint. *Veterinary Surgery* 40(2):204–210.

Rakesh V, Ducharme N, Cheetham J, Datta AK, Pease AP. 2008. Implications of different degrees of arytenoid cartilage abduction on equine upper airway characteristics. *Equine Veterinary Journal* 40:629–635.

Scherzer S, Hainisch EK. 2005. Evaluation of a canine cranial cruciate ligament repair system for use in equine laryngoplasty. *Veterinary Surgery* 34(6):548–553.

Witte TH, Cheetham J, Soderholm LV, Mitchell LM, Ducharme NG. 2010. Equine laryngoplasty sutures undergo increased loading during coughing and swallowing. *Veterinary Surgery* 39(8):949–956.

6 Biomechanics of Prosthetic Laryngoplasty

Benjamin J. Ahern

Introduction

The biomechanical principles behind prosthetic laryngoplasty (PL) are basic. Simply put, prosthetic material replaces the abductor muscle function of the larynx to achieve arytenoid abduction. Abduction of the affected arytenoid thus allows for effective airflow. However, the surgical techniques employed to achieve this function are varied and have been associated with unreliable results. As a result understanding the biomechanics involved with PL is warranted. In general, biomechanics is the study of the behavior of a biological body when subjected to forces or displacement and the subsequent effects on the system in question. In recent years, new research pertaining to equine PL has been performed. The objective of this chapter is to outline these developments and how this information is helping to improve the outcomes of PL.

What are the goals of prosthetic laryngoplasty?

Although this may seem like a basic question with an obvious answer, it is important that the under-lying principles of PL are understood. Recurrent laryngeal neuropathy (RLN) results in poor performance in equine athletes due to the inability of the cricoarytenoideus dorsalis (CAD) muscle to maintain arytenoid abduction during exercise (Dart et al. 2009; Davenport et al. 2001; Derksen et al. 1986). The loss of arytenoid abduction leads to a reduction in the cross-sectional area (CSA) of the rima glottidis resulting in decreased inspiratory flow, increased respiratory impedance, hypoxemia, exercise intolerance, and abnormal respiratory noise (Davenport et al. 2001; Derksen et al. 1986).The influence of reduction in the CSA of the rima glottidis and its effects on airflow are best understood by Poiseuille's Law regarding fluid dynamics. This law states that $R = 8 \; ul/r^4$. Interpretation of this law reveals that a unit reduction in the radius (the CSA), of a tube (e.g., the larynx) will result in an increase in the resistance to airflow by the fourth power. It follows then that optimal airflow and surgical success will likely be achieved by stable arytenoid abduction and a large airway CSA. Obtaining surgical arytenoid abduction can be achieved using a wide array of techniques. Loss of arytenoid abduction has been shown to be the most common complication following PL. In a retrospective study

Advances in Equine Upper Respiratory Surgery, First Edition. Edited by Jan Hawkins.
© 2015 ACVS Foundation. Published 2015 by John Wiley & Sons, Inc.

reported by Dixon et al. in 2003, progressive loss of abduction occurred over the first 6 weeks postoperatively with a majority (one grade of abduction loss) occurring in the first 7 days (Dixon et al. 2003). Short-term excessive loss of abduction occurred in 10 of the 200 cases reported, five due to suture migration in the cricoid, three due to broken wire, and two due to avulsion of the arytenoid.

Biomechanics of prosthetic laryngoplasty

There are four central components to a laryngoplasty construct. These are (1) the arytenoid cartilage, (2) the cricoid cartilage, (3) the cricoarytenoid (CA) articulation, and (4) the prosthetic suture/material. How these segments interact determines the effectiveness of obtaining and maintaining effective arytenoid abduction. Recent research has focused on the interplay of these central components and attempted to maximize the stability of the surgical construct.

Mechanical research of laryngoplasty has historically focused on single cycle testing to failure (Dean et al. 1990; Kelly et al. 2008; Mathews et al. 2004; Rossignol et al. 2006; Schumacher et al. 2000). A criticism of this form of research is that the forces required to cause failure of the cartilage-suture constructs appear to be vastly outside the physiological loads seen *in vivo*. Recently, cyclical models of laryngoplasty testing have been reported and are likely a more critical evaluation of traditional and novel laryngoplasty techniques (Ahern and Parente 2010; Cheetham et al. 2008b).

An important factor that is required for the evaluation of a laryngoplasty construct from a mechanical standpoint is the load is applied to the cartilage-suture construct *in vivo*. This question was examined by Witte et al. in 2010, in an experimental model using E-type buckle force transducers (Witte et al. 2010a, 2010b). In the eight horses in this *in vivo* study, the force required to achieve optimal arytenoid abduction was found to be 27.6 ± 7.5 N. During swallowing and coughing, the mean force on the suture increased by 19.0 ± 5.6 N and 12.1 ± 3.6 N, respectively. In addition, these horses were instrumented for 24 hours and it was found that the suture underwent cyclical loading due to swallowing at a mean of 1152 times in that period, a rate of 0.8 times per minute. It is important to note that in this study in one horse the force on the suture was 55% higher at surgery than in the other horses and it subsequently had complete failure of the laryngoplasty construct due to suture pullout from the arytenoid at 12 hours after surgery. From this research, it was estimated that the peak force on a laryngoplasty construct would be 46.6 N (4.75 kg). The force reported to obtain abduction was higher than the force reported to cause maximal abduction in an *in vitro* study reported by Cramp et al. in 2009 (Cramp 2009). In that study, the load required *in vitro* was only 14.7 N. However, this was an *in vitro* study on cadaveric larynges and the load may have been lower than *in vivo* due to the absence of muscular function or different suture placement positioning.

The arytenoid cartilage

The arytenoid cartilage has historically been suspected as a major cause of abduction loss post PL. Due to this belief, a majority of the laryngeal biomechanical research has been focused on the muscular process and its role in maintaining abduction (Dean et al. 1990; Kelly et al. 2008; Mathews et al. 2004; Rossignol et al. 2006). This has included evaluation of the effect of age, placement site, implantation technique, and various suture configurations (Dean et al. 1990; Herde et al. 2001; Kelly et al. 2008; Rossignol et al. 2006). Most of this research has been performed in a single cycle to failure models and have uniformly been associated with loads at failure that are much higher than those demonstrated to occur *in vivo*. As such the relevance of this early research has been called into question. However, in 2008, Kelly examined six different suture configurations in the muscular process of the arytenoid. It was concluded that sutures that sufficiently engaged the spine of the muscular process alone or in conjunction with a second suture were the most biomechanically stable. These results parallel research in dogs that found the size of the hole for the suture or the suture size had no or little effect, but those sutures that incorporated the arcuate crest were biomechanically superior (Mathews et al. 2004). The arcuate crest (*crista arcuata*) is the cartilaginous ridge that extends cranially from the apex of the muscular process along a line parallel to the orientation of the CAD muscle (Figure 6.1). This

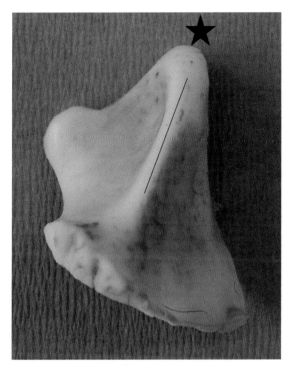

Figure 6.1   Arytenoid cartilage dissected of all soft tissue demonstrating the arcuate crest (line) extending from the muscular process (star) towards corniculate process.

research emphasizes the importance of the laryngoplasty suture(s) engaging this ridge to ensure maximum construct stability. The muscles that act to close the glottis attach to and partially obscure the arcuate crest allowing for surgical error at this point and as such it is important that when placing sutures in the muscular process, the conformation and anatomy of the cartilage are kept in mind. A recently reported technique to debride the CAJ involves transecting the CAD muscle and opening the CAJ. Utilization of this technique allows for superior identification of the muscular process and improves accurate and consistent laryngoplasty suture placement (Parente et al. 2011).

The method of suture placement into the arytenoid cartilage has not been shown to be an important factor (e.g., tunneling a hole with a hypodermic needle compared to a swaged on needle) (Rossignol et al. 2006). However, the use of a conventional cutting needle compared to a tapercut needle resulted in significantly lower peak loads at failure in a single cycle model and resulted in significantly more

distraction in a cyclical model (Ahern and Parente 2010). This was thought to result from the cutting needle creating a groove into which the suture propagated more readily than when placed with the tapercut needle. Recently, a screw placed into the arytenoid has been utilized as a point of anchorage in the arytenoid. This technique has not been utilized widely; however, it is thought to increase the stability of the arytenoid segment of the laryngoplasty construct. As a result of the previously discussed research, it would seem that placement of a prosthetic suture solidly engaging the spine of the muscular process and utilization of a tapercut or similar minimally traumatic needle for insertion will result in the most stable arytenoid suture placement for the laryngoplasty construct. Furthermore, based on the cyclical testing that has been currently performed, it appears that the arytenoid cartilage is not a major source of loss of abduction if appropriate positioning is achieved.

The cricoid cartilage

The cricoid cartilage has emerged as an important component of the laryngoplasty construct that has been underemphasized. Computed tomographic imaging of the cricoid has been found to have notable conformational differences among cricoid specimens from a group of Thoroughbred larynges (Dahlberg et al. 2009). These differences are markedly evident during dissections of the equine larynx (Figure 6.2). Logically, this variability at the caudal aspect of the cricoid cartilage may result in some variability in the ability of the cricoid to maintain a suture in the laryngoplasty construct. During anatomic dissection, the caudal aspect of the cricoid cartilage is often composed of soft, very thin cartilage that tapers to a fine edge. This area of the cartilage is readily deformed and is variably notched. Suture migration in the cricoid was identified as the cause of 50% of short-term excessive loss of abduction when it occurred in a series of 200 horses (Dixon et al. 2003). This suture migration is likely attributable to the variable shape of the caudal aspect of the cricoid cartilage.

Based on these observations on the variability of the caudal aspect of the cricoid cartilage, it has been hypothesized that this was a cause of variability in the laryngoplasty construct. Cyclical mechanical

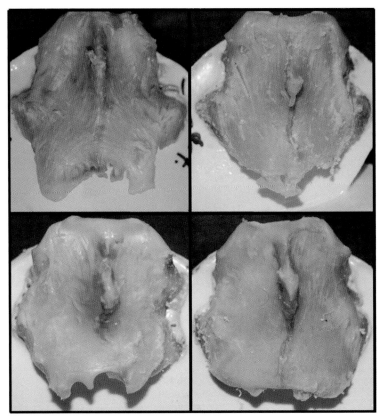

Figure 6.2   Cricoid cartilages of Thoroughbred horse larynges dissected of all soft tissues. Up is cranial and down is caudal in each image, when viewing the cricoid from a dorsal aspect. The bottom edge of each image demonstrates the marked variability of the caudal aspect of the cricoid.

testing of arytenoid and cricoid constructs from 30 to 50 N (3.06–5.1 kg) at 1 Hz for a total of 3600 cycles was performed to compare between a single strand of Ethibond and an alternate laryngoplasty system (ALPS) (Ahern 2012). The ALPS system is different in that it does not utilize the caudal aspect of the cricoid as a point of anchoring the laryngoplasty construct. In this testing the Ethibond construct had significantly more distraction than the ALPS constructs in the cricoid cartilage (5.06 ± 1.25 mm and 1.58 ± 0.19 mm, respectively). Of particular note, however, is the standard error of the mean (SEM) for the Ethibond testing of cricoid cartilage (Figure 6.3). This large SEM number translates to a very large range for the cricoid cartilages tested. This variability in the range of distraction was not evident for the ALPS or for either constructs when tested in the arytenoid cartilage. These results sup-

port the hypothesis that the variability of the caudal aspect of the cricoid cartilage is the major source of biomechanical variability in the laryngoplasty construct.

Various techniques associated with the cricoid cartilage have been proposed to reduce the loss of abduction seen in the postoperative phase. These range from sawing the suture to "seat it" before tying, placing the sutures "into" the dorsal notch when present, double loops around the caudal edge of the cricoid and novel laryngoplasty systems involving cables and washers or anchors (Schumacher et al. 2000; Ahern 2012).

It is highly likely in the author's opinion that the caudal edge of the cricoid cartilage is the most important portion and least predictable component of the equine laryngoplasty procedure. This is due to the intrinsic variability between horses and as

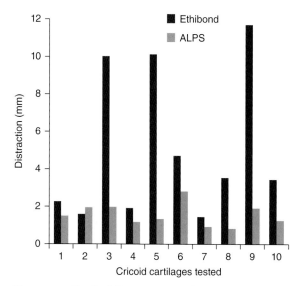

Figure 6.3 Graph of distraction (mm) during cyclical mechanical testing of cricoid cartilages tested using a single strand of Ethibond or a novel alternate laryngoplasty system. Note the variability in the amount of distraction of the Ethibond constructs.

such may be a major factor in the loss of abduction seen *in vivo* postoperatively.

The cricoarytenoid articulation

The CA articulation is an important component of a laryngoplasty construct. The distances from the longer corniculate process to the articulation and subsequently to the shorter muscular process are important components of a lever arm. As a result of this lever arm, small changes in the position of the muscular process will result in proportionally much larger changes in the positioning of the corniculate process and loss of abduction. For example, a loss of 5 mm between the arytenoid/suture/cricoid construct will lead to a 15–20 mm loss at the corniculate process and arytenoid abduction loss.

The importance of the CA articulation was examined by Cheetham et al. (2008a). In this study, the effect of stabilizing the CAJ by injecting it with polymethyl methacrylate (PMMA) was evaluated. It was found that stabilizing the joint with PMMA resisted collapse of the airway and reduced the force experienced by the suture during maxi-

mal abduction. More recently, a surgical technique to promote ankylosis of the CAJ has been published that resulted in decreased loss of abduction of the arytenoid in the postoperative period (Parente et al. 2011). When utilizing a technique to ankylose the CAJ (see Chapter 7), it is important to obtain and maintain appropriate abduction in the postoperative period during which the ankylosis matures. For example, if you have acute loss of abduction postoperatively, the ankylosis will complicate a delayed second laryngoplasty procedure and as such the repeated laryngoplasty procedure should be pursued earlier than would be commonly performed in a traditional failed laryngoplasty.

Utilization of a technique to ankylose the CAJ reduced the forces on the laryngoplasty sutures and resulted in decreased loss of abduction postoperatively and should be considered as a means to help reduce loss of arytenoid abduction (Cheetham et al. 2008a; Parente et al. 2011).

The prosthetic suture/material

Various prosthetic materials have been used for PL. Materials reported include catgut, wire, nylon, polyester, polytetrafluoroethylene, ultra-high molecular weight polyethylene, and braided cable (Ahern and Parente 2008, 2010; Ahern et al. 2012; Bohanon et al. 1990; Davenport et al. 2001; Dixon et al. 2003; Goulden and Anderson 1982; Greet et al. 1979; Kidd and Slone 2002; Kraus et al. 2003; Roberston 2000; Scherzer and Hainisch 2005; Witte et al. 2010a, b). Many of these materials are much stronger than the necessary requirements to obtain and maintain arytenoid abduction. It is broadly accepted that the use of a nonabsorbable material that is of sufficient size (e.g., No. 5 [7.0 metric]) is very unlikely to be the cause of loss of abduction in an equine laryngoplasty construct. The strength of these materials is simply so far greater than the loading seen in a laryngoplasty construct *in vivo* that so long as a reasonable suture material is selected it will suffice. Care must be taken not to damage the suture material during insertion and as such weaken its mechanical properties. Similarly, during the insertion of stainless steel wire care must be taken to prevent bending and potential weakening of the material and predisposing to acute failure. As previously mentioned, the manner in which the suture material is inserted into the cartilage may be a factor with cutting needles potentially leading to increased loss of abduction *in vitro* (Ahern and Parente 2010). It has been found that the use of two sutures in the construct is superior to a single strand (Kelly et al. 2008). This is likely due to increased cartilage stability with two strands rather than any increased strength on the part of the suture. In addition, slightly different angles of the sutures have been suggested to increase the CAJ stability *in vitro* (Dart et al. 2009).

As a result, the use of two sutures of a suitably sized prosthetic suture material attached to a minimally traumatic needle in a slightly divergent pattern at the caudal edge of the cricoid cartilage is recommended to achieve and maintain abduction.

In conclusion, the success rates that have been reported for such a commonly performed surgery are relatively modest. This is a technically demanding surgery where attention to detail and small changes are associated with large alterations of the surgical outcome. This chapter has aimed to outline the current understanding of laryngeal biomechanics associated with PL, aid in our current understanding, and improve the future results with this procedure.

References

Ahern BJ, Parente EJ. 2008. Surgical complications of the equine upper respiratory tract. *Veterinary Clinics of North America: Equine Practice* 24:465–484.

Ahern BJ, Parente EJ. 2010. Mechanical evaluation of the equine laryngoplasty. *Veterinary Surgery* 39:661–666.

Ahern BJ, Boston RC, Parente EJ. 2012. *In vitro* mechanical testing of an alternative laryngoplasty system (ALPS) for horses. *Veterinary Surgery* 41:918–923.

Bohanon T, Beard W, Robertson J. 1990. Laryngeal hemiplegia in draft horses. A review of 27 cases. *Veterinary Surgery* 19:456–459.

Cheetham J, Witte TH, Rawlinson JJ, Soderholm LV, Mohammed HO, Ducharme NG. 2008a. Intra-articular stabilisation of the equine cricoarytenoid joint. *Equine Veterinary Journal* 40:584–588.

Cheetham J, Witte TH, Soderholm LV, Hermanson JW, Ducharme NG. 2008b. In vitro model for testing novel implants for equine laryngoplasty. *Veterinary Surgery* 37:588–593.

Cramp P, Derksen FJ, Stick JA, de Feijter-Rupp H, Elvin NG, Hauptman J, Robinson NE. 2009. Effect of magnitude and direction of force on laryngeal abduction:

implications for the nerve-muscle pedicle graft technique. *Equine Veterinary Journal* 41(4):328–333.

Dahlberg JA, Valdes-Martinez A, Boston RC, Parente EJ. 2009. Analysis of conformational variations of Thoroughbred cricoid cartilages using computed tomography. *Equine Veterinary Journal* 43(2):229–234.

Dart A, Tee E, Brennan M, Dart C, Perkins N, Chapman S, Debney S. 2009. Effect of prosthesis number and position on rima glottidis area in equine laryngeal specimens. *Veterinary Surgery* 38:452–456.

Davenport C, Tulleners EP, Parente EJ. 2001. The effect of recurrent laryngeal neurectomy in conjunction with laryngoplasty and unilateral ventriculocordectomy in Thoroughbred racehorses. *Veterinary Surgery* 30:417–421.

Dean P, Nelson J, Schumacher J. 1990. Effects of age and prosthesis material on in vitro cartilage retention of laryngoplasty prostheses in horses. *American Journal of Veterinary Research* 51:114–117.

Derksen FJ, Stick JA, Scott EA, Robinson NE, Slocombe RF. 1986. Effect of laryngeal hemiplegia and laryngoplasty on airway flow mechanics in exercising horses. *American Journal of Veterinary Research* 47:16–20.

Dixon PM, McGorum BC, Railton DI, Hawe C, Tremaine WH, Dacre K, McCann J. 2003. Long-term survey of laryngoplasty and ventriculocordectomy in an older, mixed-breed population of 200 horses. Part 1: Maintenance of surgical arytenoid abduction and complications of surgery. *Equine Veterinary Journal* 35:389–396.

Goulden BE, Anderson LG. 1982. Equine laryngeal hemiplegia. III. Treatment by laryngoplasty. *New Zealand Veterinary Journal* 30:1–5.

Greet T, Baker G, Lee R. 1979. The effect of laryngoplasty on pharyngeal function in the horse. *Equine Veterinary Journal* 11:153–158.

Herde I, Boening J, Sasse H. 2001. Arytenoid cartilage retention of laryngoplasty in horses - In vitro assessment of effect of age, placement site, and implantation technique. *American Association of Equine Practitioners Proceedings* 47: 115–119.

Kelly JR, Carmalt J, Hendrick S, Wilson DG, Shoemaker R. 2008. Biomechanical comparison of six suture configurations using a large diameter polyester prosthesis in the muscular process of the equine arytenoid cartilage. *Veterinary Surgery* 37:580–587.

Kidd JA, Slone DE. 2002. Treatment of laryngeal hemiplegia in horses by prosthetic laryngoplasty, ventriculectomy and vocal cordectomy. *Veterinary Record* 150:481–484.

Kraus B, Parente EJ, Tulleners EP. 2003. Laryngoplasty with ventriculectomy or ventriculocordectomy in 104 draft horses (1992–2000). *Veterinary Surgery* 32:530–538.

Mathews KG, Roe S, Stebbins M, Barners R, Mente PL. 2004. Biomechanical evaluation of suture pullout from canine arytenoid cartilages: Effects of hole diameter, suture configuration, suture size, and distraction rate. *Veterinary Surgery* 33:191–199.

Parente EJ, Birks EK, Habecker P. 2011. A modified laryngoplasty approach promoting ankylosis of the cricoarytenoid joint. *Veterinary Surgery* 40:204–210.

Robertson J. 2000. Laryngoplasty: A novel prosthesis. *Equine Veterinary Journal* 32:5–6.

Rossignol F, Perrin R, Desbrosse F, Elie C. 2006. In vitro comparison of two techniques for suture prosthesis placement in the muscular process of the equine arytenoid cartilage. *Veterinary Surgery* 35:49–54.

Scherzer S, Hainisch EK. 2005. Evaluation of a canine cranial cruciate ligament repair system for use in equine laryngoplasty. *Veterinary Surgery* 34:548–553.

Schumacher J, Wilson AM, Pardoe C, Easter JL. (2000) In vitro evaluation of a novel prosthesis for laryngoplasty of horses with recurrent laryngeal neuropathy. *Equine Veterinary Journal* 32:43–46.

Witte TH, Cheetham J, Rawlinson JJ, Soderholm LV, Ducharme NG. 2010a. A transducer for measuring force on surgical sutures. *Canadian Journal of Veterinary Research* 74:299–304.

Witte TH, Cheetham J, Soderholm LV, Michell LM, Ducharme NG. 2010b. Equine laryngoplasty sutures undergo increased loading during coughing and swallowing. *Veterinary Surgery* 39:949–956.

7 Ablation of the Cricoarytenoid Joint

Jan Hawkins

Prosthetic laryngoplasty (PL) is the most commonly performed surgical procedure to correct recurrent laryngeal neuropathy (RLN) in the horse (Dixon et al. 2003a, b; Hawkins et al. 1997). The reported success rate of PL has ranged from 60 to 85% depending on the occupation of the horse (e.g., racing vs. low-level exercise) (Dixon et al. 2003a, b; Hawkins et al. 1997). Most horses will develop a loss of arytenoid abduction within 6 weeks of PL (Dixon et al. 2003a). Loss of arytenoid abduction results in the recurrence of exercise intolerance and upper respiratory tract noise. Reasons for suture loosening include cartilage or implant failure, soft tissue atrophy surrounding the suture material, cartilaginous anatomical abnormalities, or surgeon error (Dixon et al. 2003a). Approximately 10% of horses develop complete (failure) loss of arytenoid abduction following PL (Dixon et al. 2003a).

One possibility for minimizing the loss of arytenoid abduction following laryngoplasty would be to eliminate motion from the cricoarytenoid joint (CAJ) (Parente et al. 2011). The CAJ and the cricothyroid joints are the only articulations of the larynx. The CAJ is similar to other diarthrodial joints, consisting of articular cartilage, synovial membrane, and containing a synovial-type fluid (Kasperbauer 1998; Sellars and Sellars 1983; Wang 1998). The motion of the CAJ has been widely researched in humans and is of three types: gliding, rotational, and rocking. Pathologic fusion of the CAJ has been reported in humans (Casiano et al. 1994; Gacek and Gacek 1996; Gacek and Gacek 1999; Jurik et al. 1985; Muller and Paulsen 2002; Paulsen and Tillmann 1998). In most instances, fusion of the CAJ occurs with the affected arytenoid(s) in an adducted position. Clinical signs of the CAJ fusion in humans include inspiratory stridor and changes in voice. In horses, Parente et al. reported that ankylosis of the CAJ in combination with PL decreased the loss of arytenoid abduction after surgery (Parente et al. 2011).

Surgical debridement of the CAJ in horses can be performed with hand instrumentation and physical removal of the articular cartilage or with thermal damage supplied by surgical lasers (Parente et al. 2011; Spector and Miller 1977). The author has extensive experience with CO_2 laser debridement of the cartilaginous surfaces of the CAJ. In *in vivo* and *in vitro* studies, CO_2 laser debridement of the articular cartilage and CAJ capsule minimized

Advances in Equine Upper Respiratory Surgery, First Edition. Edited by Jan Hawkins.

postoperative loss of arytenoid abduction in combination with PL (Hawkins 2014).

Surgical technique laser debridement of CAJ

The horse is positioned in right lateral recumbency and a routine surgical approach to the larynx for PL is used. To access the CAJ, the tendon of insertion of the cricoarytenoideus dorsalis (CAD) muscle is transected with Metzenbaum scissors (Figure 7.1). It is not unusual to have a small amount of hemorrhage following transection of the CAD tendon of insertion. This can be readily controlled with pressure and suction. Once the CAD tendon has been transected, the CAJ can be digitally palpated. The joint capsule is opened with Metzenbaum scissors or No. 15 scalpel blade. Redundant joint capsule can be resected if necessary to visualize the cricoid and arytenoid facets of the CAJ (Figure 7.2). In preparation for CO_2 laser debridement of the CAJ, a sterile laser scan hand piece is inserted into a laser scan head (40C CO_2 Laser and SurgiTouch™ User interface and scanner, Lumenis, Inc., Santa Clara, CA) and the arm of the laser is covered by a sterile stockinette and adhesive wrap (Figure 7.3). The CO_2 laser is set to continuous wave, power of 15 W, with a 5-mm circular spot size (power density of 150 W/cm^2) in a noncontact

fashion delivered through a laser scan head. The hand piece of the scanner is positioned 3 cm from the articular surfaces of the CAJ. The cricoid facet is visualized by retracting the muscular process of the arytenoid rostrally with one Senn retractor or by a hemostat attached to the transected tendon of insertion of the CAD muscle and the cricopharyngeus muscle is retracted caudally with a second Senn retractor (Figure 7.4). The hand piece of the laser scanner is directed perpendicular to the articular surface whenever possible but to reach the medial aspect of the cricoid facet it is necessary to tilt the scan head ventrally approximately 45°. Following laser debridement of the cricoid facet (Figure 7.5) the Senn retractor on the muscular process is repositioned to retract the muscular process of the arytenoid rostrally to improve visualization of the arytenoid facet. The lateral aspect of the arytenoid facet is lasered by positioning the laser beam perpendicular to the facet. Even with angling of the laser medially, it is difficult to completely remove all cartilage from this facet. To remove the remaining portion of articular cartilage on the medial aspect of the arytenoid facet a 2-0 bone curette is used to manually debride the cartilage. For both the cricoid and arytenoid facets, no attempt is made to remove char secondary to the laser. Once the articular cartilage has been debrided, the CAJ capsule is lasered until charred and contracted. Smoke generated by the laser is removed with suction.

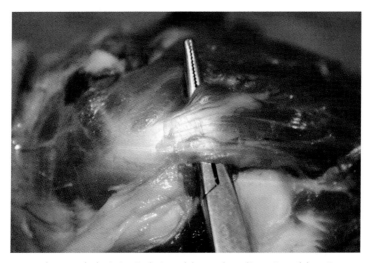

Figure 7.1 Gross postmortem photograph depicting isolation of the tendon of insertion of the cricoarytenoideus dorsalis muscle on the muscular process of the arytenoid cartilage.

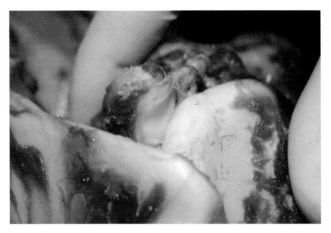

Figure 7.2 Gross postmortem photograph depicting the arytenoid facet and cricoid facet of the cricoarytenoid joint. All soft tissue has been removed for illustrative purposes only.

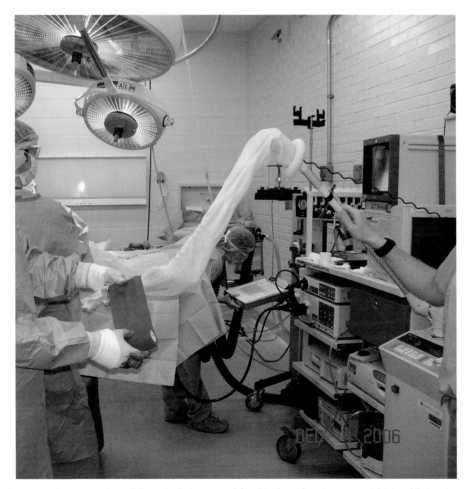

Figure 7.3 Intraoperative preparation of the articulating arm of the CO_2 laser for cricoarytenoid joint ablation. Note that specialized eyewear and endoscope have been used for intraoperative evaluation of arytenoid position.

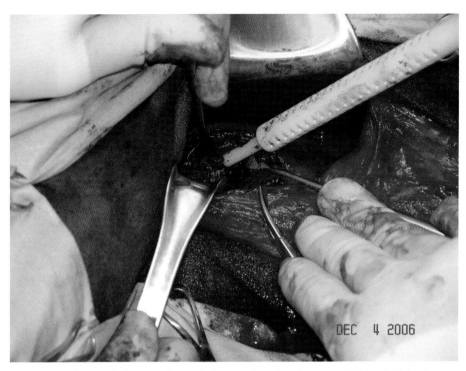

Figure 7.4   Intraoperative photograph depicting the surgical approach to the cricoarytenoid joint. A Richardson retractor is being used to pull the larynx toward the surgeon by traction on the thyroid cartilage. A Poole suction tip is used to remove blood and smoke associated with the procedure and Senn retractors are used for retraction of the muscular process rostrally and the cricopharyngeus muscle caudally.

Following laser debridement of the CAJ, a routine PL as previously described (Chapter 5) is performed. There is no specific aftercare associated with CAJ debridement. The author has not experienced any complications associated with CAJ debridement. This includes experiences with dysphagia resulting from excessive abduction following laryngoplasty. In these cases the prosthetic suture material was removed and clinical signs of dysphagia resolved despite CAJ laser debridement.

Mechanical debridement of the CAJ

Previously, Parente reported that mechanical destruction of the CAJ resulted in improved stability of the arytenoid cartilage when combined with laryngoplasty (Parente et al. 2011). Clinically, Aceto and Parente have also documented that racehorses with RLN treated with modified laryngoplasty with surgical ankylosis of the CAJ returned to a similar level of performance as their untreated cohorts (Aceto and Parente 2012).

Surgical technique mechanical destruction of CAJ

For those surgeons who do not have access to the CO_2 laser for debridement of the CAJ, mechanical destruction of the CAJ is the best option. The instrumentation for mechanical debridement of the CAJ is readily available to most surgeons in equine surgical referral centers.

The approach to the CAJ is the same as described for CO_2 laser debridement. Once the CAJ articular surfaces are exposed, a motorized hand piece (arthroscopy burr: 2-mm motorized fluted burr (Conmed Linvatec, Largo, FL) is used to debride the lateral aspects of the cricoid articular cartilage and the more lateral margin of the articular cartilage of the arytenoid facet. Using this technique it is important to avoid the creation of a longitudinal groove in the muscular process. If a longitudinal groove is created it could predispose the muscular process to fracture following suture needle placement during PL. Following articular

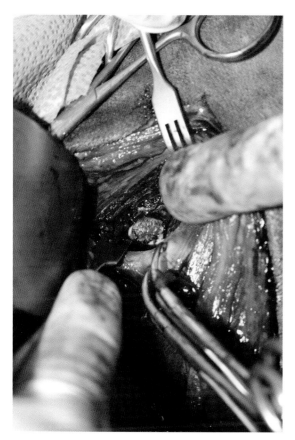

Figure 7.5   Intraoperative photograph of the cricoid facet following CO_2 laser debridement of the articular cartilage.

cartilage destruction and periarticular fibrous tissue formation to prevent arytenoid relaxation but has the disadvantage of increased cost and the concern of following laser safety procedures that require specialized eyewear and equipment. The author cannot conclude that laser ablation is better than mechanical destruction of the CAJ. Nonetheless, the author certainly recommends that surgeons performing PL for treatment of equine laryngeal hemiplegia incorporate either laser debridement or mechanical destruction of the CAJ to lessen the likelihood of arytenoid relaxation following laryngoplasty.

In conclusion, CO_2 laser or mechanical debridement of the CAJ should be considered when performing laryngoplasty in horses with RLN. No complications or negative factors have been recognized secondary to the surgical procedure. CO_2 laser or mechanical debridement of the articular cartilage and joint capsule of the CAJ prevents loss of abduction following laryngoplasty, so the extra time required to complete the procedure is well invested (Figure 7.6 and 7.7). Based on the currently available results, debridement of the CAJ in

cartilage debridement PL proceeds as previously described.

CO_2 laser and mechanical debridement of the CAJ prevent loss of arytenoid abduction following laryngoplasty (Hawkins 2014; Parente et al. 2011). CO_2 laser debridement decreases postoperative loss of abduction by altering the articulation of the CAJ in combination with PL and results in an arthrosis which prevents normal rotation, gliding, and rocking of the CAJ. Another advantage of CO_2 laser debridement as opposed to mechanical disruption is that joint capsule fibrosis occurs post laser debridement. This increases the stability around the CAJ and therefore aids in the prevention of postoperative loss of abduction when combined with PL.

The use of the laser has the advantages of causing enough alteration of the CAJ articulation via

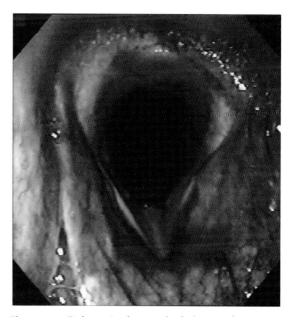

Figure 7.6   Endoscopic photograph of a horse 1 day following CO_2 laser ablation of the cricoarytenoid joint and prosthetic laryngoplasty.

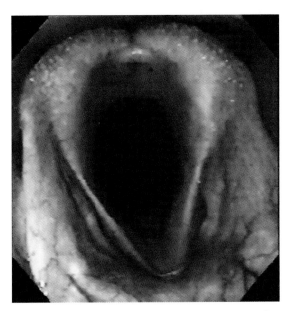

Figure 7.7   The same horse pictured in Figure 7.7 but with 45 days postoperative cricoarytenoid joint debridement and prosthetic laryngoplasty.

combination with PL should be considered in all clinical cases of RLN.

References

Aceto H, Parente EP. 2012. Using quarterly earnings to assess racing performance in 70 Thoroughbreds after modified laryngoplasty for treatment of recurrent laryngeal neuropathy. *Veterinary Surgery* 41:689–695.

Casiano RR, Ruiz PJ, Goldstein W. 1994. Histopathologic changes in the aging human cricoarytenoid joint. *Laryngoscope* 104:533–538.

Dixon PM, McGorum BC, Railton DI, Hawe C, Tremaine WH, Dacre K, McCann J. 2003a. Long-term survey of laryngoplasty and ventriculocordectomy in an older, mixed-breed population of 200 horses. Part 1: Maintenance of surgical arytenoid abduction and compli-

cations of surgery. *Equine Veterinary Journal* 35:389–396.

Dixon PM, McGorum BC, Railton DI, Hawe C, Tremaine WH, Dacre K, McCann J. 2003b. Long-term survey of laryngoplasty and ventriculocordectomy in an older, mixed-breed population of 200 horses. Part 2: Owners' assessment of the value of surgery. *Equine Veterinary Journal* 35:397–401.

Gacek M, Gacek RR. 1996. Cricoarytenoid joint mobility after chronic vocal cord paralysis. *Laryngoscope* 106:1528–1530.

Gacek RR, Gacek MR, Montgomery WW. 1999. Evidence for laryngeal paralysis in cricoarytenoid joint arthritis. *Laryngoscope* 109:279–283.

Hawkins JF, Couetil L, Miller MA. 2014. Maintenance of arytenoid abduction following carbon dioxide laser debridement of the articular cartilage and joint capsule of the cricoarytenoid joint combined with prosthetic laryngoplasty in horses: an in vivo and in vitro study. *The Veterinary Journal* 199 (2): 275–280.

Hawkins JF, Tulleners EP, Ross MW, Evans LH, Raker CW. 1997. Laryngoplasty with or without ventriculectomy for treatment of left laryngeal hemiplegia in 230 racehorses. *Veterinary Surgery* 26:484–491.

Jurik AG, Pedersen U, Noorgard A. 1985. Rheumatoid arthritis of the cricoarytenoid joints: A case of laryngeal obstruction due to acute and chronic joint changes. *Laryngoscope* 95:846–848.

Kasperbauer JL. 1998. A biomechanical study of the human cricoarytenoid joint. *Laryngoscope* 108:1704–1711.

Muller A, Paulsen FP. 2002. Impact of vocal cord paralysis on cricoarytenoid joint. *Annals of Otology, Rhinology, and Laryngology* 111:896–901.

Parente EJ, Birks EK, Habecker P. 2011. A modified laryngoplasty approach promoting ankylosis of the cricoarytenoid joint. *Veterinary Surgery* 40:204–210.

Paulsen FP, Tillmann BN. 1998. Degenerative changes in the human cricoarytenoid joint. *Laryngoscope* 108:1–17.

Sellars I, Sellars S. 1983. Cricoarytenoid joint structure and function. *The Journal of Laryngology and Otology* 97:1027–1034.

Spector GJ, Miller DW. 1977. Surgical obliteration and silastic arthroplasty of the canine cricoarytenoid joint. *Laryngoscope* 87:2049–2055.

Wang RC. 1998. Three-dimensional analysis of cricoarytenoid joint motion. *Laryngoscope* 108:1–17.

8 The Use of Partial Arytenoidectomy in the Management of Recurrent Laryngeal Neuropathy

Catherine H. Hackett

Recurrent laryngeal neuropathy (RLN) is a common cause of poor performance for horses working in a variety of athletic disciplines. As a result of abnormal innervation, dynamic arytenoid collapse into the airway interferes with respiratory function and can lead to exercise intolerance and abnormal respiratory noise. The goal of treatment for RLN is twofold: stabilize the airway and restore airflow mechanics to normal and to reduce respiratory noise associated with abnormal airflow. Although interrelated, the goals of treatment are somewhat dependent on the intended use of the affected horse (e.g., a racehorse versus a draft or show horse) and the expectations of the client.

A number of treatment options exist to correct the respiratory abnormalities caused by RLN and to date, prosthetic laryngoplasty (PL) has been the most commonly elected surgical technique (Davidson et al. 2010). PL has been successful in restoring respiratory mechanics in experimental studies to near normal values, but has variable success in returning athletic horses to full function. In general, success is higher in horses used for activities other than racing. Approximately 70% of horses are able to return to racing following laryngoplasty compared with a 90–95% return rate to other competitive activities. Therefore, although some horses return to full function, a surgical failure still exists through incomplete correction of abnormal respiratory mechanics.

PL is a technically demanding procedure leading to a large variation in results dependent on surgical expertise and technique (Beard and Waxman 2007). Most surgeons aim to attain and maintain 80–90% of maximal abduction of the arytenoid, based on experimental data (Rakesh et al. 2008), although clinical and experimental data does not support that the degree of abduction has a significant impact on performance (Barakzai et al. 2009; Brown et al. 2004). When examining horses reported to have failed to improve following laryngoplasty, horses with no abduction following surgery had laryngeal collapse at exercise (Davidson et al. 2010). The current desired outcome of PL is that airway mechanics should be sufficiently restored within 80–90% of full arytenoid abduction post-surgery; however, the degree of abduction does not correlate with return rate to performance. It is not known if the level of performance following successful PL is associated with different degrees of abduction.

Advances in Equine Upper Respiratory Surgery, First Edition. Edited by Jan Hawkins.
© 2015 ACVS Foundation. Published 2015 by John Wiley & Sons, Inc.

Coughing, aspiration, implant failure, continued noise production, seroma formation, penetration of the suture into the laryngeal lumen, implant loosening/loss of surgical abduction and exercise intolerance have all been reported as complications of PL. Collapse of ipsilateral and contralateral tissues into the airway is the most common cause of impaired respiratory function, leading to exercise intolerance following PL. In one study, seroma formation occurred in 9% of horses treated by PL, 9% of patients required additional surgery within the first 2 weeks of the procedure to either tighten or loosen the implant, 8% more horses required surgery 6 weeks or more postoperatively and coughing was noted in 43% of horses following PL either with or without signs of dysphagia (Dixon et al. 2003). Cytologic abnormalities in tracheal aspirates have been documented in nonsymptomatic horses following PL (Radcliffe et al. 2006), suggesting that subclinical levels of aspiration of feed material may be more frequent than routinely identified. Maintenance of surgical abduction post laryngoplasty has been a well-documented challenge for surgeons with a significant loss of arytenoid abduction noted in most horses during the first 6 weeks following surgery (Davidson et al. 2010; Dixon et al. 2003). Even eating can weaken the repair and lead to implant loosening or failure, as swallowing has been documented to increase pressure on the laryngoplasty suture to a greater extent than coughing (Witte et al. 2010). Loss of surgical abduction is being addressed by development of new techniques to promote ankylosis of the cricoarytenoid joint (Cheetham et al. 2008; Hawkins et al. 2014; Parente et al. 2011). In contrast to reduced abduction of the arytenoid, excessive arytenoid abduction can be associated with postoperative dysphagia and coughing in some cases (Dixon et al. 2003; Russell and Slone 1994).

Avoiding long delays in returning horses to work following respiratory surgery is an important consideration for owners and trainers. In addition to the benefits of reduced lay-up times and expense, prompt identification and correction of RLN has been shown to improve long-term clinical outcomes. A recent study showed horses affected by grade 3 RLN treated by PL returned to postoperative earnings comparable to controls while horses affected by grade 4 RLN did not restore earnings to control levels (Witte et al. 2009). This contradicted previous recommendations to delay surgery until the cricoarytenoideus dorsalis muscle is completely paralyzed (grade 4 RLN), as residual function of the laryngeal musculature has been suggested as a mechanism leading to surgical failure in some cases (Hawkins et al. 1997). Although effective in treating many horses affected by RLN, laryngoplasty is not successful in nearly a third of cases, leading to a continued search for alternate procedures to improve clinical outcomes compared to PL.

One such procedure, partial arytenoidectomy (PA), requires less experience to perform, achieves a more consistent airway diameter, and since there is no implant, has less potential for failure than PL. In an experimental study, the difference in airway mechanics between the PA and PL was modest at maximal heart rate (Radcliffe et al. 2006). This and other studies have shown that airway mechanics are returned to near normal following PA (Lumsden et al. 1994; Radcliffe et al. 2006). At submaximal intensity, PL and PA have been shown to be comparable in restoring airway function.

Complications related to PA include tracheal aspiration of feed material, coughing, and formation of intraluminal granulation tissue that may cause mechanical interference to airflow. Traditionally, veterinary surgeons have avoided PA due to fears of aspiration and concern about inferior correction of abnormal respiratory mechanics. It is true that some horses develop clinical evidence of tracheal aspiration leading to chronic coughing or life-threatening pneumonia; however, this is a rare complication (Barnes et al. 2004; Hay et al. 1993; Lumsden et al. 1994; Parente et al. 2008; Radcliffe et al. 2006; Tulleners et al. 1988a, 1988b; White and Blackwell 1980; Witte et al. 2009). In an experimental study looking at cytological abnormalities following both PL and PA surgeries, tracheal contamination was equivalent between the procedures (Radcliffe et al. 2006). If excessive granulation tissue forms intraluminally following PA, it can easily be removed using a transendoscopic laser or via the laryngotomy incision. One way to reduce the risk of excessive granulation tissue formation is to perform primary mucosal closure, using a segment of axial mucosa salvaged during the arytenoid dissection. Even without mucosal closure, complete healing of the surgical site has been documented within 8 weeks of PA (Barnes et al. 2004). An important preoperative consideration is that excessive inflammation at the arytenoidectomy site has been linked with a reduced outcome after PA (Dean and Cohen 1990); therefore, delaying PA surgery in the face of active inflammation with or without infection and managing perioperative inflammation with the use of systemic antibiotics and anti-inflammatory drugs is important for surgical success. A disadvantage of PA is that a reduction in noise postoperatively is not achieved in most horses treated by the procedure (Tulleners et al. 1988a, 1988b); therefore, PA should not be considered as a primary option in cases where the client's primary goal is noise reduction.

Evaluation of the clinical success of PA for the treatment of RLN is complicated because this technique can be used to treat a variety of conditions. In many cases, PA is elected as a second or third procedure after failed PL or as a treatment for arytenoid chondritis. Although no difference has been noted in the outcome for horses treated with PA for RLN, failed PL, or arytenoid chondritis (Parente et al. 2008; Witte et al. 2009), one can assume that the overall time out of work and the expense incurred by the owner is greater in cases requiring repeated surgeries versus primary treatment of RLN. In addition, looking at the return rate after PA, current data suggests that it might be ~10% higher than after PL (Parente et al. 2008; Witte et al. 2009). There is a population of horses for which the owner may desire a procedure that will be consistent, and will limit the overall time and expense to return the horse to work, with a slightly higher rate of return to racing, even if the resultant repair does not completely return airway mechanics to normal. In our hospital, the cost of an uncomplicated PA is slightly less than PL with a unilateral laser ventriculocordectomy, with similar hospitalization times and recovery recommendations made for both procedures.

The success of PA in horses returning to racing was 78% in one study (Barnes et al. 2004). In a study of 76 racehorses treated by PA the median time to first postoperative race was 6 months with 82% of horses able to race at least once and 63% of horses racing five or more times (Parente et al. 2008). In that study, earnings per start were not significantly different before and after surgery, leading to the conclusion that horses treated with a unilateral PA with primary mucosal closure returned to preoperative levels of performance. Other stud-

ies have shown that PA returns a high percentage of horses to racing, but their postoperative earnings are reduced compared to controls (Witte et al. 2009). Overall, one can conclude that the airway is not restored to normal patency, but the majority of racehorses treated by PA have a favorable response.

In summary, PA has been shown experimentally and clinically to produce outcomes slightly inferior to PL. In select cases, PA should be considered a viable alternative to PL in the treatment of RLN. Particularly when clients do not want to take the risk that repeated surgeries will be necessary (with concomitant expense and increased lay-up time); PA is an attractive option. Neither procedure completely restores airway mechanics to normal, but both are able to return about 70–80% of horses to racing with PA perhaps having a slightly better return rate. As a caution, both PL and PA procedures have been documented to interfere with the normal protective mechanisms of the larynx. PA has the distinct advantage of producing a more consistent airway than PL and reliable results can be dependably achieved in one procedure for treatment of RLN.

References

Barakzai SZ, Boden LA, Dixon PM. 2009. Postoperative race performance is not correlated with degree of surgical abduction after laryngoplasty in National Hunt Thoroughbred racehorses. *Veterinary Surgery* 38:934–940.

Barnes AJ, Slone DE, Lynch TM. 2004. Performance after partial arytenoidectomy without mucosal closure in 27 Thoroughbred racehorses. *Veterinary Surgery* 33:398–403.

Beard WL, Waxman S. 2007. Evidence-based equine upper respiratory surgery. *Veterinary Clinics of North America Equine Practice* 23:229–242.

Brown JA, Derksen FJ, Stick JA, Hartmann WM, Robinson NE. 2004. Effect of laryngoplasty on respiratory noise reduction in horses with laryngeal hemiplegia. *Equine Veterinary Journal* 36:420–425.

Cheetham J, Witte TH, Rawlinson JJ, Soderholm LV, Mohammed HO, Ducharme NG. 2008. Intra-articular stabilisation of the equine cricoarytenoid joint. *Equine Veterinary Journal* 40:584–588.

Davidson EJ, Martin BB, Rieger RH, Parente EJ. 2010. Exercising videoendoscopic evaluation of 45 horses with respiratory noise and/or poor performance after laryngoplasty. *Veterinary Surgery* 39:942–948.

Dean PW, Cohen ND. 1990. Arytenoidectomy for advanced unilateral chondropathy with accompanying lesions. *Veterinary Surgery* 19:364–370.

Dixon RM, McGorum BC, Railton DI, Hawe C, Tremaine WH, Dacre K, McCann J. 2003. Long-term survey of laryngoplasty and ventriculocordectomy in an older, mixed-breed population of 200 horses. Part 1: Maintenance of surgical arytenoid abduction and complications of surgery. *Equine Veterinary Journal* 35:389–396.

Hawkins JF, Tulleners EP, Ross MW, Evans LH, Raker CW. 1997. Laryngoplasty with or without ventriculectomy for treatment of left laryngeal hemiplegia in 230 racehorses. *Veterinary Surgery* 26:484–491.

Hawkins JF, Couetil L, Miller MA. 2014. Maintenance of arytenoid abduction following carbon dioxide laser debridement of the articular cartilage and joint capsule of the cricoarytenoid joint combined with prosthetic laryngoplasty in horses: An in vivo and in vitro study. *The Veterinary Journal* 199(2):275–280.

Hay WP, Tulleners EP, Ducharme NG. 1993. Partial arytenoidectomy in the horse using an extralaryngeal approach. *Veterinary Surgery* 22:50–56.

Lumsden JM, Derksen FJ, Stick JA, Robinson NE, Nickels FA. 1994. Evaluation of partial arytenoidectomy as a treatment for equine laryngeal hemiplegia. *Equine Veterinary Journal* 26:125–129.

Parente EJ, Tulleners EP, Southwood LL. 2008. Long-term study of partial arytenoidectomy with primary mucosal closure in 76 Thoroughbred racehorses (1992–2006). *Equine Veterinary Journal* 40:214–218.

Parente EJ, Birks EK, Habecker P. 2011. A modified laryngoplasty approach promoting ankylosis of the cricoarytenoid joint. *Veterinary Surgery* 40:204–210.

Radcliffe CH, Woodie JB, Hackett RP, Ainsworth DM, Erb HN, Mitchell LM, Soderholm LV, Ducharme NG. 2006. A comparison of laryngoplasty and modified partial arytenoidectomy as treatments for laryngeal hemiplegia in exercising horses. *Veterinary Surgery* 35:643–652.

Rakesh V, Ducharme NG, Cheetham J, Datta AK, Pease AP. 2008. Implications of different degrees of arytenoid cartilage abduction on equine upper airway characteristics. *Equine Veterinary Journal* 40:629–635.

Russell AP, Slone DE. 1994. Performance analysis after prosthetic laryngoplasty and bilateral ventriculectomy for laryngeal hemiplegia in horses: 70 cases (1986–1991). *Journal of the American Veterinary Medical Association* 204:1235–1241.

Tulleners EP, Harrison IW, Raker CW. 1988a. Management of arytenoid chondropathy and failed laryngoplasty in horses: 75 cases (1979–1985). *Journal of the American Veterinary Medical Association* 192:670–675.

Tulleners EP, Harrison IW, Mann P, Raker CW. 1988b. Partial arytenoidectomy in the horse with and without mucosal closure. *Veterinary Surgery* 17:252–257.

White NA, Blackwell RB. 1980. Partial arytenoidectomy in the horse. *Veterinary Surgery* 9:5–12.

Witte TH, Mohammed HO, Radcliffe CH, Hackett RP, Ducharme NG. 2009. Racing performance after combined prosthetic laryngoplasty and ipsilateral ventriculocordectomy or partial arytenoidectomy: 135 Thoroughbred racehorses competing at less than 2400 m (1997–2007). *Equine Veterinary Journal* 41:70–75.

Witte TH, Cheetham J, Soderholm LV, Mitchell LM, Ducharme NG. 2010. Equine laryngoplasty sutures undergo increased loading during coughing and swallowing. *Veterinary Surgery* 39:949–956.

9 Evaluation and Management of the Horse Following Failed Laryngoplasty

Jan Hawkins

Introduction

The reported success of prosthetic laryngoplasty (PF) has ranged from 65% to 90%. The reported success has been dependent on the horse's intended use with racehorses having a lower prognosis for success compared to nonracehorses (Hawkins et al. 1997). In one retrospective study of racehorses with recurrent laryngeal neuropathy (RLN) treated with PL 5% experienced a failed laryngoplasty (Hawkins et al. 1997). Possible causes for failed laryngoplasty include cartilage failure, suture pullout through the muscular process of the arytenoid cartilage, postoperative infection, and surgeon error (Dixon et al. 2003). The most common cause of PL failure, the author has observed, is fracture of the muscular process of the arytenoid cartilage following prosthetic suture placement. Options for failed laryngoplasty include retirement from athletic use, repeat laryngoplasty, and partial arytenoidectomy (PA).

Evaluation of the horse with failed laryngoplasty

All horses with a history of exercise intolerance or upper respiratory tract noise following PL should have a physical and endoscopic examination performed. Other pertinent historical information includes the extent of any complications following the surgical procedure, including coughing or signs of surgical site infection following PL. Incisional complications can lead to implant failure and subsequent loss of arytenoid abduction (Figure 9.1). In the majority of cases the cause of laryngoplasty failure cannot be determined. In some instances there is no history of previous surgery. This occurs most frequently when racehorses have had multiple owners. Clinical signs associated with previous surgery include thickening of the left aspect of the larynx as assessed by laryngeal palpation and the presence of an incisional scar ventral to the linguofacial vein (Figure 9.2). This can usually only be determined following clipping of the hair and close examination. Endoscopic examination of the horse suspected of a failed laryngoplasty typically reveals complete (grade 4) laryngeal hemiplegia, although occasionally some horses will have mild ability to abduct or move the arytenoid (Figure 9.3). If the horse has had a previous, known history of PL, it is straightforward to determine that the procedure has failed when the endoscopic examination reveals grade 4 laryngeal

Advances in Equine Upper Respiratory Surgery, First Edition. Edited by Jan Hawkins.
© 2015 ACVS Foundation. Published 2015 by John Wiley & Sons, Inc.

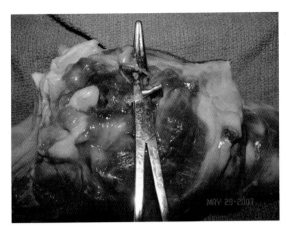

Figure 9.1   A gross postmortem specimen of cartilage failure following an incisional infection secondary to inadvertent penetration of the laryngeal lumen during prosthetic laryngoplasty.

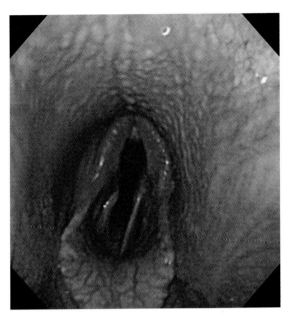

Figure 9.3   Endoscopic photograph of a horse with a failed right-sided prosthetic laryngoplasty. Note the fibrosis associated with right laser ventriculocordectomy site.

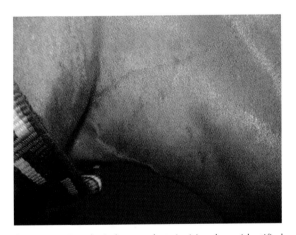

Figure 9.2   Prosthetic laryngoplasty incisional scar identified following the removal of the hair from the left aspect of the larynx.

hemiplegia. However, if some degree of abduction is present postlaryngoplasty, even though it is not ideal, high-speed treadmill examination should be considered (Davidson et al. 2010). In a study by Davidson et al. (2010) evaluating horses following left laryngoplasty with clinical signs of respiratory noise and poor performance, a variety of abnormalities were identified on the high-speed treadmill. These abnormalities included dynamic collapse of the arytenoid cartilage, billowing of the left and sometimes the right vocal fold, aryepiglottic folds, corniculate process of the left arytenoid cartilage, dorsal displacement of the soft palate, and pharyngeal collapse. This emphasizes the importance of dynamic examination prior to deciding on definitive surgical treatment.

Preoperative planning

A frank discussion of what the expectations would be following additional surgery should be discussed with the owner. Without corrective surgery the horse will most likely not be a successful athlete. Treadmill endoscopy may also alter the preoperative plan because other surgical procedures in addition to or instead of repeat laryngoplasty may be required. In the study by Davidson et al. (2010) collapse of other upper airway structures was common and including left (if not previously removed) and right vocal cord, aryepiglottic fold, corniculate process of the arytenoid, soft palate, and pharynx. These collapsing structures must be addressed in addition to the dynamic collapse of the left arytenoid.

Decision making repeat laryngoplasty versus PA

Therefore, if an athletic career is desired for the horse the author generally recommends that an attempt be made to repeat the laryngoplasty as long as there is no previous history of incisional infection. Following incisional infection there is typically an abundance of fibrous connective tissue which makes repeat laryngoplasty difficult. If repeat laryngoplasty cannot be successfully performed then PA should be considered (Parente 2008; Tulleners 1988). This should be discussed with the owner prior to surgery. Some owners are concerned about the possibility that the repeat laryngoplasty will fail as well and would rather proceed with PA. All of these options should be discussed prior to surgery.

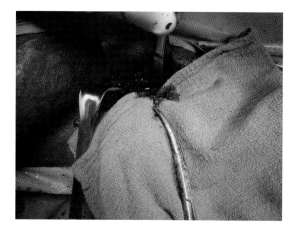

Figure 9.4   Intraoperative photograph of prosthetic suture material removal following a failed prosthetic laryngoplasty. The hemostat in the photograph is grasping the knots of the suture material.

Repeat PL

If an attempt at repeat PL is going to be made the horse is positioned as previously described (Chapter 5). If PA is chosen the horse is positioned in dorsal recumbency. For repeat PL, the videoendoscope should be positioned within the left nasal passage so that the larynx can be visualized. The skin incision follows the previously performed incision for the initial PL. A variable amount of fibrous connective tissue is located ventral to the linguofacial vein and dorsal to the larynx. This connective tissue can be difficult to dissect through and hemorrhage associated with this tissue is typical. The amount of scar tissue between the cricopharyngeus and thyropharyngeus muscles and the perilaryngeal region is variable. Suction is required for hemorrhage control. The cricopharyngeus and thyropharyngeus muscle bellies are divided along the previous incision. Following division of these two muscle bellies it is not unusual for there to be a scar tissue between the muscular process and the thyroid cartilage. In some cases it can be difficult to divide this scar tissue between the two as the knot(s) of the prosthetic suture material is located within this scar tissue. If possible the knot(s) of the previously placed suture should be located and removed (Figure 9.4). If the suture has pulled

through the muscular process a loop of suture may be embedded in the scar tissue behind the muscular process. In the majority of cases the cause for laryngoplasty failure cannot be determined. Once the previous suture material has been removed repeat laryngoplasty proceeds as previously described for routine PL. Once the prosthetic sutures are positioned in the cricoid and muscular process the first suture is tightened and tied under endoscopic guidance. If the surgeon is satisfied with the security of the tied suture and the position of the arytenoid, the second suture is tied. If at any point the surgeon does not feel that the sutures will maintain arytenoid abduction, then PA should be considered. In some horses abduction is maintained initially and then over a period of minutes of observation it becomes apparent that abduction is being lost. If this occurs it is not likely that abduction will be maintained despite the hopes of the surgeon that it will. The most likely cause for this is muscular process failure. If repeat PL is deemed unsuccessful, the suture material should be removed and the horse positioned in dorsal recumbency for PA.

PA proceeds as described in Chapters 35 and 36. If repeat laryngoplasty is chosen, follow-up endoscopy should be performed at 1–3 day intervals to ensure that successful arytenoid abduction is being maintained following laryngoplasty.

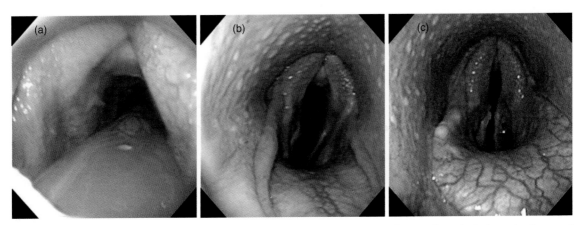

Figure 9.5   (a) Intraoperative photograph of right arytenoid abduction following repeat laryngoplasty. (b) Endoscopic photograph 1 day following right repeat laryngoplasty. (c) Endoscopic photograph 3 days following right repeat laryngoplasty. Note complete loss of abduction. This horse was subsequently treated with partial arytenoidectomy.

For some horses, gradual loss of abduction can be observed if the repeat laryngoplasty is unsuccessful in maintaining arytenoid abduction (Figures 9.5a–9.5c). The only alternative for these horses is PA. This emphasizes the importance of open communication with the owner because a failed repeat laryngoplasty means additional expense and hospitalization.

Complications

The most common complication following repeat laryngoplasty is incisional seroma and/or surgical site infection. Mild seromas are managed with benign neglect, pressure bandaging, and antimicrobial and anti-inflammatory therapy. Large seromas which interfere with swallowing or contribute to airway obstruction should be drained. This is accomplished by removing skin sutures and establishing drainage. The risk for surgical site infection does increase with the establishment of incisional drainage. The other complication which can develop as has been previously discussed is failure of arytenoid abduction following repeat laryngoplasty.

The prognosis following successful repeat laryngoplasty is at least as good as that for successful first time PL. The prognosis following PA is good.

References

Davidson EJ, Martin BB, Rieger RH, Parente EJ. 2010. Exercising videoendoscopic evaluation of 45 horses with respiratory noise and/or poor performance after laryngoplasty. *Veterinary Surgery* 39(8):342–348.

Dixon RM, McGorum BC, Railton DI, Hawe C, Tremaine WH, Dacre K, McCann J. 2003. Long-term survey of laryngoplasty and ventriculocordectomy in an older, mixed-breed population of 200 horses. Part 1: Maintenance of surgical arytenoid abduction and complications of surgery. *Equine Veterinary Journal* 35:389–396.

Hawkins JF, Tulleers EP, Ross MW, Evans LH, Raker CW. 1997. Laryngoplasty with or without ventriculectomy for treatment of left laryngeal hemiplegia in 230 racehorses. *Veterinary Surgery* 26(6):484–491.

Parente EJ, Tulleners EP, Southwood LL. 2008. Long-term study of partial arytenoidectomy with primary mucosal closure in 76 Thoroughbred racehorses (1992–2006). *Equine Veterinary Journal* 40(3):214–248.

Tulleners EP, Harrsion IW, Raker CW. 1988. Management of arytenoid chondropathy and failed laryngoplasty in horses: 75 cases (1979–1985). *Journal of the American Veterinary Medical Association* 192(5):670–675.

10 Evaluation and Management of the Horse with Dysphagia Following Prosthetic Laryngoplasty

Jan Hawkins

Introduction

Dysphagia following prosthetic laryngoplasty (PL) occurs in approximately 5–10% of horses and coughing occurs in approximately 25% of horses (Hawkins et al. 1997). Some degree of coughing and in some instances dysphagia in the immediate postoperative period is not uncommon and usually resolves over the first couple of weeks following surgery. Persistent dysphagia and coughing is relatively rare but is seen most commonly in horses with hyperabduction of the arytenoid cartilage (Dixon et al. 2003), although some horses experience dysphagia post laryngoplasty in the absence of hyperabduction (Figure 10.1). Although the cause of postoperative dysphagia has not been definitively determined the author believes that the presence of the prosthetic suture material interferes with normal swallowing during mastication of food material (Dixon et al. 2003; Greet et al. 1979; Hawkins et al. 1997; Raker 1975). This could be due to adhesions dorsal to the larynx involving the esophagus or abnormal function of the crico and thyropharyngeus muscles. The only sure method of resolving the dysphagia is removal of the prosthetic suture material.

Evaluation

Horses with dysphagia following PL cough while eating and frequently have nasal discharge of feed material. Abnormal physical examination findings include low-grade fever (<101°F), mucopurulent nasal discharge, or feed material at the nares (Figure 10.2). Coughing may be observed during the examination or following manual manipulation of the trachea. Endoscopic examination findings include feed material in the nares, wall of the nasopharynx, and trachea, and abduction of the arytenoid cartilage associated with laryngoplasty (Figure 10.3).

Management

Conservative

All horses with postoperative dysphagia should be initially treated conservatively. This should involve feeding the horse from the ground, wetting the hay, or trying pelleted feeds. Conservative management also includes the administration of antimicrobials and anti-inflammatory therapy. Antimicrobial

Advances in Equine Upper Respiratory Surgery, First Edition. Edited by Jan Hawkins.
© 2015 ACVS Foundation. Published 2015 by John Wiley & Sons, Inc.

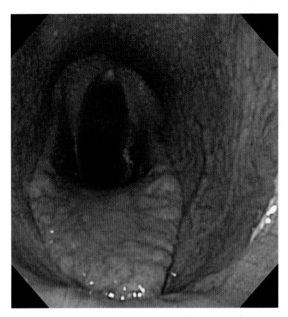

Figure 10.1   A horse with dysphagia following prosthetic laryngoplasty. Note moderate abduction of the left arytenoid cartilage.

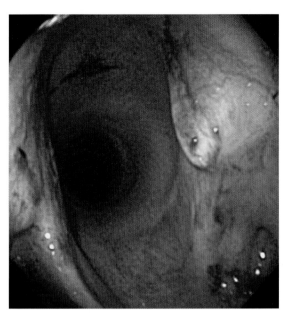

Figure 10.3   Endoscopic photograph of horse with aspiration of feed material following prosthetic laryngoplasty.

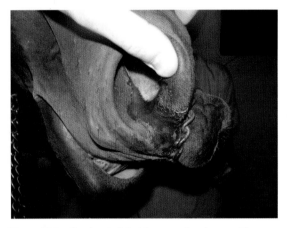

Figure 10.2   Feed material at the nares in a horse with clinical signs of dysphagia post prosthetic laryngoplasty.

degree of arytenoid abduction or laryngoplasty suture removal. Some surgeons have managed postoperative dysphagia secondary to hyperabduction of the arytenoid with loosening or replacement of the suture material so that the arytenoid is no longer hyperabducted. The only sure way to resolve postoperative dysphagia is to remove the suture material. The decision for suture removal becomes one of timing? If the suture is removed before fibrous connective tissue has stabilized the muscular process of the arytenoid cartilage loss of abduction will occur and an unsuccessful result in regards to return to athletic performance will be obtained.

Surgery

Dixon et al. have described loosening of prosthetic suture 3–10 days following PL to manage postoperative dysphagia (Dixon et al. 2003). However, he uses stainless steel suture, so to loosen the prosthesis the steel is untwisted to decrease the amount of abduction. If more traditional suture materials are used then the previously placed suture is removed

therapy is indicated to lessen the chance for aspiration pneumonia. The most common antimicrobials used include trimethoprim or sulfamethoxazole (30 mg/kg, PO, q12h), procaine or potassium penicillin G (22 000 U/kg, IM or IV, q6–12h), and gentamicin sulfate (6.6 mg/kg, IV, q24h). Horses nonresponsive to conservative management are candidates for replacement of the prosthesis and reducing the and replaced. The degree of relaxation would be determined with intraoperative endoscopy.

The author prefers to remove the prosthetic suture material rather than replace the suture in the immediate postoperative period. If at all possible the author prefers to wait at least 60 days before considering removal of the prosthetic suture material. This is done for two reasons: some horses will improve over time and the dysphagia will resolve

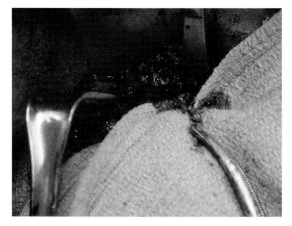

Figure 10.4 Intraoperative photograph depicting removal of prosthetic suture material in a horse with postoperative dysphagia. No effort is made to transect adhesions associated with the prosthetic suture material.

without additional surgery and waiting for at least 60 days allows enough fibrous connective tissue to form around the muscular process to prevent loss of abduction post suture removal. However, the surgeon could be forced into removing the prosthetic suture material earlier than 60 days if the horse develops severe aspiration pneumonia. The author was initially taught that when removing the suture material, all adhesions around the muscular process and thyroid cartilage be transected to allow for relaxation of the degree of arytenoid abduction. Typically when this is done athletic use is generally lost but the signs of dysphagia will resolve. It is a commonly held belief that the degree of arytenoid abduction is what causes postoperative dysphagia. But it has been the author's experience that even horses with less than ideal arytenoid abduction can be dysphagic. This has led the author to believe that it is the presence of the suture material and its interference with normal swallowing that leads to postoperative dysphagia (Greet et al. 1979) although others have questioned this and have reported that dysphagia does not always resolve with suture removal (Greet et al. 1979; Raker 1975). Structures which could be involved in postoperative dysphagia include the esophagus and abnormal function of the pharyngeal constrictor muscles.

Once the decision has been made to remove the prosthetic suture material the larynx is approached

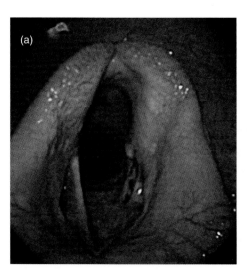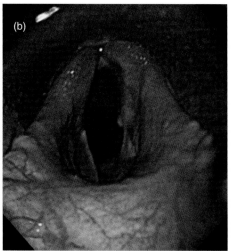

Figure 10.5 (a) Preoperative endoscopic photograph and (b) Postoperative endoscopic photograph following prosthetic suture removal in a horse experiencing postoperative dysphagia. Also note the minimal loss of abduction. This also had laser ablation of the cricoarytenoid joint performed at the time of initial prosthetic laryngoplasty.

by incising along the previous surgical incision. A variable amount of fibrous connective tissue is typically present between the linguofacial vein and the dorsal aspect of the larynx. Some horses have minimal scar tissue and some have a moderate amount. Hemorrhage associated with dissection is not unusual and is more than expected compared to a first time laryngoplasty. The crico and thyropharyngeus muscle bellies are divided along the previous scar and an attempt is made to palpate the knots of the suture material. Frequently, the knots are not that easy to palpate and dissection with a hemostat and/or scissors is required to identify the suture material. As little scar tissue as possible is disrupted to expose the suture material. The knots of the suture material are typically located just beneath the dorsal wing of the thyroid cartilage so the dissection should be centered there. Once identified, the knots are secured within a hemostat and the suture material is transected and removed (Figure 10.4). No attempts are made to decrease the amount of abduction previously obtained from the initial laryngoplasty. The crico and thyropharyngeus muscle bellies are closed routinely as is the remainder of the incision. Postoperatively seroma formation is not uncommon and occasionally an incisional infection results. Seroma or incisional infection should be treated with drainage if swelling is excessive.

Outcome

It generally takes 3–5 days following suture removal for signs of dysphagia to improve. In general,

signs promptly resolve following suture removal (Figures 10.5a and 10.5b). The author currently performs cricoarytenoid joint ankylosis in all horses treated with PL. I have had the opportunity to remove the suture material of horses with postoperative dysphagia following cricoarytenoid joint ankylosis and the dysphagia resolved in all cases following suture removal and without disruption of the cricoarytenoid joint (CAJ) ankylosis. The prognosis for athletic use following suture removal should be favorable as long as the desired amount of arytenoid abduction has been maintained following suture removal. Horses that have lost arytenoid abduction and show poor performance results should be considered surgical candidates for partial arytenoidectomy.

References

Dixon PM, McGorum BC, Railton DI, Hawe C, Tremaine WH, Dacre K, McGann J. 2003. Long-term survey of laryngoplasty and ventriculocordectomy in an older, mixed-breed population of 200 horses. Part 1: Maintanence of surgical arytenoid abduction and complications of surgery. *Equine Veterinary Journal* 35:389–396.

Greet TR, Baker GJ, Lee R. 1979. The effect of laryngoplasty on pharyngeal function in the horse. *Equine Veterinary Journal* 11:153–158.

Hawkins JF, Tulleners EP, Ross MW, Evans LH, Raker CW. 1997. Laryngoplasty with or without ventriculectomy for treatment of left laryngeal hemiplegia in 230 racehorses. *Veterinary Surgery* 26:484–491.

Raker CW. 1975. Complications related to the insertion of a suture to retract the arytenoid cartilage to correct laryngeal hemiplegia in the horse. *Veterinary Surgery* 4:64–66.

11 Treatment of Recurrent Laryngeal Neuropathy in Racehorses

Eric J. Parente

Prognosis and postoperative evaluation of horses after treatment of recurrent laryngeal neuropathy: evaluation of the racehorse

Achieving a consistent successful outcome for treatment of recurrent laryngeal neuropathy (RLN) in the racehorse continues to be a challenge. The majority of horses are treated by one of three surgical approaches and each with their own prognosis. The treatments are resection of the vocal cord and laryngeal ventricle, partial arytenoidectomy (PA), or prosthetic laryngoplasty (PL) with ventriculocordectomy. Because none of the procedures have proven to yield a uniformly positive outcome, the selection of the procedure to be performed is based on the surgeon's preference and sometimes relative to the degree of arytenoid dysfunction.

Ventriculocordectomy

Resection of the vocal cord and saccule has been advocated for treatment of RLN because it has very limited complications and has yielded positive racing results in retrospective studies (Henderson et al. 2007; Robinson et al. 2006; Taylor et al. 2006), but it is generally employed for horses that retain some function of the arytenoid at rest and have presumed maintenance of some abduction during exercise. There is evidence that laser ventriculocordectomy can mitigate respiratory obstruction in an experimental RLN model, but ventriculocordectomy alone is not generally accepted as a definitive treatment for racehorses by most clinicians. Furthermore, if ventriculocordectomy is performed in a horse that is initially not experiencing complete dynamic collapse of the arytenoid during exercise, the progressive nature of the disease will likely result in greater dynamic collapse in the future and more significant respiratory compromise that will warrant techniques that yield greater arytenoid stabilization. High-speed treadmill examination can be useful in evaluating the horse with grade 3a or 3b arytenoid abduction at rest.

Partial arytenoidectomy

PA is also considered a surgical option for the treatment of RLN. It is only considered for horses

Advances in Equine Upper Respiratory Surgery, First Edition. Edited by Jan Hawkins.
© 2015 ACVS Foundation. Published 2015 by John Wiley & Sons, Inc.

with unilateral disease since it is very unlikely that a racehorse with any degree of bilateral chondropathy will be able to race after surgery. While the respiratory mechanics in an experimental model of RLN were not dramatically different in horses undergoing a PA or PL (Radcliffe et al. 2006), subsequent retrospective clinical evaluations demonstrated that horses undergoing PA can perform well (Parente et al. 2008) but not as well as horses undergoing PL (Witte et al. 2009). Potential reasons for limited improved performance after arytenoidectomy are dynamic obstruction of the glottis from aryepiglottic folds or residual corniculate mucosa, and lower airway inflammation secondary to decreased ability to protect the lower airway. There have been no long-term studies on racehorses after an arytenoidectomy determining causes of diminished performance.

Prosthetic laryngoplasty

PL is the treatment option most often employed for racehorses with RLN. Clinical success after laryngoplasty in racehorses has been modest, ranging from 45% to 70% (Davenport et al. 2001; Hammer et al. 1998; Hawkins et al. 1997; Kidd and Slone 2002). There is no evidence that the preoperative degree of arytenoid dysfunction limits the success of the surgery. Postoperative loss of abduction likely has the greatest impact on the limited success. Loss of abduction after PL has been documented both clinically (Davenport et al. 2001; Dixon et al. 2003; Hawkins et al. 1997; Kidd and Slone 2002) and experimentally (Brown et al. 2004; Radcliffe et al. 2006). The most dramatic loss is within the first few weeks but can continue as long as 6 weeks or more, and the amount of abduction loss is not uniform for every horse (Dixon et al. 2003). There is also controversial evidence that the resting degree of abduction after surgery has any bearing on the stability of the arytenoid during exercise or on postoperative performance (Barakzai et al. 2009a; Davidson et al. 2010). A conclusion made by some clinicians that stability is more important than the amount of abduction is misleading since these two factors are not exclusive of each other, and ideally a stable opening with greater abduction is the most favorable physiologic condition that will provide the greatest airflow.

Resting postoperative endoscopic evaluations are recommended 1 day and 4 weeks after surgery to assess the resting position of the arytenoid, healing of the cordectomy (if performed), and any unanticipated abnormalities. A target of approximately 80% of full abduction is desirable. Greater abduction will increase the risk of aspiration, but the amount of abduction is not directly correlated to the amount of aspiration. Greater than 80% abduction will also increase the risk of long-term chondropathy even without any gross evidence of aspiration.

Coughing secondary to aspiration is another potential complication postoperatively. Gross feed material should never be seen within the nasopharynx or larynx, yet some clinicians expect horses will cough for several days after surgery associated with maximal arytenoid abduction from the time of surgery, and anticipate the coughing will stop as the horse loses some abduction. While this may be true, postoperative coughing can virtually be eliminated by minimizing surgical trauma during the laryngoplasty, by more deliberate positioning of arytenoid abduction with intraoperative endoscopy, and employing a technique that minimizes postoperative abduction loss. Thus "overabduction" is avoided at surgery. If abduction appears excessive on resting endoscopic examination and coughing persists beyond several weeks, revision is recommended.

The modified laryngoplasty was developed to minimize abduction loss in the immediate postoperative period as well as to enhance the long-term stability of the abduction created at surgery (Parente et al. 2011). In earlier studies only 70–80% of horses treated by traditional laryngoplasty returned to racing (Barakzai et al. 2009b; Davenport et al. 2001; Hawkins et al. 1997; Witte et al. 2009), and even those that raced had limited career lengths. In a recent retrospective using quarterly earnings to assess success (Aceto and Parente 2011), the results showed that 100% of the horses undergoing a modified laryngoplasty returned to racing; they had similar earnings over all quarters (except the first during the immediate postoperative period), and had a competitive career of similar length to cohort controls. This is in contrast to other studies (Barakzai et al. 2009b; Witte et al. 2009) which demonstrated a shortened career length of the traditional laryngoplasty horses versus controls, and this refutes a common perception that horses having undergone a laryngoplasty will have a shorter racing career with decreased earnings relative to their peers.

Horses that continue to make abnormal respiratory noise or experience continued poor performance after PL should warrant further diagnostic examinations to determine the cause. A resting endoscopic examination should be performed first to assess the amount of arytenoid abduction and shape/appearance of the corniculate. Horses with well-abducted arytenoids (>70%) should undergo exercising endoscopy over ground or on a treadmill to determine if there is dynamic collapse of the arytenoid or other soft tissues (Davidson et al. 2010). If the left arytenoid is not collapsing, the other likely potential offenders are the right aryepiglottic fold or right vocal cord (assuming the left vocal cord is no longer present).

If the glottic opening is obviously compromised at rest, from an unabducted arytenoid or arytenoid chondropathy then revision surgery or retirement from racing must be considered.

References

Aceto H, Parente EJ. 2011. Using quarterly earnings to assess racing performance in 70 Thoroughbreds after modified laryngoplasty for treatment of recurrent laryngeal neuropathy. *Veterinary Surgery* 41:689–695.

Barakzai SZ, Boden LA, Dixon PM. 2009a. Postoperative race performance is not correlated with degree of surgical abduction after laryngoplasty in National Hunt Thoroughbred racehorses. *Veterinary Surgery* 38(8):934–940.

Barakzai SZ, Boden LA, Dixon PM. 2009b. Race performance after laryngoplasty and ventriculocordectomy in National Hunt racehorses. *Veterinary Surgery* 38(8):941–945.

Brown JA, Derksen FJ, Stick JA, Hartmann WM, Robinson NE. 2004. Effect of laryngoplasty on respiratory noise reduction in horses with laryngeal hemiplegia. *Equine Veterinary Journal* 36(5):420–425.

Davenport CL, Tulleners EP, Parente EJ. 2001. The effect of recurrent laryngeal neurectomy in conjunction with laryngoplasty and unilateral ventriculocordectomy in Thoroughbred racehorses. *Veterinary Surgery* 30:417–421.

Davidson EJ, Martin BB, Rieger RH, Parente EJ. 2010. Exercising videoendoscopic evaluation of 45 horses

with respiratory noise and/or poor performance after laryngoplasty. *Veterinary Surgery* 39(8):942–948.

Dixon PM, McGorum BC, Railton DI, Hawe C, Tremaine WH, Dacre K, McGann J. 2003. Long-term survey of laryngoplasty and ventriculocordectomy in an older, mixed-breed population of 200 horses. Part 1: Maintenance of surgical arytenoid abduction and complications of surgery. *Equine Veterinary Journal* 35:389–396.

Hammer EJ, Tulleners EP, Parente EJ, Martin BB Jr. 1998. Videoendoscopic assessment of dynamic laryngeal function during exercise in horses with grade-III left laryngeal hemiparesis at rest: 26 cases (1992–1995). *Journal American Veterinary Medical Association* 212(3):399–403.

Hawkins JF, Tulleners EP, Ross MW, Evans LH, Raker CW. 1997. Laryngoplasty with or without ventriculectomy for treatment of left laryngeal hemiplegia in 230 racehorses. *Veterinary Surgery* 26:484–491.

Henderson CE, Sullins KE, Brown JA. 2007. Transendoscopic, laser-assisted ventriculocordectomy for treatment of left laryngeal hemiplegia in horses: 22 cases (1999–2005). *Journal American Veterinary Medical Association* 231(12):1868–1872.

Kidd JA, Slone DE. 2002. Treatment of laryngeal hemiplegia in horses by prosthetic laryngoplasty, ventriculectomy, and vocal cordectomy. *Veterinary Record* 150:481–484.

Parente EJ, Birks EK, Habecker PA. 2011. Modified laryngoplasty approach promoting ankylosis of the cricoarytenoid joint. *Veterinary Surgery* 40(2):204–210.

Parente EJ, Tulleners EP, Southwood LL. 2008. Long-term study of partial arytenoidectomy with primary mucosal closure in 76 Thoroughbred racehorses (1992–2006). *Equine Veterinary Journal* 40:214–218.

Radcliffe CH, Woodie JB, Hackett RP, Ainsworth DM, Erb HN, Mitchell LM, Soderholm LV, Ducharme NG. 2006. A comparison of laryngoplasty and modified partial arytenoidectomy as treatments for laryngeal hemiplegia in exercising horses. *Veterinary Surgery* 35:643–652.

Robinson P, Derksen FJ, Stick JA, Sullins KE, Detolve PG, Robinson NE. 2006. Effects of unilateral laser-assisted ventriculocordectomy in horses with laryngeal hemiplegia. *Equine Veterinary Journal* 38(6):491–496.

Taylor SE, Barakzai SZ, Dixon P. 2006. Ventriculocordectomy as the sole treatment for recurrent laryngeal neuropathy: Long-term results from ninety-two horses. *Veterinary Surgery* 35(7):653–657.

Witte TH, Mohammed HO, Radcliffe CH, Hackett RP, Ducharme NG. 2009. Racing performance after combined prosthetic laryngoplasty and ipsilateral ventriculocordectomy or partial arytenoidectomy: 135 Thoroughbred racehorses competing at less than 2400 m (1997–2007). *Equine Veterinary Journal* 41:70–75.

12 Treatment of Recurrent Laryngeal Neuropathy in Draft Horses

Warren Beard

Introduction

Recurrent laryngeal neuropathy (RLN) in draft horses shares many of the characteristics of the condition seen in other breeds. It is an idiopathic, principally left-sided condition resulting in increased inspiratory resistance, exercise intolerance, and respiratory noise (Derksen et al. 1986). Due to their increased size and intended uses, there are differences that the practitioner needs to be aware of when working on draft horses.

The size of the horse has long been recognized as a risk factor for RLN with larger breeds more at risk. Hospital data from North American teaching hospitals have shown that draft horses have the highest risk of developing RLN with an odds ratio of 2.5–2.9 (Beard and Hayes 1993), and one survey found the prevalence of RLN to be 35% in Michigan show horses (Brackenhoff et al. 2006). Similarly, it has been shown that the prevalence of RLN is higher for larger animals within the same breed, with increasing height recognized as a risk factor in Belgian and Percheron horses. This would explain the observation that RLN appears to be more common in show horses used in hitch competitions than

in the smaller-sized work horses commonly used by the Amish, although referral bias may also play a role. Anecdotally, it seems that the wheel team horses, the largest pair in a hitch, are more commonly affected. Draft horses tend to develop RLN at an older age than other horses with a peak age of diagnosis of 7–9 years compared to 2–3 years for Thoroughbreds and 4–6 years for Standardbreds (Beard and Hayes 1993).

Diagnosis

Most draft horses presented for RLN will be show horses used in hitch or pulling competitions. The owners or trainers are usually professional horsemen or at a minimum very knowledgeable. Given the high incidence of RLN in draft breeds, it is common for owners to have had a horse with RLN in the past. Consequently, most owners are able to make a tentative diagnosis based on clinical signs.

The primary complaint is usually respiratory noise which is exacerbated by the upright head carriage desired in show horses. The owners rightly or wrongly feel that competition judges discriminate

Advances in Equine Upper Respiratory Surgery, First Edition. Edited by Jan Hawkins.
© 2015 ACVS Foundation. Published 2015 by John Wiley & Sons, Inc.

against horses making respiratory noise. Owners place a lesser emphasis on exercise intolerance, likely because the respiratory impairment does not lead to an inability to perform. Realistically, it is not taxing for eight very large horses to pull an empty wagon. Endoscopic examination of the upper airway will confirm the diagnosis of RLN as well as the presence or absence of other upper airway abnormalities. Grading of laryngeal function in draft breeds is no different from light breeds of horses regardless of the grading scale chosen. The overwhelming majority of draft horses present with grade IV/IV laryngeal function (Hackett 1991). It seems paradoxical, in light of the fact that draft horse owners are so familiar with RLN that there would not be more horses diagnosed in the early stages. In the author's experience there will be a higher incidence of prior surgical procedures in draft breeds presenting for RLN. Particular attention should be paid to evidence of prior surgery such as scarring of the ventricles or vocal cords, or an arytenoid cartilage that is not moving but also not hanging vertically in the position typical of grade IV paralysis. These findings would indicate that the horse may have undergone previous attempts at surgical correction. If there is reason to suspect prior surgery, it is indicated to clip the hair from the laryngoplasty and laryngotomy sites to examine for scars. Prior attempts at surgery should be noted and factored into decision making process for surgical procedure and prognosis. A repeat prosthetic laryngoplasty (PL) is more difficult because of scar tissue from the previous surgical approach. The prognosis for a successful outcome is somewhat dependent on why the first procedure failed, such as splitting of the muscular process as opposed to suture loosening, and this cannot be determined until the time of surgery. A vocal cordectomy may be performed if a ventriculectomy (VE) alone was performed at the first procedure.

Anesthesia

There is abundant anecdotal evidence that draft horses have more intraoperative and postoperative anesthetic complications than light breed horses. There are many locales today where it is widely believed that general anesthesia in draft horses is an ill-advised undertaking. Recent retrospective studies in draft breeds undergoing colic surgery (Rothenbuhler et al. 2006) and laryngoplasty (Kraus et al. 2003) highlight the fact that anesthetic complications are more frequent in draft horses and the complication rate increases with the increasing size of the horse (Kraus et al. 2003; Rothenbuhler et al. 2006). The most common intraoperative complications are hypotension and hypoxemia which are predisposing causes to the principal postoperative complications of myopathy and neuropathy. General anesthesia can be safely performed in draft horses; however, to ignore the hard-learned lessons of the past is an invitation to disaster.

Following are some suggestions to facilitate general anesthesia in draft breeds. Anesthetic complications increase with increasing length of the anesthetic procedure so it follows that anything that may be done to expedite the procedure will pay benefits in decreasing perioperative complications. Speed does not result from hurrying; rather it comes from efficiency borne of forethought and clear purpose. Time-saving measures include but are not limited to: having adequate help available and making sure everyone knows their job, clipping of the surgical site prior to induction, and having the surgical table, gowns, gloves, and equipment laid out prior to anesthetic induction. The anesthetic management should be entrusted to skilled personnel that have at their disposal anesthetic monitoring equipment that allows them to measure arterial blood gases and arterial pressures. Use adequate padding (two 6-inch thick foam pads) and be especially attentive to positioning. Be aware that many horses are too large for some surgery tables and many times the hoists may not be rated for the weights of the largest horses.

Selection of surgical procedure(s)

There are two components to successful treatment of RLN: normalization of upper airway mechanics and elimination of the respiratory noise. A careful history is required to determine if the horse is exercise intolerant, makes an objectionable noise, or both. The owners always notice the respiratory noise but are sometimes hesitant to decide that performance is impaired. An owner may believe that there is no performance limitation because the horse is able to complete the desired activity yet still complain about increased respiratory effort and increased recovery time following exercise. The aforementioned signs are evidence of exercise impairment and suggest that the horse would benefit from a PL as well as a procedure, such as ventriculocordectomy (VCE), to decrease noise.

Prosthetic laryngoplasty

Treadmill studies have convincingly demonstrated that a PL is effective at restoring airway mechanics to normal or approaching normal values (Derksen et al. 1986; Shappell et al. 1988; Tetens et al. 1996). A criticism of the early studies was that the treadmill speeds used were not fast enough to extrapolate the results to racehorses (Derksen et al. 1986). It is worth noting that the speed used (7.2 m/s) is generally faster than the speeds at which most draft horses perform making it reasonable to extrapolate these results to draft horses. A PL will reduce respiratory noise but will not eliminate it altogether (Brown et al. 2004). Further reductions in noise beyond that provided by a PL require either a VE or VCE; however, addition of these procedures results in no measurable improvement in airway mechanics compared to the PL alone (Tetens et al. 1996).

The technique of PL is essentially unchanged since the original description and is performed the same in draft horses as in other breeds. One would think that their larger size would provide more working space and allow better visualization of the process. Unfortunately, the reverse is true as the tissues are less pliable and the large mandible makes for less exposure than in a Thoroughbred less than half the size. Surgeons with small hands may have difficulty reaching the muscular process for suture placement. The larynx can be rotated ventrally toward the surgeon to facilitate suture placement in the muscular process by placing a Senn or similar retractor on the dorsal border of the thyroid cartilage. The author prefers to place the endoscope in the nasopharynx intraoperatively to provide visual confirmation that the arytenoid is being abducted during suture tightening. The endoscope is positioned such that the surgeon can look along the left side of the endotracheal tube to confirm that the arytenoid cartilage is being abducted off of the tube. To this end, it is helpful to use an endotracheal tube at least one size smaller than typical for the size of

horse being operated; because if the endotracheal tube is forcing the arytenoid into an abducted position, it can be difficult to tell if suture tightening is moving the arytenoid. For most large draft horses a 26-mm inner diameter endotracheal tube is usually appropriate.

Draft breeds subjectively appear to be narrower in their nasopharynx than the typical Thoroughbred. Consequently, there is usually not enough space to achieve the maximal abduction of the arytenoid that the surgeon usually strives for in racing breeds. Although the surgeon usually aims for greater abduction, a successful outcome can result if the arytenoid is abducted away from the midline and fixed such that it cannot collapse during inspiration as long as the laryngoplasty is coupled with one of the VE procedures discussed later. In the author's hands it is uncommon to be able to overabduct an arytenoid cartilage in a draft horse.

Ventriculectomy and ventriculocordectomy

Respiratory noise associated with RLN is best eliminated with either a VCE or a VE (Brown et al. 2003; Cramp et al. 2009). Research studies using sound intensity as the objective outcome variable concluded that a VCE is superior to a VE when the procedures are performed without a PL (Cramp et al. 2009). It is not known if this superiority persists when these procedures are combined with PL. It has been demonstrated that no further improvement in airway mechanics is obtained following laryngoplasty by the addition of a VCE (Tetens et al. 1996). Interestingly, a retrospective study in a large series of draft horses found that more horses were able to perform successfully following a VE than following a VCE; however, numerous confounding variables present in a retrospective study prohibit making any firm inferences (Kraus et al. 2003). There is no evidence to suggest whether there is an advantage to performing the procedure transendoscopically or via a laryngotomy. A unilateral cordectomy alone is not efficacious in eliminating respiratory noise (Brown 2005).

Both bilateral VE and bilateral VCE result in a small improvement in airway mechanics when performed alone (Cramp et al. 2009). The author is firmly of the opinion that PL will yield the most satisfactory result. However, performing the VCE alone would be appropriate for a horse in which the only complaint is respiratory noise. Currently the author's treatment of choice is a PL combined with a bilateral VE, based principally on years of favorable experience with this combination. The most recent estimates of prognosis for a return to athletic activity following a combined PL and VCE or VE are approximately 90% (Kraus et al. 2003). The author would choose a VCE over a VE if a PL were not being performed or if the PL was not as successful as desired.

References

Beard WL, Hayes HM. 1993. Risk factors for laryngeal hemiplegia in the horse. *Preventive Veterinary Medicine* 17:57–63.

Brakenhoff JE, Holcombe SJ, Hauptman JG, Smith HK, Nickels FA, Caron JP. 2006. The prevalence of laryngeal disease in a large population of competition draft horses. *Veterinary Surgery* 35:579–583.

Brown JA, Derksen FJ, Stick JA, Hartmann WM, Robinson NE. 2003. Ventriculocordectomy reduces respiratory noise in horses with laryngeal hemiplegia. *Equine Veterinary Journal* 35:570–574.

Brown JA, Derksen FJ, Stick JA, Hartmann WM, Robinson NE. 2004. Effect of laryngoplasty on respiratory noise reduction in horses with laryngeal hemiplegia. *Equine Veterinary Journal* 36:420–425.

Brown JA, Derksen FJ, Stick JA, Hartmann WM, Robinson NE. 2005. Laser vocal cordectomy fails to effectively reduce respiratory noise in horses with laryngeal hemiplegia. *Veterinary Surgery* 34:247–252.

Cramp P, Derksen FJ, Stick JA, Nickels FA, Brown KE, Robinson P, Robinson NE. 2009. Effect of ventriculectomy versus ventriculocordectomy on upper airway noise in draught horses with recurrent laryngeal neuropathy. *Equine Veterinary Journal* 41:729–734.

Derksen FJ, Stick JA, Scott EA, Robinson NE, Slocombe RF. 1986. Effect of laryngeal hemiplegia and laryngoplasty on airway flow mechanics in exercising horses. *American Journal of Veterinary Research* 47:16–20.

Hackett RP, Ducharme NG, Fubini SL, Erb HN. 1991. The reliability of endoscopic examination in assessment of arytenoid cartilage movement in horses. Part I: Subjective and objective laryngeal evaluation. *Veterinary Surgery* 20:174–179.

Kraus BM, Parente EJ, Tulleners EP. 2003. Laryngoplasty with ventriculectomy or ventriculocordectomy in 104 draft horses (1992–2000). *Veterinary Surgery* 32:530–538.

Rothenbuhler R, Hawkins JF, Adams SB, Lescum TB, Weil AB, Glickman LT, Fessler JF, Glickman NG. 2006. Evaluation of surgical treatment for signs of acute abdominal pain in draft horses: 72 Cases (1983–2002). *Journal of American Veterinary Medical Association* 228:1546–1550.

Shappell KK, Derksen FJ, Stick JA, Robinson NE. 1988. Effects of ventriculectomy, prosthetic laryngoplasty, and exercise on upper airway function in horses with induced left laryngeal hemiplegia. *American Journal of Veterinary Research* 49:1760–1765.

Tetens J, Derksen FJ, Stick JA, Lloyd JW, Robinson NE. 1996. Efficacy of prosthetic laryngoplasty with and without bilateral ventriculocordectomy as treatments for laryngeal hemiplegia in horses. *American Journal of Veterinary Research* 57:1668–1673.

13 Evaluation and Treatment of the Horse with Fourth Branchial Arch Defects

Katherine Garrett

Description and etiology

Fourth branchial arch congenital abnormalities are an uncommon but important cause of upper airway dysfunction. Fourth branchial arch abnormalities are presumed to result from errors in the development of the laryngeal cartilages and associated musculature. During embryonic development, the branchial arches are formed from mesodermal tissue (Wilson 1979). In humans, the thyroid, cricoid, and arytenoid cartilages are formed from the fourth and possibly the sixth branchial arches (Hester et al. 1994; Mandell 2000; Wilson 1979). Although the embryonic origins of the equine larynx have not been specifically elucidated, they are generally assumed to be analogous to the human larynx. The specific mechanism of disease has not been determined for fourth branchial yyarch disorders. However, the functional abnormalities and clinical signs in this disease appear to be at least partly the result of the anatomic abnormalities.

Reports of fourth branchial arch abnormalities in the equine literature consist of isolated case reports or case series (Blikslager et al. 1999; Cook 1974; Crabill et al. 1994; Deegen 1987; Dixon et al. 1993; Garrett et al. 2009; Goulden et al. 1976; Kannegieter et al. 1986; Klein et al. 1989; Lane 2001; Smith and Mair 2009; Wilson et al. 1986). The disorder appears to be present along a spectrum; horses are affected to varying degrees, both in regards to the severity of the anatomic abnormalities present and the specific clinical signs manifested by the patient. Horses may be affected unilaterally (left or right sides) or bilaterally (either symmetrically or asymmetrically). Historically, unilateral right-sided disease has been the most commonly reported.

Pathologic anatomic features

The anatomic abnormalities characteristic of this condition generally involve the thyroid and cricoid cartilages. The most consistent features are a lack of a cricothyroid articulation and a rostrocaudally shortened and dorsoventrally elongated thyroid cartilage. Additional pharyngeal muscular abnormalities have also been described.

The lack of a cricothyroid articulation is the result of combined abnormalities of the cricoid and thyroid cartilages (Dixon et al. 1993; Garrett et al. 2009; Goulden et al. 1976; Kannegieter et al. 1986; Klein et al. 1989; Lane 2001; Wilson et al. 1986). On the

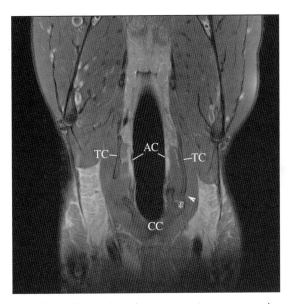

Figure 13.1   Dorsal plane short tau inversion recovery turbo spin echo magnetic resonance image at the level of the cricothyroid articulation. The left side of the horse is to the right side of the image. The asterisk (∗) indicates the normal left cricoid articular process and the white arrowhead indicates the normal caudal cornu of the left thyroid cartilage which forms the normal left cricothyroid articulation. The right side of the thyroid and cricoid cartilages do not articulate. The caudal cornu of the right thyroid cartilage lamina and the right cricoid articular process are absent. There is an abnormal gap between the cricoid and thyroid cartilages on the right. TC, thyroid cartilage; AC, arytenoid cartilage; CC, cricoid cartilage. Reprinted from Garrett et al. (2009) with permission from Wiley-Blackwell.

affected side, the cricoid cartilage articular process is absent or hypoplastic. In addition, the thyroid lamina fails to extend caudally to form the caudal cornu of the thyroid cartilage (Figure 13.1). The lack of the normal caudal extension of the thyroid cartilage results in the palpable gap between the thyroid and cricoid cartilages. Another consequence of the lack of caudal extension of the thyroid cartilage is that the arytenoid cartilage assumes an abnormally caudal-relative position to the thyroid cartilage. As a result, the cricoarytenoideus lateralis and vocalis muscles are positioned in the gap between the thyroid and cricoid cartilages rather than between the thyroid and arytenoid cartilages (Figures 13.2a and 13.2b).

In normal horses, the thyroid lamina extends to a level slightly ventral to the dorsal extent of the muscular process of the arytenoid cartilage. In horses

with fourth branchial arch disorder, the abnormal dorsal extension of the thyroid cartilage lamina leads to its extension dorsal to the muscular process of the arytenoid cartilage (Figure 13.3) (Dixon et al. 1993; Garrett et al. 2009; Goulden et al. 1976; Lane 2001). It has also been noted that the muscular process of the arytenoid cartilage on the affected side is smaller than normal in some cases.

Rotation and/or widening of the cricoid cartilage spine are present in some cases (Figure 13.4) (Garrett et al. 2009; Klein et al. 1989). Rotation of the cricoid cartilage may lead to an abnormal anatomic course of the cricoarytenoideus dorsalis muscle, with its origin on the cricoid cartilage positioned more ventrally than is typical. In the author's opinion, the abnormal course of the arytenoid abductor resulting in altered biomechanics may be a cause for incomplete arytenoid abduction as opposed to incomplete abduction resulting from recurrent laryngeal neuropathy. This is supported by the finding of normal echogenicity of the cricoarytenoideus lateralis muscles in horses with fourth branchial arch abnormalities when assessed ultrasonographically, as increased echogenicity of the cricoarytenoideus lateralis muscle has been associated with abnormal arytenoid abduction characteristic of recurrent laryngeal neuropathy (Garrett et al. 2011).

Pharyngeal muscle abnormalities have also been described, the most common of which is the absence or hypoplasia of the cricopharyngeus muscle(s) (Figure 13.4) (Garrett et al. 2009; Goulden et al. 1976; Klein et al. 1989; Lane 2001; Wilson et al. 1986). The thyropharyngeus muscles have also been reported to be hypoplastic, absent, or hyperplastic (Dixon et al. 1993; Lane 2001; Wilson et al. 1986). These pharyngeal muscle abnormalities have been suggested as a cause of dysphagia and aeroesophagus (Dixon et al. 1993; Wilson et al. 1986).

Diagnosis

History

Horses may present for evaluation of abnormal upper airway noise, exercise intolerance, poor performance, dyspnea, dysphagia, or chronic colic (Blikslager et al. 1999; Cook 1974; Crabill et al. 1994; Garrett et al. 2009; Goulden et al. 1976; Kannegieter et al. 1986; Klein et al. 1989; Lane 2001; Smith and

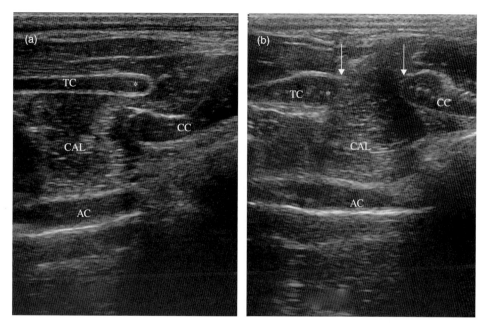

Figure 13.2 (a) Longitudinal ultrasound image of a normal larynx at the mid portion of the arytenoid cartilage. Cranial is to the left of the image. The cricoarytenoideus lateralis muscle is positioned in its normal location deep to the thyroid cartilage. The caudal cornu of the thyroid cartilage (∗) is imaged close to its articulation with the cricoid cartilage. (b) Longitudinal image of the right side of the larynx of a horse with fourth branchial arch disorder at the midportion of the arytenoid cartilage. Cranial is to the left of the image. The cricoarytenoideus lateralis muscle is positioned between the thyroid cartilage and the cricoid cartilage in an abnormal space (between arrows). The caudal aspect of the thyroid cartilage (∗) is abnormally shaped and does not articulate with the cricoid cartilage. TC, thyroid cartilage; CAL, cricoarytenoideus lateralis muscle; AC, arytenoid cartilage; CC, cricoid cartilage. Reprinted from Garrett et al. (2009) with permission from Wiley-Blackwell.

Mair 2009). Alternatively, horses may have no overt signs of an upper airway problem and may be identified during upper airway endoscopy for other reasons (e.g., prepurchase examination) (Blikslager et al. 1999; Garrett et al. 2009; Lane 2001).

Physical examination

General physical examination is unremarkable. However, laryngeal palpation reveals a unilateral or bilateral gap between the thyroid and cricoid cartilages (Garrett et al. 2009; Lane 2001; Smith and Mair 2009).

Resting upper airway endoscopy

The classically described findings of fourth branchial arch disorder include rostral displacement of the palatopharyngeal arch (Figure 13.5) and/or abnormal right arytenoid cartilage move-

ment (Blikslager et al. 1999; Garrett et al. 2009; Goulden et al. 1976; Kannegieter et al. 1986; Klein et al. 1989; Lane 2001; Smith and Mair 2009; Wilson et al. 1986). However, abnormal left arytenoid cartilage movement, abnormal bilateral arytenoid cartilage movement, and dorsal displacement of the soft palate have also been described in horses with fourth branchial arch abnormalities (Blikslager et al. 1999; Cook 1974; Dixon et al. 1993; Garrett et al. 2009; Lane 2001). Horses with arytenoid cartilage movement abnormalities may have partial abduction of the arytenoid cartilage(s) or complete loss of arytenoid abduction. Horses with abnormal left arytenoid movement may appear identical endoscopically to horses with left recurrent laryngeal neuropathy. Abnormal arytenoid movement, if present, is generally ipsilateral to the anatomic abnormalities.

Rostral displacement of the palatopharyngeal arch may be present to varying degrees of severity and symmetry. In other cases, the palatopharyngeal arch has a normal anatomic position (Dixon et al.

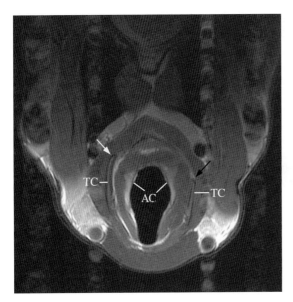

Figure 13.3   Transverse proton density turbo spin echo magnetic resonance image at the level of the arytenoid cartilages. The left side of the horse is to the right side of the image. The lamina of the right side of the thyroid cartilage extends dorsal to the muscular process of the arytenoid cartilage (white arrow). The left side of the larynx is normal with the muscular process of the arytenoid extending dorsal to the thyroid lamina (black arrow). TC, thyroid cartilage; AC, arytenoid cartilage. Reprinted from Garrett et al. (2009) with permission from Wiley Blackwell.

1993; Kannegieter et al. 1986). Rostral displacement of the palatopharyngeal arch can also be intermittent in nature.

Dynamic upper airway endoscopy

Dynamic upper airway endoscopy may confirm abnormal arytenoid movement. The affected arytenoid cartilage may collapse into the airway or may simply maintain a partially abducted position while failing to achieve full abduction (Garrett et al. 2009; Lane 2001). In other cases, normal arytenoid abduction is present, even in the face of abnormal arytenoid movement during resting upper airway endoscopy (Garrett et al. 2009; Smith and Mair 2009).

Rostral displacement of the palatopharyngeal arch may be constant, intermittent, or absent (Lane 2001). Some horses with rostral displacement of the

palatopharyngeal arch during resting upper airway endoscopy have a normally positioned palatopharyngeal arch during exercise and vice versa (Garrett et al. 2009). However, further rostral displacement of the palatopharyngeal arch during exercise leading to substantial obstruction of the rima glottidis has not been observed in the author's experience.

A variety of additional upper airway abnormalities have been diagnosed during dynamic upper airway endoscopy, including dorsal displacement of the soft palate, axial deviation of the aryepiglottic folds, axial deviation of the vocal folds, dorsal pharyngeal collapse, and palate billowing (Garrett et al. 2009; Lane 2001; Smith and Mair 2009).

Due to the varying degrees and ways in which horses are clinically affected by this condition, a dynamic upper airway examination is extremely helpful in determining the particular anatomic structures contributing to airway obstruction and/or noise production during exercise and the extent to which each is contributing. This knowledge is important when designing a treatment plan.

Diagnostic imaging

Radiography, ultrasonography, and magnetic resonance imaging have all been used to assist with the diagnosis of this condition. Radiographically, a standard lateral–lateral projection of the larynx is typically the most useful. In many cases, the laryngeal region appears normal. In horses with rostral displacement of the palatopharyngeal arch, the displacing tissue can be imaged rostral to the corniculate process of the arytenoid cartilage (Figure 13.6) (Crabill et al. 1994; Lane 2001). The presence of aeroesophagus can be determined in some cases (Dixon et al. 1993; Goulden et al. 1976; Klein et al. 1989; Lane 2001; Smith and Mair 2009). As the cricopharyngeus muscles form the cranial esophageal sphincter, absence or hypoplasia of these muscles has been postulated to be the reason for the aeroesophagus.

Recently, ultrasonography and magnetic resonance imaging have been used to image the characteristic anatomic abnormalities found in disorders of the fourth branchial arch (Garrett et al. 2009). Both of these modalities are able to demonstrate the abnormal dorsal extension of the thyroid lamina, absence of the cricoid cartilage articular process

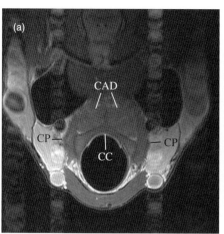
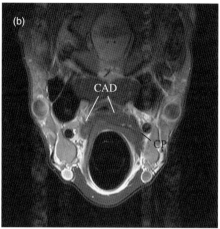

Figure 13.4   (a) Transverse proton density turbo spin echo magnetic resonance image of a normal larynx at the level of the cricoid cartilage. The left side of the horse is to the right side of the image. (b) Transverse proton density turbo spin echo magnetic resonance image of a horse with fourth branchial arch disorder at the level of the cricoid cartilage. The left side of the horse is to the right side of the image. Note the widening and rotation to the right of the spine of the cricoid cartilage and subsequent abnormal positioning of the left and right cricoarytenoideus dorsalis muscles. The left cricopharyngeus muscle is present while the right cricopharyngeus muscle and cricoid articular process are absent. CAD, cricoarytenoideus dorsalis muscle; CP, cricopharyngeus muscle; CC, cricoid cartilage. Reprinted from Garrett et al. (2009) with permission from Wiley Blackwell.

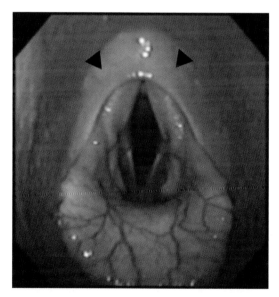

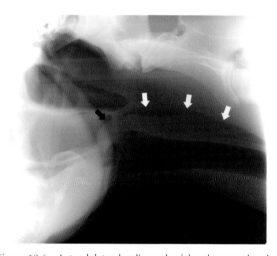

Figure 13.6   Lateral–lateral radiograph of the pharyngeal and laryngeal region of a horse with fourth branchial arch abnormality. Rostral is to the left of the image. The rostrally displaced palatopharyngeal arch can be seen as a teardrop-shaped soft tissue opacity (black arrow). Air is present within the esophagus (white arrows).

Figure 13.5   Resting upper airway examination of a horse with fourth branchial arch abnormality. Note the rostrally displaced position of the palatopharyngeal arch (black arrowheads).

and caudal cornu of the thyroid cartilage, and the lack of the cricothyroid articulation manifesting as a gap between the thyroid and cricoid cartilages (Figures 13.1–13.4). As would be expected, magnetic resonance imaging allows a more thorough evaluation of this region. Abnormalities of the pharyngeal muscles and the degree of cricoid cartilage rotation can be better appreciated using magnetic resonance imaging (Figure 13.4). However, magnetic resonance imaging can be costly and, for evaluation of the laryngeal region, requires general anesthesia. In the author's experience, in nearly all cases, ultrasonography is sufficient to confirm the diagnosis and assist in determining the extent of the abnormalities.

Accurate diagnosis is extremely important when considering various causes of abnormal arytenoid movement, as the treatments and prognoses may differ. Horses with unilateral left-sided fourth branchial arch abnormality with abnormal left arytenoid movement have been misdiagnosed with left recurrent laryngeal neuropathy or arytenoid chondritis. In some cases, the abnormal anatomy consistent with fourth branchial arch abnormality was discovered only during attempted prosthetic laryngoplasty during which the abnormal laryngeal anatomy was encountered. Inclusion of ultrasonography (or magnetic resonance imaging) as part of the diagnostic evaluation of upper airway disorders can help reduce these types of errors.

Treatment

Currently, no treatment exists to restore normal anatomy to an affected animal, as is typical for a congenital condition. When possible, treatment is focused on modifying the clinical signs of the condition and their impact on performance, but results have been mixed. Generally, this involves improving airway dynamics to improve exercise tolerance and/or to reduce or eliminate upper airway noise. To the author's knowledge, there have been no controlled clinical trials in evaluating treatment of this disorder. Treatment has been based upon the outcome of clinical cases described in case series and case reports. Additional complicating factors in assessing the success of various treatments are the spectrum of clinical signs and differing degrees of anatomic malformation that affected horses exhibit.

When considering potential treatments, the use of the horse is an important consideration. For some breeds and uses (e.g., show horses) elimination of noise is usually the primary goal of the client if the horse does not exhibit exercise intolerance. For other breeds (e.g., racehorses), improvement of airway dynamics is the major goal of treatment,

as these horses must perform at or near maximal intensity.

Although one of the endoscopic hallmarks of fourth branchial arch disorder is rostral displacement of the palatopharyngeal arch, laser ablation or surgical resection of this tissue did not improve performance in a case series (three Thoroughbred racehorses and one western pleasure Quarter Horse) and in an individual case report, although these methods did resolve the clinical sign of rostral displacement of the palatopharyngeal arch (Blikslager et al. 1999; Crabill et al. 1994). The lack of improvement in performance is perhaps unsurprising, as in the author's experience, the palatopharyngeal arch does not displace further into the airway and presents minimal obstruction to airflow during dynamic upper airway endoscopy.

If abnormal arytenoid movement is a feature of the condition in a particular patient and elimination of noise is the primary goal of the client, resection of the laryngeal saccule and vocal cord on the affected side(s) has been effective in some clinical cases (Garrett et al. 2009).

If restoring airway dynamics as close to normal as possible is the primary goal in a horse with abnormal arytenoid movement, prosthetic laryngoplasty combined with ventriculocordectomy can be undertaken. In this situation, the surgeon should be cognizant that the abnormal anatomy makes prosthetic laryngoplasty a more challenging procedure. A smaller than normal muscular process of the arytenoid cartilage that is partially obscured by a more dorsal extension of the thyroid cartilage lamina than is normal complicates the placement of the laryngoplasty suture. Resection of the dorsal aspect of the thyroid lamina has been helpful in gaining access to the muscular process of the arytenoid cartilage. In addition, the abnormal anatomy of the cricoid cartilage may preclude ideal suture placement around the caudal aspect of the cricoid cartilage. Nonideal suture placement may lead to an inadequate or suboptimal degree of abduction postoperatively. The surgeon should attempt to determine preoperatively if the expected degree of abduction postoperatively would be an improvement over the preoperative state. In these cases, dynamic upper airway examination is extremely helpful to determine the degree of arytenoid abduction that can be achieved. If the arytenoid is unable to completely abduct, but is able to be maintained in a mostly (at least 70–80%) abducted position and does not collapse into the rima glottidis, prosthetic laryngoplasty may be unable to improve significantly upon the airway dynamics existing preoperatively. Arytenoidectomy may also be a viable option in these cases.

In one case (a Tennessee Walking Horse) that had dorsal displacement of the soft palate as a feature of this condition, a tie-forward procedure eliminated abnormal upper airway noise and exercise intolerance. Interestingly, this horse was affected bilaterally symmetrically and had normal arytenoid movement during dynamic upper airway examination (Garrett et al. 2009).

Additional airway disorders (e.g., vocal cord collapse, axial deviation of the aryepiglottic folds, pharyngeal collapse) may be seen during dynamic upper airway examination and can be treated as they would be in the absence of a fourth branchial arch abnormality.

As was previously noted, fourth branchial arch abnormalities appear to present as a spectrum of abnormalities, so no single treatment can be recommended for all cases. An individualized treatment program that takes into account the clinical signs, resting and dynamic upper airway endoscopic findings, and goals of the client is of paramount importance. In some cases, benign neglect may be an appropriate treatment. For example, the author is aware of a Thoroughbred racehorse who was able to race successfully without clinical signs of an upper airway disorder but was later diagnosed with a fourth branchial arch abnormality (at age 6 years).

Conclusion

The true prevalence of fourth branchial arch defects is unknown, as there are likely many affected horses that have no obvious clinical signs so have never undergone upper airway evaluation and remain undiagnosed. Hopefully, increased use of diagnostic imaging will lead to increased recognition of this condition. The clinician should be cognizant that fourth branchial arch defect remains a differential diagnosis for horses with a variety of endoscopic abnormalities and clinical signs. Sur-gical intervention may reduce the clinical signs in some patients, but an accurate evidence-based prognosis remains unknown.

References

Blikslager AT, Tate LP, Tudor R. 1999. Transendoscopic laser treatment of rostral displacement of the palatopharyngeal arch in four horses. *Journal of Clinical Laser Medicine Surgery* 17:49–52.

Cook WR. 1974. Some observations on diseases of the ear, nose and throat in the horse, and endoscopy using a flexible fibreoptic endoscope. *Veterinary Record* 94:533–541.

Crabill M, Schumacher J, Walker M. 1994. What is your diagnosis? Rostral displacement of the palatopharyngeal arch. *Journal of the American Veterinary Medical Association* 204:1347–1348.

Deegen E, Klein HJ. 1987. Rostrale verlagerung des arcus palatopharygicus beim pferd. *Pferdeheilkunde* 3:303–308.

Dixon PM, McGorum BC, Else RW. 1993. Cricopharyngeal-laryngeal dysplasia in a horse with sudden clinical onset idiopathic laryngeal hemiparesis. *New Zealand Veterinary Journal* 41:134–138.

Garrett KS, Woodie JB, Embertson RM, Pease AP. 2009. Diagnosis of laryngeal dysplasia in five horses using magnetic resonance imaging and ultrasonography. *Equine Veterinary Journal* 41:766–771.

Garrett KS, Woodie JB, Embertson RM. 2011. Association of treadmill upper airway endoscopic evaluation with results of ultrasonography and resting upper airway endoscopic evaluation. *Equine Veterinary Journal* 43:365–371.

Goulden BE, Anderson LJ, Davies AS, Barnes GR. 1976. Rostral displacement of the palatopharyngeal arch: A case report. *Equine Veterinary Journal* 8:95–98.

Hester TO, Jones RO, Haydon RC. 1994. Anomalies of the branchial apparatus: A case report and review of embryology, anatomy and development. *Journal of the Kentucky Medical Association* 92:358–362.

Kannegieter NJ, Goulden BE, Anderson LJ. 1986. Right-sided laryngeal dysfunction in a horse. *New Zealand Veterinary Journal* 34:66–68.

Klein HJ, Deegen E, Stockhofe N, Wissdorf H. 1989. Rostral displacement of the palatopharyngeal arch in a seven-month-old Hanoverian colt. *Equine Veterinary Journal* 21:382–383.

Lane JG. 2001. Fourth branchial arch defects in Thoroughbred horses: A review of 60 cases. In: Viel L, Robinson NE, Ducharme NG, McGorum BC, eds. *Proceedings of the Second World Equine Airways Symposium*. Edinburgh.

Mandell DL. 2000. Head and neck anomalies related to the branchial apparatus. *Otolaryngology Clinics North America* 33:1309–1332.

Smith LJ, Mair TS. 2009. Fourth branchial arch defect in a Welsh section A pony mare. *Equine Veterinary Education* 21:364–366.

Wilson DB. 1979. Embryonic development of the head and neck: Part 2, the branchial region. *Head & Neck Surgery* 2:59–66.

Wilson RG, Sutton RH, Groenendyk S. 1986. Rostral displacement of the palato pharyngeal arch in a Thoroughbred yearling. *Australian Veterinary Journal* 63:99–100.

14 Future Developments in the Management and Treatment of Recurrent Laryngeal Neuropathy

Jonathan Cheetham

Introduction

The future of the management of recurrent laryngeal neuropathy (RLN) is likely to advance through four main themes: (1) incremental improvements to existing techniques through the identification of a solvable problem; (2) earlier and better diagnosis; (3) novel surgical techniques; and (4) improved follow-up and assessment of success.

In the last few years progress has been made toward tackling one of the major problems associated with prosthetic laryngoplasty (PL), that of arytenoid abduction loss in the early postoperative period. It is well documented that the majority of horses experience some degree of arytenoid abduction loss in the first 6 weeks after surgery (Barakzai et al. 2009; Dixon et al. 2003). Emerging work suggests that arytenoid position at 6 weeks postoperatively is likely to represent long-term arytenoid position. A number of studies have worked toward tackling this common problem experienced by all upper airway surgeons. This work has identified an increase in load on the prosthetic suture through the ventromedial force produced by the pharyngeal

constrictors during swallowing (Witte et al. 2010) and has suggested solutions through increased stabilization of the arytenoid in an abducted position either through curettage of the cricoarytenoid joint or curettage combined with additional stabilization through the use of polymethyl methacrylate or bone cement (Cheetham et al. 2008; Parente 2004). Other incremental improvements have been made through improved understanding of the relationship between airway pressures and arytenoid abduction (Rakesh et al. 2008).

Traditionally the diagnosis of RLN has been made using high-speed treadmill videoendoscopy, (Lane et al. 2006; Parente et al. 2002; Rakestraw et al. 1991) by determining the degree of arytenoid abduction. One major limitation of this method is that it only detects disease once it has become severe enough to affect arytenoid function. The ability to identify young horses affected by RLN prior to expensive sales preparation would be of considerable value to the equine industry. Early diagnosis of RLN would also allow the use of more physiological surgical techniques, such as reinnervation, to restore muscle function before extensive

Advances in Equine Upper Respiratory Surgery, First Edition. Edited by Jan Hawkins.
© 2015 ACVS Foundation. Published 2015 by John Wiley & Sons, Inc.

muscle atrophy and fibrosis have occurred. Restoration of physiological function through reinnervation and nerve–muscle pedicle transplant techniques have produced positive results. However, there is a delay of up to 12 months before any improvement in arytenoid function is seen (Ducharme et al. 1989; Fulton et al. 1991; Fulton et al. 1992) and as a result these techniques have not been widely adopted. Early diagnosis of RLN would allow the use of these more physiological techniques based on surgical reinnervation. Reinnervation is most likely to be successful if it is accomplished before terminal changes of disuse atrophy and fibrosis occur in the laryngeal muscles. Attempts to diagnose the condition at an earlier stage have included electromyography and nerve conduction studies (Curtis et al. 2005; Hawe et al. 2001; Moore et al. 1988; Steiss et al. 1989). Recently a number of noninvasive imaging techniques have emerged which may allow the early diagnosis of disease (Chalmers et al. 2006a,b; Garrett et al. 2010). These techniques and other neurodiagnostic methods hold great promise for early diagnosis and intervention before irreversible fibrosis and dysfunction occur.

A number of novel surgical techniques have been explored in the last few years for the treatment of RLN. These have focused on the use of functional electrical stimulation (FES) of laryngeal muscle (Cheetham et al. 2011; Scheuch et al. 2002). FES is a technique that may be applied for the treatment of lower motor neuron injury (Kern et al. 2002; Neil et al. 2007; Salmons et al. 2005). It has been shown that FES can have a marked positive influence in human patients, even after chronic denervation (Kern et al. 2002). FES of the intrinsic laryngeal musculature has been studied in both humans and in animal models (Broniatowski et al. 1985; Broniatowski et al. 2008; Katada et al. 2008; Kim et al. 1987; Ptok and Strack 2008; Sanders 1991; Zealear et al. 1996; Zrunek et al. 1991). The goal of laryngeal pacing is to produce FES of the posterior cricoarytenoid (PCA) muscle with the goal of restoring muscle mass and function. Although clinical trials in horses with naturally occurring disease are currently underway this work is still at an early stage and its widespread application remains something of an unknown. Other tissue engineering and gene therapy techniques will undoubtedly emerge over the next few years.

The last area of anticipated improvement in upper airway surgery is improved assessment of postoperative success. Until recently, postoperative "success" has been judged using indirect or proxy measures such as racing performance or owner opinion of reduction in respiratory noise, all of which may be influenced by numerous other factors. These methods may under- or overestimate success and are unable to determine the precise cause of perceived surgical "failure." A number of studies are beginning to emerge in which clinical cases are evaluated with postoperative exercising endoscopy (Barnett et al. 2011a,b; Davidson et al. 2010; Davidson and Parente 2011). These studies have been crucial in identifying and quantifying causes of surgical failure, thus providing feedback to improve surgical treatments. Other such studies providing followup on the upper respiratory tract surgery are in progress and are crucial for assessing surgical procedures using an objective and accurate approach. It has previously been extremely difficult to obtain definitive followup of cases which have undergone respiratory surgery; however, it is hoped that increased owner acceptance of overground endoscopy systems as compared to treadmill examination will mean that such cross-sectional studies are now much more achievable.

References

Barakzai SZ, Boden LA, Dixon PM. 2009. Race performance after laryngoplasty and ventriculocordectomy in national hunt racehorses. *Veterinary Surgery* 38(8):941–945.

Barnett TP, Dixon PM, Parkin TDH, Barakzai SZ. 2011a. *A Prospective Study of Horses Undergoing Videoendoscopic Dynamic Assessment of the Upper Airway Following Laryngoplasty*. Presented at European College of Veterinary Surgeons Annual Congress. Ghent, Belgium.

Barnett TP, Dixon PM, Parkin TDH, Barakzai SZ. 2011b. *Long-Term Abduction and Stability of Arytenoid Cartilages Following Laryngoplasty*. Presented at British Equine Veterinary Association Annual Congress. Liverpool, UK.

Broniatowski MS, Kaneko S, Jacobs G, Nose Y, Tucker HM. 1985. Laryngeal pacemaker. II. electronic pacing of reinnervated posterior cricoarytenoid muscles in the canine. *The Laryngoscope* 95(10):1194–1198.

Broniatowski MS, Grundfest-Broniatowski S, Zobenica NS, Tyler DJ. 2008. Artificial manipulation of voice in the human by an implanted stimulator. *The Laryngoscope* 118(10):1889–1893.

Chalmers HJ, Cheetham J, Yeager AE, Ducharme NG. 2006a. Ultrasonography of the equine larynx. *Veterinary Radiology and Ultrasound.* 47(5):476–481.

Chalmers HJ, Cheetham J, Mohammed HO, Ducharme NG. 2006b. Ultrasonography as an aid in the diagnosis of recurrent laryngeal neuropathy in horses. Abstract. *Proceedings of the 2006 American College of Veterinary Surgeons Veterinary Symposium.* p. 3.

Cheetham J, Witte TH, Rawlinson JJ, Soderholm LV, Proudman HO, Ducharme NG. 2008. Intra-articular stabilisation of the equine cricoarytenoid joint. *Equine Veterinary Journal* 40(6):584–588.

Cheetham J, Regner A, Jarvis JC, Priest D, Sanders I, Soderholm LV, Mitchell LM, Ducharme NG. 2011. Functional electrical stimulation of intrinsic laryngeal muscles under varying loads in exercising horses. *PLoS ONE* 6(8):e24258.

Curtis RA, Hahn CN, Evans DL, Williams T, Begg L. 2005. Thoracolaryngeal reflex latencies in Thoroughbred horses with recurrent laryngeal neuropathy. *Veterinary Journal* 170(1):67–76.

Davidson EJ, Parente EJ. 2011. Exercising videoendoscopic evaluation of 7 horses with abnormal respiratory noise and poor performance following partial arytenoidectomy. *Equine Veterinary Education* 23(12): 626–629.

Davidson EJ, Martin BB, Rieger RH, Parente EJ. 2010. Exercising videoendoscopic evaluation of 45 horses with respiratory noise and/or poor performance after laryngoplasty. *Veterinary Surgery* 39(8):942–948.

Dixon PM, McGorum BC, Railton DI, Hawe C, Tremaine WH, Dacre K, McCann J. 2003. Long-term survey of laryngoplasty and ventriculocordectomy in an older, mixed-breed population of 200 horses. Part 1: Maintenance of surgical arytenoid abduction and complications of surgery. *Equine Veterinary Journal* 35(4):389–396.

Ducharme NG, Horney FD, Hulland TJ, Partlow GD, Schnurr D, Zutrauen K. 1989. Attempts to restore abduction of the paralyzed equine arytenoid cartilage. II. Nerve implantation (Pilot study). *Canadian Journal of Veterinary Research=Revue Canadienne De Recherche Veterinaire* 53(2):210–215.

Fulton IC, Derksen FJ, Stick JA, Robinson NE, Walshaw R. 1991. Treatment of left laryngeal hemiplegia in standardbreds, using a nerve muscle pedicle graft. *American Journal of Veterinary Research* 52(9):1461–1467.

Fulton IC, Derksen FJ, Stick JA, Robinson NE, Duncan ID. 1992. Histologic evaluation of nerve muscle pedicle graft used as a treatment for left laryngeal hemiplegia in Standardbreds. *American Journal of Veterinary Research* 53(4):592–596.

Garrett KS, Woodie JB, Embertson RM. 2010. Association of treadmill upper airway endoscopic evaluation with results of ultrasonography and resting upper airway endoscopic evaluation. *Equine Veterinary Journal* 52(4):365–371.

Hawe C, Dixon PM, Mayhew IG. 2001. A study of an electrodiagnostic technique for the evaluation of equine recurrent laryngeal neuropathy. *Equine Veterinary Journal* 33(5):459–465.

Katada A, Van Himbergen D, Kunibe I, Nonaka S, Harabuchi Y, Huang S, Billante CR, Zealear DL. 2008. Evaluation of a deep brain stimulation electrode for laryngeal pacing. *The Annals of Otology, Rhinology, and Laryngology* 117(8):621–629.

Kern H, Hofer C, Modlin M, Forstner C, Raschka-Hogler D, Mayr W, Stohr H. 2002. Denervated muscles in humans: limitations and problems of currently used functional electrical stimulation training protocols. *Artificial Organs* 26(3):216–218.

Kim KM, Choi HS, Kim GR, Hong WP, Chun YM, Park YJ. 1987. Laryngeal pacemaker using a temperature sensor in the canine. *The Laryngoscope* 97(10):1207–1210.

Lane JG, Bladon B, Little DR, Naylor JR, Franklin SH. 2006. Dynamic obstructions of the equine upper respiratory tract. Part 2: Comparison of endoscopic findings at rest and during high-speed treadmill exercise of 600 Thoroughbred racehorses. *Equine Veterinary Journal* 38(5):401–407.

Moore MP, Andrews F, Reed SM, Grant BD. 1988. Electromyographic evaluation of horses with laryngeal hemiplegia. *Journal of Equine Veterinary Science* 8(6):424–427.

Neil KM, Axon JE, Todhunter PG, Adams PL, Caron JP, Adkins AR. 2007. Septic osteitis of the distal phalanx in foals: 22 cases (1995–2002). *Journal of the American Veterinary Medical Association* 230(11):1683–1690.

Parente EJ. 2004. *Improvements in laryngoplasty.* Stratford-upon-Avon, London: R & W Publication (Newmarket) Ltd.

Parente EJ, Martin BB, Tulleners EP, Ross MW. 2002. Dorsal displacement of the soft palate in 92 horses during high-speed treadmill examination (1993–1998). *Veterinary Surgery* 31(6):507–512.

Ptok M, Strack D. 2008. Electrical stimulation-supported voice exercises are superior to voice exercise therapy alone in patients with unilateral recurrent laryngeal nerve paresis: Results from a prospective, randomized clinical trial. *Muscle and Nerve* 38(2):1005–1011.

Rakesh V, Ducharme NG, Cheetham J, Datta AK, Pease AP. 2008. Implications of different degrees of arytenoid cartilage abduction on equine upper airway characteristics. *Equine Veterinary Journal* 40(7):629–635.

Rakesh V, Rakesh NG, Datta AK, Cheetham J, Pease AP. 2008. Development of equine upper airway fluid mechanics model for Thoroughbred racehorses. *Equine Veterinary Journal* 40(3):272–279.

Rakestraw PC, Hackett RP, Ducharme NG, Nielan GJ, Erb HN. 1991. Arytenoid cartilage movement in resting and exercising horses. *Veterinary Surgery* 20(2): 122–127.

Salmons S, Ashley Z, Sutherland H, Russold MF, Li F, Jarvis JC. 2005. Functional electrical stimulation of denervated muscles: Basic issues. *Artificial Organs* 29(3):199–202.

Sanders I. 1991. Electrical stimulation of laryngeal muscle. *Otolaryngologic Clinics of North America* 24(5):1253–1274.

Scheuch BC, Van Hoogmoed LM, Wilson WD, Snyder JR, MacDonald MH, Watson ZE, Steffey EP. 2002. Comparison of intraosseous or intravenous infusion for delivery of amikacin sulfate to the tibiotarsal joint of horses. *American Journal of Veterinary Research* 63(3):374–380.

Steiss JE, Marshall AE, Humburg JM. 1989. Electromyographic evaluation of conduction time of the recurrent laryngeal nerve: Findings in clinically normal horses and ponies. *Equine Veterinary Journal* 21(3):218–220.

Witte TH, Cheetham J, Soderholm LV, Mitchell LM, Ducharme NG. 2010. Equine laryngoplasty sutures undergo increased loading during coughing and swallowing. *Veterinary Surgery* 39(8):949–956.

Zealear DL, Rainey CL, Herzon GD, Netterville JL, Ossoff RH. 1996. Electrical pacing of the paralyzed human larynx. *The Annals of Otology, Rhinology, and Laryngology* 105(9):689–693.

Zrunek M, Bigenzahn W, Mayr W, Unger E, Feldner-Busztin H. 1991. A laryngeal pacemaker for inspiration-controlled, direct electrical stimulation of the denervated posterior cricoarytenoid muscle in sheep. *European Archives of Oto-Rhino-Laryngology* 248(8):445–448.

15 Objective Evaluation Following Surgical Correction of Upper Airway Abnormalities

Jonathan Cheetham

Introduction

The objective assessment of postoperative athletic performance following upper airway surgery in both racehorses and sports horses is very important to owners, trainers, and veterinarians. Performance can be assessed on either a horse level or on a population basis and assessment may be either direct, using postoperative endoscopy at rest or exercise, or indirect through the assessment of proxy measures such as racing performance.

At an individual horse level, the best assessment of postoperative outcome is direct evaluation of the upper airway through dynamic video endoscopy either on a treadmill or using an overground endoscope. Dynamic video endoscopy has rightly gained widespread acceptance for the diagnosis of upper respiratory disorders (Allen and Franklin 2010; Desmaiziers et al. 2009; Franklin et al. 2008; Pollock and Reardon 2009; Pollock et al. 2009; Tamzali et al. 2008; Van Erck 2011; Witte et al. 2011) and reports using them to assess upper airway function after surgical intervention are starting to emerge (Barnett et al. 2011; Bassage and Richardson 1998).

As direct endoscopic evaluation provides an actual evaluation of upper airway function, it should be encouraged in horses that are not performing as anticipated after surgery. Exercising endoscopy should be viewed as cost-effective because the losses sustained by incorrect or incomplete assessment are considerable (Lane 2012). These include the costs of incorrect treatment, costs of convalescence and retraining, costs of additional surgery, loss of earnings, and devaluation of horses which have had multiple surgeries (Lane 2012).

Overground endoscopy has a number of practical advantages over high-speed treadmill endoscopy, in particular that the horse does not need to travel to a referral center and can be exercised under normal training conditions. In sport horses, a further advantage is the ability of the rider to manipulate head position to replicate performance conditions. This is especially important in this group of horses as upper airway obstructions may not manifest without poll flexion (Davidson et al. 2011; Van Erck 2011). Poll flexion is not unique to the ridden animal and can also be successfully induced in horses exercising on treadmills (Davidson et al. 2011; Franklin et al.

Advances in Equine Upper Respiratory Surgery, First Edition. Edited by Jan Hawkins.
© 2015 ACVS Foundation. Published 2015 by John Wiley & Sons, Inc.

2006; Strand and Skjerve 2012; Strand et al. 2012; Van Erck 2011).

The major limitation of overground endoscopy is the potential for an inadequate level of exercise intensity during the test and hence a false-negative diagnosis of "no abnormality detected." To avoid this, it is crucial that there is clear communication between veterinarian, trainer, and rider prior to the examination to determine the length and intensity of the test. Currently overground exercise tests tend not to be standardized and this can produce considerable variability in results.

A number of studies evaluating noise as a diagnostic tool, and comparing owner-reported noise to direct assessment of upper airway function, have shown that diagnosis of upper respiratory tract obstructions based solely on owner-reported noise and performance history may result in incomplete diagnoses (Witte et al. 2011) and conclude that endoscopy should be performed in horses with abnormal respiratory noise to rule out complex conditions of the upper portion of the respiratory tract (Witte et al. 2011). A similar principle applies to postoperative assessment.

When assessing performance following a surgical intervention at a population level, it is important to consider the level of evidence that a particular study provides (Kapatkin 2007; Parkin et al. 2005; Weiner 2006). Randomized controlled trials (RCTs) and systematic reviews represent the highest level of evidence (Altman et al. 2001; Phillips et al. 2005). Equine RCTs are sparse and there are none assessing upper airway function. These trials are particularly difficult in equine surgical practice as many "connections" are often involved with one animal, making obtaining informed consent complex. There is one meta-analysis of existing studies which assesses the efficacy of a variety of treatments for dorsal displacement of the soft palate (DDSP) (Allen et al. 2012). Several cohort studies are available to assess the effects of upper airway surgery on performance. These have focused on the efficacy of interventions for DDSP (Barakzai et al. 2009; Cheetham et al. 2008) and recurrent laryngeal neuropathy (RLN) (Witte et al. 2009).

There is no consensus on indirect objective outcome measures that can be used to determine if a medical or surgical treatment affects a racehorse's performance. There are several ways in which authors strive to measure the rate of return to

racing and a variety of parameters have been used. These include the number of starts (Laws et al. 1993; Schnabel et al. 2006; Schnabel et al. 2007), the presence of at least one postoperative start (Bassage and Richardson 1998; Cheetham et al. 2008; Lucas et al. 1999; Schnabel et al. 2007; Zekas et al. 1999), lifetime earnings (Laws et al. 1993), race class level (Cervantes et al. 1992; Yovich and McIlwraith 1986; Zekas et al. 1999), and earnings per start (Barakzai et al. 2004; Cervantes et al. 1992; Hawkins et al. 1997; Schnabel et al. 2006, Schnabel et al. 2007; Woodie et al. 2005). There are also more complex means of analysis for assessing the performance including performance index (Barakzai et al. 2004; Barnes et al. 2004; Cheetham et al. 2008; Hawkins et al. 1997; Reardon et al. 2008a; Woodie et al. 2005) and regression models aimed at standardizing racing performance to uniform conditions (Martin 2000; Martin et al. 2000).

In upper airway surgery, a wide variety of outcome measures are used and some studies use many outcomes (Allen et al. 2012). There is some evidence that the outcome measure may have a substantial effect on the reported results (Allen et al. 2012; Barakzai et al. 2009). Return to racing (i.e., a postoperative start) may not be the most appropriate indicator of a successful surgical outcome. Several authors have reported the proportion of horses that return to racing and then provided a more stringent definition of success, that is, increased earnings (Barakzai and Dixon 2005; Barakzai et al. 2004; Barakzai et al. 2009; Duncan 1997; Dykgraaf et al. 2005; Franklin et al. 2009). In all cases, the proportion of horses considered to be successfully treated was substantially lower than the proportion that returned to racing, suggesting that a postoperative start may be an optimistic measure of success. The way race performance is assessed may also substantially affect the apparent success rates (Barakzai et al. 2009; Franklin et al. 2009; Reardon et al. 2008a, 2008b). Success rates may be affected by the race parameter used as well as the number of races. Reardon showed a significant, but very weak correlation between ratings and earnings and found significant differences between ratings and performance index and earnings and performance index. This resulted in variation in success rates (28–51% and 42–67%) when different parameters were examined over the same time period (Reardon et al. 2008a, 2008b). The number of races assessed before and after an intervention also had an effect on the reported success rates (Barakzai et al. 2009; Franklin et al. 2009).

One issue in the indirect assessment of postoperative function in cohort studies is the selection of an appropriate "control" group. Most studies in this field are before-and-after studies reporting pre- and postintervention data. The ideal "control" group for intervention studies is cases affected by the problem that undergo no treatment. As this is difficult to achieve, horses that are presumed to be unaffected are often selected as a "control" group. The clear limitation here is that these "control" horses cannot usually be confirmed as unaffected.

In addition to varying outcome measures of success, there is no standardization among data sampling or data classification schemes. Some studies separate Thoroughbred and Standardbred racehorses, while others do not, and few studies separate horses by sex or age at the time of diagnosis, treatment, or return to racing.

There is also little available data on the background rate of loss of horses in racing. Three studies have accurately analyzed the factors associated with failure of Thoroughbred horses to train and race (Bailey et al. 1997; Jeffcott et al. 1982; Wilsher et al. 2006). Two of these studies were performed in the United Kingdom (Jeffcott et al. 1982; Wilsher et al. 2006) and one in Australia (Bailey et al. 1997). Lameness and respiratory problems were identified as major causes of wastage in all the three studies.

There are a small number of longitudinal studies examining the racing careers of Thoroughbred horses. In Australia, high-performing horses were more likely to be male and 40% of horses that started, earned no money at all (More 1999). Of the horses that first started as 2- or 3-year olds, only 71% continued racing for at least 1 year and 46% for 2 years after their first start. Studies in Canada have previously examined the influence of age, gait, and sex among Canadian Standardbreds (Physick-Sheard 1986a, 1986b). A similar study in the United States identified variation in age, sex, and gait between Thoroughbreds and Standardbreds (Cheetham et al. 2010).

Determining natural trends in earnings and the number of starts is important because if earnings do decline with age, then it would be important to include age as a covariate in an outcome analysis of performance after upper airway surgery.

In summary, while the indirect assessment of postoperative function through proxy measures such as race performance will necessarily continue for some time, there is likely to be an increasing emphasis of direct assessment using dynamic endoscopy.

References

Allen KJ, Franklin SH. 2010. Comparisons of overground endoscopy and treadmill endoscopy in UK Thoroughbred racehorses. *Equine Veterinary Journal* 42(3):186–191.

Allen KJ, Christley RM, Birchall MA, Franklin SH. 2012. A systematic review of the efficacy of interventions for dynamic intermittent dorsal displacement of the soft palate. *Equine Veterinary Journal* 44(3):259–266.

Altman DG, Schulz KF, Moher D, Egger M, Davidoff F, Elbourne D, Gotzsche PC, Lang T, CONSORT GROUP. 2001. The revised CONSORT statement for reporting randomized trials: Explanation and elaboration. *Annals of Internal Medicine* 134(8):663–694.

Bailey CJ, Rose RJ, Reid SW, Hodgson DR. 1997. Wastage in the Australian Thoroughbred racing industry: A survey of Sydney trainers. *Australian Veterinary Journal* 75(1):64–66.

Barakzai SZ, Dixon PM. 2005. Conservative treatment for Thoroughbred racehorses with intermittent dorsal displacement of the soft palate. *Veterinary Record* 157(12):337–340.

Barakzai SZ, Johnson VS, Baird DH, Bladon B, Lane JG. 2004. Assessment of the efficacy of composite surgery for the treatment of dorsal displacement of the soft palate in a group of 53 racing Thoroughbreds (1990–1996). *Equine Veterinary Journal* 36(2):175–179.

Barakzai SZ, Boden LA, Hillyer MH, Marlin DJ, Dixon PM. 2009. Efficacy of thermal cautery for intermittent dorsal displacement of the soft palate as compared to conservatively treated horses: Results from 78 treadmill diagnosed horses. *Equine Veterinary Journal* 41(1):65–69.

Barnes AJ, Slone DE, Lynch TM. 2004. Performance after partial arytenoidectomy without mucosal closure in 27 Thoroughbred racehorses. *Veterinary Surgery* 33(4):398–403.

Barnett TP, Dixon PM, Barakzai SZ. 2011. Long-term abduction and stability of arytenoid cartilages following laryngoplasty. *Proceedings of the 50th British Equine Veterinary Association Annual Congress.* Liverpool, England. p. 174.

Bassage LH, Richardson DW. 1998. Longitudinal fractures of the condyles of the third metacarpal and metatarsal bones in racehorses: 224 cases (1986–1995). *Journal of the American Veterinary Medical Association* 212(11):1757–1764.

Cervantes C, Madison JB, Ackerman N, Reed WO. 1992. Surgical treatment of dorsal cortical fractures of the third metacarpal bone in Thoroughbred racehorses: 53 cases (1985–1989). *Journal of the American Veterinary Medical Association* 200(12):1997–2000.

Cheetham J, Pigott JH, Thorson LM, Mohammed HO, Ducharme NG. 2008. Racing performance following the laryngeal tie-forward procedure: A case-controlled study. *Equine Veterinary Journal* 40(5):501–507.

Cheetham J, Riordan AS, Mohammed HO, McIlwraith CW, Fortier LA. 2010. Relationships between race earnings and horse age, sex, gait, track surface and number of race starts for Thoroughbred and standardbred racehorses in North America. *Equine Veterinary Journal* 42(4):346–350.

Davidson EJ, Martin BB, Boston RC, Parente EJ. 2011. Exercising upper respiratory videoendoscopic evaluation of 100 nonracing performance horses with abnormal respiratory noise and/or poor performance. *Equine Veterinary Journal* 43(1):3–8.

Desmaiziers LM, Serraud N, Plainfosse B, Michel A, Tamzali Y. 2009. Dynamic respiratory endoscopy without treadmill in 68 performance standardbred, Thoroughbred and saddle horses under natural training conditions. *Equine Veterinary Journal* 41(4):347–352.

Duncan DW. 1997. Retrospective study of 50 Thoroughbred racehorses subjected to radical myectomy for treatment of dorsal displacement of the soft palate. *Proceedings of the American Association of Equine Practitioners* 43:237–238.

Dykgraaf S, McIlwraith CW, Baker VA, Byrd WJ, Daniel RC. 2005. Sternothyroideus tenectomy combination surgery for treatment of dorsal displacement of the soft palate in 96 Thoroughbred racehorses (1996–2004). *Proceedings of the 51st Annual Convention of the American Association of Equine Practitioners* 323–326.

Franklin H, Burnt JF, Allen KJ. 2008. Clinical trials using a telemetric endoscope for use during over-ground exercise: A preliminary study. *Equine Veterinary Journal* 40(7):712–715.

Franklin SH, Naylor JR, Lane JG. 2006. Videoendoscopic evaluation of the upper respiratory tract in 93 sport horses during exercise testing on a high-speed treadmill. *Equine Veterinary Journal* 36:540–545.

Franklin SH, McCluskie LK, Woodford NS, Tremaine WH, Lane JG, Bladon BM, Barakzai SZ, Dixon PM, Hillyer MH, Allen KJ. 2009. A comparison of the efficacy of soft palate cautery and the laryngeal tie-forward procedure in Thoroughbred racehorses with a definitive diagnosis of palatal dysfunction. *Proceedings of the 48th British Equine Veterinary Association Congress.* (p. 168). Fordham, Cambridgeshire, UK: Equine Veterinary Journal, Ltd.

Hawkins JF, Tulleners EP, Ross MW, Evans LH, Raker CW. 1997. Laryngoplasty with or without ventriculectomy for treatment of left laryngeal hemiplegia in 230 racehorses. *Veterinary Surgery* 26(6):484–491.

Jeffcott LB, Rossdale PD, Freestone JC, Frank J, Towers-Clark PF. 1982. An assessment of wastage in Thoroughbred racing from conception to 4 years of age. *Equine Veterinary Journal* 14(3):185–198.

Kapatkin AS. 2007. Outcome-based medicine and its application in clinical surgical practice. *Veterinary Surgery* 36(6):515–518.

Lane JG. 2012. Complications of wind surgery and what to do about them. *Association of Racecourse Veterinary Surgeons Summer Meeting*. Loughborough, UK.

Laws EG, Richardson DW, Ross MW, Moyer W. 1993. Racing performance of standardbreds after conservative and surgical treatment for tarsocrural osteochondrosis. *Equine Veterinary Journal* 25(3):199–202.

Lucas JM, Ross MW, Richardson DW. 1999. Postoperative performance of racing standardbreds treated arthroscopically for carpal chip fractures: 176 cases (1986–1993). *Equine Veterinary Journal* 31(1):48–52.

Martin GS. 2000. Factors associated with racing performance of Thoroughbreds undergoing lag screw repair of condylar fractures of the third metacarpal or metatarsal bone. *Journal of the American Veterinary Medical Association* 217(12):1870–1877.

Martin BB, Reef VB, Parente EJ, Sage AD. 2000. Causes of poor performance of horses during training, racing, or showing: 348 cases (1992–1996). *Journal of the American Veterinary Medical Association* 216(4):554–558.

More SJ. 1999. A longitudinal study of racing Thoroughbreds: Performance during the first years of racing. *Australian Veterinary Journal* 77(2):105–112.

Parkin TD, Brown PE, French NP, Morgan KL. 2005. Cooking the books or simply getting the best out of the data? Assessing the nature of the relationship between variables. *Equine Veterinary Journal* 37(3):189–191.

Phillips B, Ball C, Sackett D, Badenoch D, Straus S, Haynes B, Dawes M. 2005. Levels of evidence and grades of recommendation. Oxford, UK: Oxford Centre for Evidence-Based Medicine. www.cebm.net/levels_of_evidence.asp ed

Physick-Sheard PW. 1986a. Career profile of the Canadian standardbred. I. Influence of age, gait and sex upon chances of racing. *Canadian Journal of Veterinary Research* 50(4):449–456.

Physick-Sheard PW. 1986b. Career profile of the Canadian standardbred. II. Influence of age, gait and sex upon number of races, money won and race times. *Canadian Journal of Veterinary Research* 50(4):457–470.

Pollock PJ, Reardon RJ. 2009. Dynamic respiratory endoscopy without a treadmill: Initial experiences. *Equine Veterinary Education* 21(7):367–370.

Pollock PJ, Reardon RJ, Parkin TD, Johnston MS, Tate J, Love S. 2009. Dynamic respiratory endoscopy in 67 Thoroughbred racehorses training under normal ridden exercise conditions. *Equine Veterinary Journal* 41:354–360.

Reardon RJ, Fraser BS, Bladon BM. 2008a. Laryngeal tie-forward combined with thermocautery as treatment of horses with signs associated with intermittent dorsal displacement of the soft palate: A case-control study in British racing Thoroughbreds. *Proceedings of the 47th British Equine Veterinary Association Congress* p. 340.

Reardon RJ, Fraser BS, Heller J, Lischer C, Parkin R, Bladon BM. 2008b. The use of race winnings, ratings and a performance index to assess the effect of thermocautery of the soft palate for treatment of horses with suspected intermittent dorsal displacement. A case-control study in 110 racing Thoroughbreds. *Equine Veterinary Journal* 40(5):508–513.

Schnabel LV, Bramlage LR, Mohammed HO, Embertson RM, Ruggles AJ, Hopper SA. 2006. Racing performance after arthroscopic removal of apical sesamoid fracture fragments in Thoroughbred horses age > or = 2 years: 84 cases (1989–2002). *Equine Veterinary Journal* 38(5):446–451.

Schnabel LV, Bramlage LR, Mohammed HO, Embertson RM, Ruggles AJ, Hopper SA. 2007. Racing performance after arthroscopic removal of apical sesamoid fracture fragments in Thoroughbred horses age < 2 years: 151 cases (1989–2002). *Equine Veterinary Journal* 39(1):64–68.

Strand E, Skjerve E. 2012. Complex dynamic upper airway collapse: Associations between abnormalities in 99 harness racehorses with one or more dynamic disorders. *Equine Veterinary Journal* 44(5):524–528.

Strand E, Fjordbakk CT, Sundberg K, Spangen L, Lunde LH, Hanche-Olsen S. 2012. Relative prevalence of upper respiratory tract obstructive disorders in two breeds of harness racehorses (185 cases: 1998–2006). *Equine Veterinary Journal* 44(5):518–523.

Tamzali Y, Serraud N, Baup B, Desmaiziers LM. 2008. How to perform endoscopy during exercise without a treadmill. *Proceedings of the American Association of Equine Practitioners* 54:24–28.

Van Erck E. 2011. Dynamic respiratory videoendoscopy in ridden sport horses: Effect of head flexion, riding and airway inflammation in 129 cases. *Equine Veterinary Journal* 43(40):18–24.

Weiner SJ. 2006. From research evidence to context: The challenge of individualising care. *Equine Veterinary Journal* 38(3):195–196.

Wilsher S, Allen WR, Wood JL. 2006. Factors associated with failure of Thoroughbred horses to train and race. *Equine Veterinary Journal* 38(2):113–118.

Witte TH, Mohammed HO, Radcliffe CH, Hackett RP, Ducharme NG. 2009. Racing performance after combined prosthetic laryngoplasty and ipsilateral ventriculocordectomy or partial arytenoidectomy: 135 Thoroughbred racehorses competing at less than 2400 m (1997–2007). *Equine Veterinary Journal* 41(1): 70–75.

Witte SH, Witte TH, Harriss F, Kelly G, Pollock P. 2011. Association of owner-reported noise with findings during dynamic respiratory endoscopy in Thoroughbred racehorses. *Equine Veterinary Journal* 43(1):9–17.

Woodie JB, Ducharme NG, Kanter P, Hackett RP, Erb HN. 2005. Surgical advancement of the larynx (laryngeal tie-forward) as a treatment for dorsal displacement of the soft palate in horses: A prospective study 2001–2004. *Equine Veterinary Journal* 37(5):418–423.

Yovich JV, McIlwraith CW. 1986. Arthroscopic surgery for osteochondral fractures of the proximal phalanx of the metacarpophalangeal and metatarsophalangeal (fetlock) joints in horses. *Journal of the American Veterinary Medical Association* 188(3):273–279.

Zekas LJ, Bramlage LR, Embertson RM, Hance SR. 1999. Results of treatment of 145 fractures of the third metacarpal/metatarsal condyles in 135 horses (1986–1994). *Equine Veterinary Journal* 31(4):309–313.

Section II

Dorsal Displacement of the Soft Palate

16 Dorsal Displacement of the Soft Palate: Pathophysiology and New Diagnostic Techniques

Jonathan Cheetham

Introduction

Dorsal displacement of the soft palate (DDSP) results in upper airway expiratory obstruction at exercise. It is a common cause of poor performance in racehorses and has a prevalence of 10–20% (Dart et al. 2001; Ducharme 2006; Lane 2006a; Tan et al. 2005). Most affected horses make a loud, vibrant respiratory "gurgling or snoring" noise which is caused by fluttering of the caudal margin of the soft palate (Barakzai et al. 2004; Parente et al. 2002). In approximately 20–30% of horses with DDSP, noise is not reported (Franklin et al. 2006; Parente et al. 2002). A definitive diagnosis is made during high-speed treadmill examination, if the caudal border of the soft palate is seen dorsal to the epiglottis for more than 8 seconds (Rehder et al. 1995). Endoscopic examination of the upper airway at rest is a poor predictor of DDSP at exercise (Barakzai and Dixon 2011; Lane 2006b). DDSP is more common in racehorses, especially 2–4-year olds. Exercise intolerance is often described by trainers and riders or drivers as "choking down" or "hitting a wall" because DDSP causes significant expiratory obstruction that limits minute ventilation. Mouth breathing during exhalation is recognized by fluttering of the cheeks as air is diverted underneath the soft palate through the mouth, and is a specific sign that a horse has displaced its soft palate dorsal to the epiglottis. Occasionally coughing during exercise is reported in association with the disease; this complaint is more common in sport horses.

Etiology

The consequence of DDSP in both naturally and experimentally induced DDSP is expiratory obstruction with increased expiratory trachea pressure, deviation of airflow through the mouth with reduced nasopharyngeal expiratory pressure, billowing of the cheeks, reduced ventilation, and poor performance (Cheetham et al. 2009; Pigott et al. 2010; Rehder et al. 1995).

The etiology of DDSP is multifactorial and not completely understood. Physical obstruction due to subepiglottic palatal masses, granulomas, or cysts can interfere with the subglottic position of the soft palate and produce DDSP (Ducharme 2006; Tulleners et al. 1997).

Advances in Equine Upper Respiratory Surgery, First Edition. Edited by Jan Hawkins.
© 2015 ACVS Foundation. Published 2015 by John Wiley & Sons, Inc.

Experimentally, three methods have been used to induce DDSP: local blockade of the pharyngeal branch of the vagus nerve (X) producing DDSP at rest (Holcombe et al. 1998), bilateral resection of the paired thyrohyoid muscles producing DDSP at slow-speed exercise (Ducharme et al. 2003), and bilateral local anesthetic blockade of the hypoglossal nerve producing DDSP during high-speed exercise (Cheetham et al. 2009). These experimental models relate to the anatomy and etiology of naturally occurring disease.

The pharyngeal branch of the vagus nerve innervates three of the four intrinsic muscles of the soft palate. The soft palate completely divides the pharynx into nasal and oral compartments in horses. Because the horse is an obligate nasal breather, it is critically important that the soft palate remains ventral to the epiglottis, except during swallowing, to allow unimpeded nasal breathing. The soft palate extends caudally from the hard palate to the base of the larynx and consists of the oral mucous membrane, which contains ductile openings of the palatine glands, the palatine glands, the palatine aponeurosis, palatinus and palatopharyngeus muscles, and the nasopharyngeal mucous membrane (Sisson 1975a). The caudal free margin of the soft palate continues dorsally, on either side of the larynx, forming the lateral pillars of the soft palate. These pillars unite dorsally, forming the posterior pillar of the soft palate or the palatopharyngeal arch.

The position of the soft palate is determined by the coordinated activity of groups of antagonistic muscles which include the levator veli palatini, tensor veli palatini, palatinus, and palatopharyngeus muscles (Table 16.1) (Kuehn et al. 1982; Moon et al. 1994).

All apart from the tensor veli palatine muscle are innervated by the pharyngeal branch of the vagus nerve (Sisson 1975b) and this mechanism is believed to be important in young horses in which inflammation of this nerve branch occurs in association with pharyngeal lymphoid hyperplasia.

The *levator veli palatini* muscle attaches to the petrous part of the temporal bone and the lateral lamina of the guttural pouch. It travels along the lateral wall of the nasopharynx and terminates within the soft palate. It acts to elevate the soft palate during swallowing, vocalization, and dilation of the ostia of the auditory tube diverticula.

The *tensor veli palatini* is a flat, fusiform muscle that, like the levator, attaches to the petrous part of the temporal and pterygoid bones, and the lateral lamina of the guttural pouch (Sisson 1975b). Its tendon is reflected around the hamulus of the pterygoid bone, where it is lubricated by a bursa. The tendon then ramifies in the palatine aponeurosis (Sisson 1975b). It receives motor innervation from the mandibular branch of the trigeminal nerve. Contraction of this muscle tenses the palatine aponeurosis and, therefore, the rostral portion of the soft palate, and depresses this portion of the soft palate toward the tongue (Kuehn et al. 1982; Moon et al. 1994; Sisson 1975b). Contraction of the tensor veli palatini muscle also aids in opening the pharyngeal opening of the guttural pouch (Baptiste 1997). Bilateral transection of the tendon of the tensor veli palatini muscle in horses causes instability of the rostral portion of the soft palate resulting in inspiratory obstruction during intense exercise (Holcombe et al. 1997).

The *palatinus* muscle (uvula retractor muscle) consists of two fusiform muscles that lie on either side of the midline of the soft palate, beneath the nasopharyngeal mucosa, extending caudally from the hard palate (Sisson 1975b). The muscles attach to the caudal aspect of the palatine aponeurosis and terminate near the caudal free margin of the soft palate. A small muscle bundle arising from the lateral aspect of each muscle continues a short distance caudodorsally into the palatopharyngeal arch (Sisson 1975b). Contraction of the palatinus muscle shortens the soft palate (Kuehn et al. 1982; Moon et al. 1994; Sisson 1975b).

The *palatopharyngeus* muscle originates from the palatine aponeurosis and the lateral border of the palatinus muscle (Sisson 1975b). It travels caudally along the lateral wall of the nasopharynx to the pharyngeal raphe, forming part of the superior constrictor muscle group. Contraction of this muscle shortens the soft palate and draws the larynx and esophagus toward the root of the tongue.

As discussed, bilateral local anesthesia of the pharyngeal branches of the vagus nerve induces persistent DDSP and dysphasia in horses (Holcombe et al. 1998). Horses can become dysphasic, with or without persistent soft palate dysfunction, following guttural pouch lavage with caustic solutions, guttural pouch empyema, trauma, or mycosis (DeLahunta 1977; Mayhew 1989). These

Table 16.1   Function and innervation of muscles controlling the tone of the equine soft palate

Muscle	Function	Innervation
Tensor veli palatini	Tenses the rostral aspect of the soft palate	Mandibular branch of the trigeminal nerve
Levator veli palatini	Elevates the palate during swallowing and closes the nasopharynx	Pharyngeal branch of the vagus
Palatinus	Shorten and depress the palate	Pharyngeal branch of the vagus
Palatopharyngeus	Shorten and depress the palate	Pharyngeal branch of the vagus

data suggest that dysfunction of the neuromuscular group, including the pharyngeal branch of the vagus nerve, palatinus, and palatopharyngeus muscles may be involved in the pathogenesis of intermittent DDSP in exercising horses.

Electromyographic measurements of the palatinus and palatopharyngeus muscles in normal horses exercising on a treadmill showed that these muscles are active, synchronous with respiration, and their activity increases as exercise intensifies (Holcombe et al. 2007; Morello et al. 2008). Palatinus muscle EMG activity is diminished in horses with DDSP and EMG activity does not significantly increase as treadmill speed increases (Holcombe et al. 2007). The muscles of the soft palate tend to have a predominantly fast fiber type (type 2) with a low proportion of type 1 muscle fibers (Hawkes et al. 2010; Holcombe 2001). The majority of these type 2 fibers are type 2 A, which suggests that these fibers have increased endurance relative to most skeletal muscle fast-twitch fibers (Holcombe 2001).

Bilateral resection of the paired thyrohyoid muscles also produces DDSP at slow-speed exercise (Ducharme et al. 2003). The thyrohyoid muscle is a flat rectangular muscle attached to the lateral surface of the thyroid cartilage lamina that inserts on the caudal part of the thyrohyoid bone (Sisson 1975b). The hypoglossal nerve innervates the thyrohyoid muscle, which draws the larynx rostrally and dorsally and the root of the tongue caudally through its attachment to the thyrohyoid and basihyoid bones (Chan and Tize 2003; Chang and Mortola 1981; Fulton et al. 1992). Laryngeal elevation is essential for airway projection during the pharyngeal phase of swallowing and reduced laryngeal elevation is a common cause of aspiration in dysphagic human patients (Duncan et al. 1974; Fulton et al. 1991; Holcombe et al. 2002; Kannegieter and Dore 1995; King et al. 2001;

Kirkham and Vasey 2002; Linford et al. 1983; Lumsden et al. 1994). The equine thyrohyoid is predominantly active during expiration (Ducharme et al. 2003). These findings formed the basis for the laryngeal "tie-forward" in which a prosthetic suture is placed to mimic the action of the thyrohyoid muscles and move the larynx rostrally and dorsally (Cheetham et al. 2008; Woodie et al. 2005).

Finally, bilateral local anesthetic blockade of the distal portion of the hypoglossal nerve also produces DDSP during high-speed exercise. The mechanism here may be through induced dysfunction of the rostral hyoid muscles which move the larynx forward when they contract. The equine larynx is suspended from the skull petrous part of the temporal bone by a chain of hyoid bones. The hyoid apparatus consists of the paired stylohyoid, epihyoid, ceratohyoid, and thyrohyoid bones, and the central basihyoid bone. The stylohyoid bone articulates with the petrous part of the temporal bone, allowing the stylohyoid bones to move cranial to caudal, in a pendulous manner. The ceratohyoid bone attaches to the distal end of the stylohyoid bone. The base or root of the tongue is attached to the lingual process of the basihyoid bone.

The genioglossus, hyoglossus, and styloglossus muscles are extrinsic muscles of the tongue that, in part, control the position and function of the tongue and provide attachments to the hyoid apparatus (Sisson 1975b). The rostral hyoid muscles (hyoglossus, styloglossus, genioglossus, and geniohyoideus) are innervated by the hypoglossal nerve and attach to the hyoid apparatus (the hyoglossus to the basihyoid and thyrohyoid bones, the styloglossus to the stylohyoid bone, the genioglossus to the basihyoid and ceratohyoid bones, and the geniohyoideus to the lingual process of the basihyoid bone), which suspend the larynx from the petrous part of the temporal bone.

Contraction of the genioglossus muscle protracts the tongue and pulls the basihyoid bone rostrally. Genioglossus also acts with the hyoglossus muscle to depress and retract the tongue. Hyoglossus and genioglossus activity are synchronous with respiration, and activity of these muscles correlates well with increases in the pharyngeal airway size during breathing (Brouillette and Thach 1980; Fregosi and Fuller 1997; Fuller et al. 1999; Van de Graaff et al. 1984).

Collectively, the muscles that control laryngeal position through their attachment to the hyoid apparatus appear to play an important part in nasopharyngeal stability at exercise. Associations have been shown between laryngeal position and nasopharyngeal stability in horses (Cheetham et al. 2008; Ortved et al. 2010). For example, horses with DDSP during treadmill examination have a more ventral basihyoid bone at rest, although the magnitude of this difference is small (Chalmers et al. 2009). Horses with a more dorsal postoperative basihyoid position are associated with an increased probability of racing following postoperatively laryngeal "tie-forward"(Cheetham et al. 2008). The position of the larynx at rest has been shown to be related to the occurrence of obstructive sleep apnea (OSA), a sleep disorder in humans (Shahar et al. 2001; Young et al. 1993), and changes in laryngeal position are associated with variable airway stability in patients with OSA (Riha et al. 2005; Sforza et al. 2000).

In a clinical population of horses with DDSP, the frequency of swallowing increases immediately prior to the onset of DDSP (Pigott et al. 2010). This study suggested that the drive to swallow is diminished in normal horses as they run faster, but that this mechanism may be overridden in horses affected by DDSP. Elucidation of this mechanism might provide insight into the etiology of DDSP. An alternate interpretation is that swallowing directly results in DDSP. The observation of DDSP as an immediate sequel to a swallow (Franklin et al. 2002; Lane 2006a; Parente et al. 2002; Rehder et al. 1995) could support either interpretation.

The normal phasic inspiratory descent of the larynx seen in humans (Collett et al. 1986) may be amplified in the horse and seen as caudal retraction of the larynx during exercise. Swallowing can be produced by a variety of sensory inputs including pressure, tactile, and liquid stimulation (Filaretov

and Filimonova 1969; Mathew et al. 1982; Miller 1982; Storey 1968). In addition, stretch receptors in the geniohyoid, mylohyoid, and thyrohyoid muscles may also play a role (Filaretov and Filimonova 1969). It is possible that decreased function of the tongue musculature at exercise, similar to that seen in OSA patients (Fogel et al. 2005; Gumery et al. 2005), may allow increased caudal retraction of the larynx, increased firing of tongue muscle proprioceptive fibers (Filaretov and Filimonova 1969), and hence increased swallowing. The use of a tongue-tie may prevent this caudal laryngeal retraction (Barakzai and Dixon 2005; Barakzai et al. 2009).

The traditional diagnosis of DDSP is performed using dynamic endoscopy either during treadmill examination or using an over ground scope as the correlation between resting and exercising endoscopic findings is poor (Barakzai and Dixon 2011; Lane 2006b). More recently, other techniques have emerged which may be useful for the diagnosis of DDSP. These include laryngeal ultrasound (see Chapter 18) to determine the depth of the basihyoid bone (Chalmers et al. 2009). In this study, a significant relationship was found between the depth of the basihyoid bone at rest and the occurrence of DDSP at exercise with a more ventral location of the basihyoid bone was present in horses with DDSP. The mechanism for this difference is unknown.

Radiographic assessment of laryngeal position and nasopharyngeal stability has also been used (Cheetham et al. 2008; Ortved et al. 2010). These studies assessed the position of the caudal aspect of the basihyoid bone, thyrohyoid–thyroid articulation, and the ossification at the epiglottic base against a reference framework based on laryngeal position. This method was found to be repeatable and a more dorsal postoperative position of the body of the thyroid was associated with an increased probability of racing postoperatively (Cheetham et al. 2008). Similarly, horses with a more dorsal postoperative thyroid position were also more likely to race postoperatively. In a second study, horses with persistent DDSP were found to have a more caudal larynx (ossification of the thyroid cartilage), a more caudal and dorsal basihyoid bone, and a more dorsal thyrohyoid–thyroid articulation than horses with intermittent DDSP. These techniques are currently being evaluated for the early diagnosis of DDSP in a clinical population.

References

Baptiste K. 1997. Functional anatomy observations of the pharyngeal orifice of the equine guttural pouch (auditory tube diverticulum). *The Veterinary Journal* 153(3):311–319.

Barakzai SZ, Dixon PM. 2005. Conservative treatment for Thoroughbred racehorses with intermittent dorsal displacement of the soft palate. *The Veterinary Record* 157(12):337–340.

Barakzai SZ, Dixon PM. 2011. Correlation of resting and exercising endoscopic findings for horses with dynamic laryngeal collapse and palatal dysfunction. *Equine Veterinary Journal* 43(1):18–23.

Barakzai SZ, Finnegan C, Boden LA. 2009. Effect of 'tongue tie' use on racing performance of Thoroughbreds in the United Kingdom. *Equine Veterinary Journal* 41(8):812–816.

Barakzai SZ, Johnson VS, Baird DH, Bladon B, Lane JG. 2004. Assessment of the efficacy of composite surgery for the treatment of dorsal displacement of the soft palate in a group of 53 racing Thoroughbreds (1990–1996). *Equine Veterinary Journal* 36(2):175–179.

Brouillette RT, Thach BT. 1980. Control of genioglossus muscle inspiratory activity. *Journal of Applied Physiology: Respiratory, Environmental and Exercise Physiology* 49(5):801–808.

Chalmers HJ, Yeager AE, Ducharme N. 2009. Ultrasonographic assessment of laryngohyoid position as a predictor of dorsal displacement of the soft palate in horses. *Veterinary Radiology & Ultrasound* 50(1):91–96.

Chan RW, Tize IR. 2003. Effect of postmortem changes and freezing on the viscoelastic properties of vocal fold tissues. *Annals of Biomedical Engineering* 31(4):482–491.

Chang HK, Mortola JP. 1981. Fluid dynamic factors in tracheal pressure measurement. *Journal of Applied Physiology: Respiratory, Environmental and Exercise Physiology* 51(1):218–225.

Cheetham J, Pigott JH, Thorson LM, Mohammed HO, Ducharme NG. 2008. Racing performance following the laryngeal tie-forward procedure: A case-controlled study. *Equine Veterinary Journal* 40(5):501–507.

Cheetham J, Pigott JH, Hermanson JW, Campoy L, Soderholm LV, Thorson LM, Ducharme NG. 2009. Role of the hypoglossal nerve in equine nasopharyngeal stability. *Journal of Applied Physiology* 107(2):471–477.

Collett PW, Brancatisano AP, Engel LA. 1986. Upper airway dimensions and movements in bronchial asthma. *The American Review of Respiratory Disease* 133(6):1143–1149.

Dart AJ, Dowling BA, Hodgson DR, Rose RJ. 2001. Evaluation of high-speed treadmill videoendoscopy for diagnosis of upper respiratory tract dysfunction in horses. *Australian Veterinary Journal* 79(2):109–112.

DeLahunta A. 1977. *Veterinary Neuroanatomy and Clinical Neurology*. Philadelphia, PA: W.B. Saunders Company.

Ducharme NG. 2006. Pharynx. In: Auer JA, Stick JA, eds. *Equine Surgery*, 3rd ed (pp. 544–565). St. Louis, MO: Elsevier Health Sciences.

Ducharme NG, Hackett RP, Woodie JB, Dykes N, Erb HN, Mitchell LM, Soderholm L V. 2003. Investigations into the role of the thyrohyoid muscles in the pathogenesis of dorsal displacement of the soft palate in horses. *Equine Veterinary Journal* 35(3):258–263.

Duncan ID, Griffths IR, McQueen A, Baker GO. 1974. The pathology of equine laryngeal hemiplegia. *Acta Neuropathologica* 27(4):337–348.

Filaretov AA, Filimonova AB. 1969. Proprioception in the muscles of deglutition. *Fiziologicheskii Zhurnal SSSR Imeni* 55(5):552–557.

Fogel RB, Trinder J, White DP, Malhotra A, Raneri J, Schory K, Kleverlaan D, Pierce RJ. 2005. The effect of sleep onset on upper airway muscle activity in patients with sleep apnea versus controls. *The Journal of Physiology* 564(Pt 2):549–562.

Franklin SH, Naylor JR, Lane JG. 2002. Effect of dorsal displacement of the soft palate on ventilation and airflow during high-intensity exercise. *Equine Veterinary Journal. Supplement* (34):379–383.

Franklin SH, Naylor JR, Lane JG. 2006. Videoendoscopic evaluation of the upper respiratory tract in 93 sport horses during exercise testing on a high-speed treadmill. *Equine Veterinary Journal. Supplement* (36): 540–545.

Fregosi RF, Fuller DD. 1997. Respiratory-related control of extrinsic tongue muscle activity. *Respiration Physiology* 110(2–3):295–306.

Fuller DD, Williams JS, Janssen PL, Fregosi RF. 1999. Effect of co-activation of tongue protrudor and retractor muscles on tongue movements and pharyngeal airflow mechanics in the rat. *The Journal of Physiology* 519(Pt 2):601–613.

Fulton IC, Derksen FJ, Stick JA, Robinson NE, Walshaw R. 1991. Treatment of left laryngeal hemiplegia in standardbreds, using a nerve muscle pedicle graft. *American Journal of Veterinary Research* 52(9):1461–1467.

Fulton IC, Derksen FJ, Stick JA, Robinson NE, Duncan ID. 1992. Histologic evaluation of nerve muscle pedicle graft used as a treatment for left laryngeal hemiplegia in standardbreds. *American Journal of Veterinary Research* 53(4):592–596.

Gumery PY, Roux-Buisson H, Meignen S, Comyn FL, Dematteis M, Wuyam B, Pepin JL, Levy P. 2005. An adaptive detector of genioglossus EMG reflex using Berkner transform for time latency measurement in OSA pathophysiological studies. *IEEE Transactions on Bio-Medical Engineering* 52(8):1382–1389.

Hawkes CS, Hahn CN, Dixon PM. 2010. Histological and histochemical characterisation of the equine soft palate muscles. *Equine Veterinary Journal* 42(5):431–437.

Holcombe SJ. 2001. New thoughts on URT anatomy: Relevancy. *Proceedings of the 29th Annual Surgical Forum*.

American College of Veterinary Surgeons.Chicago, IL. pp. 59–62.

Holcombe SJ, Derksen FJ, Stick JA, Robinson NE. 1997. Effect of bilateral tenectomy of the tensor veli palatini muscle on soft palate function in horses. *American Journal of Veterinary Research* 58(3):317–321.

Holcombe SJ, Derksen FJ, Stick JA, Robinson NE. 1998. Effect of bilateral blockade of the pharyngeal branch of the vagus nerve on soft palate function in horses. *American Journal of Veterinary Research* 59(4):504–508.

Holcombe SJ, Cornelisse CJ, Berney C, Robinson NE. 2002. Electromyographic activity of the hyoepiglotticus muscle and control of epiglottis position in horses. *American Journal of Veterinary Research* 63(12):1617–1621.

Holcombe SJ, Derksen FJ, Robinson NE. 2007. Electromyographic activity of the palatinus and palatopharyngeus muscles in exercising horses. *Equine Veterinary Journal* 39(5):451–455.

Kannegieter NJ, Dore ML. 1995. Endoscopy of the upper respiratory tract during treadmill exercise: A clinical study of 100 horses. *Australian Veterinary Journal* 72(3):101–107.

King DS, Tulleners EP, Martin BB Jr, Parente EJ, Boston R. 2001. Clinical experiences with axial deviation of the aryepiglottic folds in 52 racehorses. *Veterinary Surgery* 30(2):151–160.

Kirkham LE, Vasey JR. 2002. Surgical cleft soft palate repair in a foal. *Australian Veterinary Journal* 80(3):143–146.

Kuehn DP, Folkins JW, Cutting CB. 1982. Relationships between muscle activity and velar position. *The Cleft Palate Journal* 19(1):25–35.

Lane JG, Bladon B, Little DR, Naylor JR, Franklin SH. 2006a. Dynamic obstructions of the equine upper respiratory tract. Part 1: Observations during high-speed treadmill endoscopy of 600 thoroughbred racehorses. *Equine Veterinary Journal* 38(5):393–399.

Lane JG, Bladon B, Little DR, Naylor JR, Frankin SH. 2006b. Dynamic obstructions of the equine upper respiratory tract. Part 2: Comparison of endoscopic findings at rest and during high-speed treadmill exercise of 600 thoroughbred racehorses. *Equine Veterinary Journal* 38(5):401–407.

Linford RL, O'Brien TR, Wheat JD, Meagher DM. 1983. Radiographic assessment of epiglottic length and pharyngeal and laryngeal diameters in the thoroughbred. *American Journal of Veterinary Research* 44(9):1660–1666.

Lumsden JM, Derksen FJ, Stick JA, Robinson NE, Nickels FA. 1994. Evaluation of partial arytenoidectomy as a treatment for equine laryngeal hemiplegia. *Equine Veterinary Journal* 26(2):125–129.

Mathew OP, Abu-Osba YK, Thach BT. 1982. Genioglossus muscle responses to upper airway pressure changes: Afferent pathways. *Journal of Applied Physiology: Respiratory, Environmental and Exercise Physiology* 52(2):445–450.

Mayhew IG. 1989. *Large Animal Neurology: A Handbook for Veterinary Clinicians*. Philadelphia, PA: Lea and Febiger.

Miller AJ. 1982. Deglutition. *Physiological Reviews* 62(1):129–184.

Moon JB, Smith AE, Folkins JW, Lemke JH, Gartlan M. 1994. Coordination of velopharyngeal muscle activity during positioning of the soft palate. *The Cleft Palate-Craniofacial Journal* 31(1):45–55.

Morello SL, Ducharme NG, Hackett RP, Warnick LD, Mitchell LM, Soderholm LV. 2008. Activity of selected rostral and caudal hyoid muscles in clinically normal horses during strenuous exercise. *American Journal of Veterinary Research* 69(5):682–689.

Ortved KF, Cheetham J, Mitchell LM, Ducharme NG. 2010. Successful treatment of persistent dorsal displacement of the soft palate and evaluation of laryngohyoid position in 15 racehorses. *Equine Veterinary Journal* 42(1):23–29.

Parente EJ, Martin BB, Tulleners EP, Ross MW. 2002. Dorsal displacement of the soft palate in 92 horses during high-speed treadmill examination (1993–1998). *Veterinary Surgery* 31 (6):507–512.

Pigott JH, Ducharme NG, Mitchell LM, Soderholm LV, Cheetham J. 2010. Incidence of swallowing during exercise in horses with dorsal displacement of the soft palate. *Equine Veterinary Journal* 38(5):393–399.

Rehder RS, Ducharme NG, Hackett RP, Nielan GJ. 1995. Measurement of upper airway pressures in exercising horses with dorsal displacement of the soft palate. *American Journal of Veterinary Research* 56(3):269–274.

Riha RL, Brander P, Vennelle M, Douglas NJ. 2005. A cephalometric comparison of patients with the sleep apnea/hypopnea syndrome and their siblings. *Sleep* 28(3):315–320.

Sforza E, Bacon W, Weiss T, Thibault A, Petiau C, Krieger J. 2000. Upper airway collapsibility and cephalometric variables in patients with obstructive sleep apnea. *American Journal of Respiratory and Critical Care Medicine* 161(2 Pt 1):347–352.

Shahar E, Whitney CW, Redline S, Lee ET, Newman AB, Nieto FJ, O'Connor GT, Boland LL, Schwartz JE, Samet JM. 2001. Sleep-disordered breathing and cardiovascular disease: Cross-sectional results of the sleep heart health study. *American Journal of Respiratory and Critical Care Medicine* 163(1):19–25.

Sisson S. 1975a. Equine digestive system. In: Getty R, ed. *Sisson and Grossman's the Anatomy of the Domestic Animals Volumes 1 and 2*, 5th ed. (pp. 454–497). Philadelphia, PA: W.B. Saunders Company.

Sisson S. 1975b. Equine myology. In: Getty R, ed. *Sisson and Grossman's the Anatomy of the Domestic Animals Volumes 1 and 2*, 5th ed. (pp. 386–387). Philadelphia, PA: W.B. Saunders Company.

Storey AT. 1968. Laryngeal initiation of swallowing. *Experimental Neurology* 20:359–365.

Tan RH, Dowling BA, Dart AJ. 2005. High-speed treadmill videoendoscopic examination of the upper respiratory tract in the horse: The results of 291 clinical cases. *Veterinary Journal* 170(2):243–248.

Tulleners EP, Stick JA, Leitch M, Trumble TN, Wilkerson JP. 1997. Epiglottic augmentation for treatment of dorsal displacement of the soft palate in racehorses: 59 Cases (1985–1994). *Journal of the American Veterinary Medical Association* 211(8):1022–1028.

Van de Graaff WB, Gottfried SB, Mitra J, van Lunteren E, Cherniack NS, Strohl KP. 1984. Respiratory function of hyoid muscles and hyoid arch. *Journal of Applied Physiology: Respiratory, Environmental and Exercise Physiology* 57(1):197–204.

Woodie JB, Ducharme NG, Kanter P, Hackett RP, Erb HN. 2005. Surgical advancement of the larynx (laryngeal tie-forward) as a treatment for dorsal displacement of the soft palate in horses: A prospective study 2001–2004. *Equine Veterinary Journal* 37(5):418–423.

Young T, Palta M, Dempsey J, Skatrud J, Weber S, Badr S. 1993. The occurrence of sleep-disordered breathing among middle-aged adults. *The New England Journal of Medicine* 328(17):1230–1235.

17 Dorsal Displacement of the Soft Palate: Standing and Dynamic Endoscopic Examination

Elizabeth Davidson

Introduction

Dorsal displacement of the soft palate (DDSP) is one of the most common upper respiratory dysfunctions in performance horses (Lane et al. 2006a; Martin et al. 2000; Morris 1990). Affected horses have exercise intolerance and are often described by their owners or trainers as "hitting a wall," "choking down," or "swallowing their tongue." Upper airway endoscopy confirms the diagnosis by visualization of the entire soft palate because the epiglottis is no longer visible being ventral to the soft palate (Figure 17.1). In this configuration, the soft palate reduces the cross-sectional area of the nasopharynx, causing a functional obstruction to airflow (Franklin et al. 2002; Holcombe et al. 1998). Noise is produced by vibration of the caudal free margin of the soft palate as air flows beneath the soft palate. This fluttering of the soft palate creates an expiratory "gurgling," "fluttering," or "snoring" respiratory noise. Some horses with DDSP will not make an abnormal respiratory noise during displacement. Horses without abnormal respiratory noise are identified as "silent displacers" and may represent 30% of affected horses (Derksen et al. 2001; Franklin et al. 2004; Parente et al. 2002).

Because DDSP is an intermittent dynamic event that occurs during high-intensity exercise, making an accurate diagnosis is difficult and the actual prevalence of DDSP in performance horses is unknown. In many instances a diagnosis of DDSP is based on historical or clinical signs such as a sudden deterioration in performance (i.e., abrupt decrease in speed), gurgling upper respiratory noise, and standing endoscopic findings. However, because this sporadic upper airway obstruction occurs while the horse is exercising, exercising endoscopy is the most definitive way to diagnose DDSP.

Endoscopic examination at rest

Resting endoscopic examination is performed to assess nasopharyngeal function and to rule in or out other causes of abnormal airway noise and exercise intolerance. Epiglottic aberrations such as hypoplasia, flaccidity (Figure 17.2), or deviation to one side may support a diagnosis of DDSP. Bruising of the roof of the nasopharynx near the guttural pouch openings (choke ring) and ulcers on the dorsal aspect of the caudal free edge of the soft

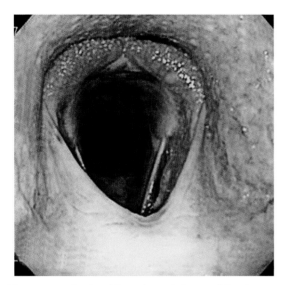

Figure 17.1   Resting videoendoscopic image of the pharynx of a horse with dorsal displacement of the soft palate.

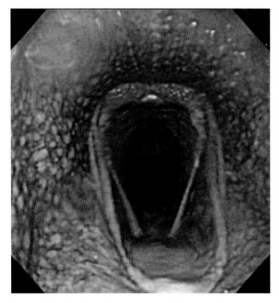

Figure 17.2   Resting videoendoscopic image of the pharynx during nasal occlusion. Note the "flaccid" appearance of the epiglottis and soft palate instability.

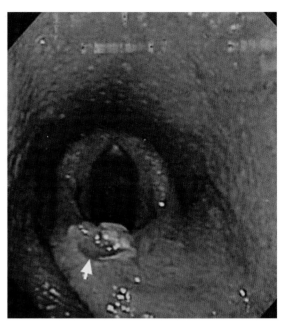

Figure 17.3   Dorsal displacement of the soft palate. Note the ulcer (arrow) along the dorsal aspect of the caudal free edge.

palate (Figure 17.3) may also be noted in horses with DDSP. Other anatomical abnormalities such as subepiglottic masses or cysts or masses on the soft palate may impede the normal position of the soft palate. Epiglottic entrapment can contribute

to intermittent or persistent DDSP (see Chapter 24) in horses. Endoscopic evaluation of the guttural pouches should be performed in young horses or horses with concurrent respiratory infections since enlarged retropharyngeal nodes maybe associated with neuropathy of the pharyngeal branch of the vagus predisposing horses to exercise-induced DDSP (Holcombe et al. 1998). Evidence of previous upper respiratory surgery such as a "notched" appearance of the caudal free edge of the palate (previous staphylectomy) or dermal scar over the ventral aspect of the cricoid cartilage (laryngotomy or sternothyrohyoideus myectomy) should also be noted.

Endoscopic examination at rest should include diagnostic techniques that encourage soft palatal displacement. Gently bumping the epiglottis with the endoscope, spraying the pharynx with water, or applying pressure to the external aspect of the larynx may cause the horse to displace the soft palate. Occluding the external nares, introducing the endoscope into the trachea and slowly withdrawing it, or flexing the head and neck may induce soft palate displacement. These maneuvers allow complete visualization of the dorsal portion of the caudal soft palate. It should be noted that DDSP during these maneuvers, particularly the ease of displacement and prolonged displacement despite swallowing, have been considered strong indicators of soft palate dysfunction. However, these maneuvers commonly induce DDSP in most horses and as such endoscopic findings at rest should be viewed with caution with respect to exercising palatal function or dysfunction.

Endoscopic examination during exercise

The current gold standard for diagnosis of intermittent DDSP is exercising examination via treadmill or overground endoscopy (see Chapter 2). Diagnosis is based on visualization of the entire soft palate, positioned dorsal to epiglottis, for longer than 8 seconds (Rehder et al. 1995; Woodie et al. 2005). This expiratory obstruction typically occurs when the horse is fatigued at the end of

exercise or during changes in exercise intensities. Exercising DDSP can occur as a spontaneous single event during speed (Figure 17.4) or may be preceded by a wide range of anatomical events. In some horses, progressive dorsoventral oscillatory movement (billowing) of the caudal half of the soft palate (aka palatal instability) (Figure 17.5) is noted immediately before DDSP. In others, frequent or inappropriate swallowing or axial deviation of the aryepiglottic folds may be observed prior to DDSP (Figure 17.6). Head gear, head and neck flexion, pressure on the bit, and effect of the rider/driver can also be predisposing factors.

Given the multitude of conditions and events that contribute to displacement, the exercising endoscopic testing protocol should accurately mimic the racing/showing conditions under which the horse is making abnormal respiratory noise or exhibiting exercise intolerance. Dynamic tests that include exercising the horse to the point of fatigue

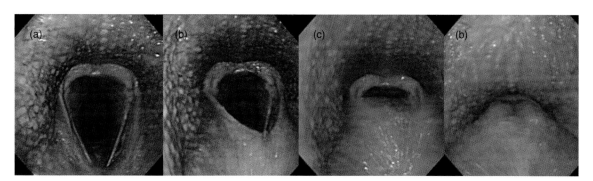

Figure 17.4   Exercising images of spontaneous dorsal displacement of the soft palate. (a) Inspiration, (b–d) progressive upper airway obstruction of the soft palate during expiration.

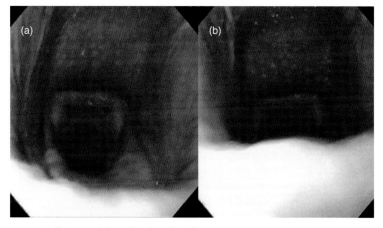

Figure 17.5   (a, b) Progressive billowing of the soft palate dorsally.

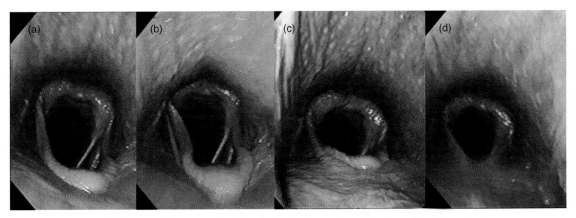

Figure 17.6   (a–d) Axial deviation of the aryepiglottic immediately prior to dorsal displacement of the soft palate.

or altering the speed, for example, exercising at maximal speed then rapid decrease in speed then return to maximal speed, should be performed when appropriate. Additional maneuvers that may increase the likelihood of diagnosis include exercise with and without head gear, tension on the bit, and enforced poll flexion. Even with an adequate stress test, DDSP is not always visualized during exercising endoscopy making accurate diagnosis difficult in every horse. Some clinicians will reach the diagnosis when the horse's history is highly suggestive of DDSP and alternative causes of dynamic upper respiratory obstruction have been eliminated with exercising endoscopy (Lane et al. 2006b; Parente et al. 2002)

Resting versus exercising endoscopic examination

Before the widespread use of dynamic endoscopy during exercise, endoscopic findings in the standing, resting horse have been used to "predict" which horses will dorsally displace their soft palates during exercise. While resting endoscopy is helpful for physical causes of palate dysfunction such as pharyngeal cysts or epiglottic entrapment, there is weak to no correlation between resting and exercising palatal function (Barakzai and Hawkes 2010; Lane et al. 2006a, 2006b; Parente and Martin 1995; Parente et al. 2002). Horses that displace the soft palate at rest are often normal during dynamic endoscopy and, conversely, many horses that are normal during resting endoscopic exam-

ination develop DDSP at exercise. The results of four retrospective studies of horses with confirmed DDSP during exercising endoscopy are tabulated in Table 17.1; most horses with exercising DDSP have normal palate function at rest.

Epiglottic hypoplasia and flaccidity observed during resting endoscopy have been suggested as etiological factors in horses with intermittent DDSP (Haynes 1981; Robertson 1991) because an abnormal epiglottis may be physically or functionally unable to hold the soft palate in its normal position (Figure 17.7). However, significant associations between epiglottic length and exercising DDSP have not been reported. In addition, clinical and experimental data indicate contact between the epiglottis and the soft palate is not essential for soft palate position or function (Holcombe et al. 1997; Parente et al. 1998). Horses with retroversion of the epiglottis do not dorsally displace their soft palates; normal soft palate position is maintained. It has also been reported that hypoplasia and flaccidity observed during nasal occlusion may simply be due to contraction of the hyoepiglotticus muscle and not an underlying conformational abnormality (Holcombe et al. 2002) that may predispose affected horse to displace.

Ulceration involving the dorsal aspect of the caudal soft palate is often associated with intermittent DDSP. However, there are many horses with palate ulceration that do not displace during treadmill endoscopy (Parente and Martin 1995), and most horses with exercising DDSP do not have ulceration (Table 17.1). Although it seems logical that friction between the ventral surface of the epiglottis and the free border of the soft palate will lead to ulceration, this presumption has not been corroborated with high-speed treadmill (HSTM) endoscopy.

Despite historical and anecdotal rhetoric, resting endoscopic findings often do not accurately reflect exercising palate function. While spontaneous DDSP during resting endoscopy may be highly specific for exercising DDSP, it is also extremely insensitive (Barakzai and Dixon 2011; Lane et al. 2006b). In fact, a diagnosis of DDSP based solely on characteristic history and resting endoscopic findings results in false negative diagnosis in 85% of race horses with respiratory noise or exercise intolerance (Lane et al. 2006b). Exercising endoscopy remains the gold standard for diagnosis.

Persistent DDSP

Persistent DDSP (see Chapter 24) is a rare condition characterized by the inability to visualize the epiglottis at any time during endoscopic evaluation of the upper airway including after repeated swallowing or nasal occlusion. Affected horses make a loud rattling noise and often have some degree of dysphagia, coughing, and aspiration pneumonia. It is usually secondary to underlying pathology such as pharyngeal cysts, pharyngeal paresis, or epiglottic abnormalities (Holcombe and Ducharme 2004; Ortved et al. 2010). To assess the epiglottis for structural or functional abnormalities, removal of the twitch or sedation may relax the horse and permit

Table 17.1   Endoscopic findings in horses with DDSP during exercise

| No. of horses | Exercising endoscopy | | | Resting endoscopy | | | | | | |
	DDSP	PI prior to DDSP	Concurrent URT obstruction	Abnormal epiglottis	Ulceration on caudal border	DDSP with nasal occlusion	Excessive pharyngitis	History of noise	Reference
46	24	5	3	0	1	2	8	20	Courouce-Malblanc et al. (2010)
92	92	–	35	13	9	46	9	57	Parente et al. (2002)
600	237	237	60	14	18	–	–	202	Lane et al. (2006a), (2006b)
100	20	–	6	4	1	–	1	20	Kannegieter and Dore (1995)

DDSP, dorsal displacement of the soft palate; PI, palatal instability; URT, upper respiratory tract.

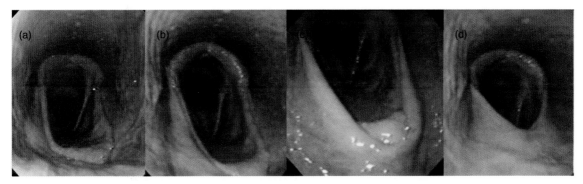

Figure 17.7   Exercising videoendoscopic images of the pharynx. (a) flaccid epiglottis, (b–d) progressive loss of the normal subepiglottic position of the soft palate.

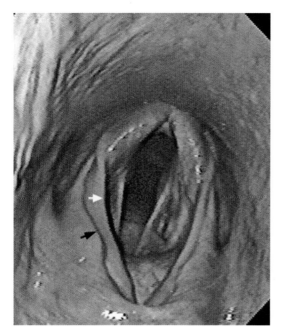

Figure 17.8   Concurrent epiglottic entrapment and persistent dorsal displacement of the soft palate. Entrapping aryepiglottic tissue (white arrow) is ventral to the soft palate (black arrow).

replacement of the soft palate to its subepiglottic position. After desensitization with local anesthetic, bronchoesophageal forceps may be used to reposition the soft palate or to pull the free edge of the palate to one side. Alternatively, oral endoscopic examination can be performed with general anesthesia or sedation and a mouth speculum.

The most commonly associated structural abnormality is epiglottic entrapment (Haynes 1981; Tate et al. 1990). It is important to differentiate those horses that are entrapped and displaced from those that are just displaced. The displaced and entrapped horses usually have dorsal bulging of the soft palate and two edges of tissue may be seen at the caudal edge of the palate (Figure 17.8). Less commonly there is extensive subepiglottic pathology from primary ulceration and fibrosis or from previous surgery for epiglottic entrapment (Aitken and Parente 2011; Haynes 1981; Ortved et al. 2010; Tate et al. 1990).

DDSP in show horses

DDSP has also been reported in show horses (Davidson et al. 2011; Franklin et al. 2006). In these horses, exercise that requires a flexed head and neck position can be a contributing factor and exercising endoscopic examination should be performed with and without enforced poll flexion. As in racehorses, there is weak correlation between resting DDSP and exercising DDSP in show horses. In one study, DDSP was more prevalent in dressage horses than jumpers (Van Erck 2011).

References

Aitken MR, Parente EJ. 2011. Epiglottic abnormalities in mature nonracehorses: 23 cases (1990–2009). *Journal of the American Veterinary Medical Association* 238:1634–1638.

Barakzai SZ, Dixon PM. 2011. Correlation of resting and exercising endoscopic findings for horses with dynamic laryngeal collapse and palatal dysfunction. *Equine Veterinary Journal* 43:18–23.

Barakzai SZ, Hawkes CS. 2010. Dorsal displacement of the soft palate and palatal instability. *Journal of Equine Veterinary Education* 22:253–264.

Courouce-Malblanc A, Deniau V, Rossignol R, Corde R, Leleu R, Maillard K, Pitel PH, Pronost S, Fortier G. 2010. Physiological measurements and prevalence of lower airway diseases in Trotters with dorsal displacement of the soft palate. *Equine Veterinary Journal Supplement* 42:246–255.

Davidson EJ, Martin BB, Boston RC, Parente EJ. 2011. Exercising upper respiratory videoendoscopic evaluation of 100 nonracing performance horses with abnormal noise and/or poor performance. *Equine Veterinary Journal* 43:3–8.

Derksen FJ, Holcombe SJ, Hartmann W, Robinson NE, Stick JA. 2001. Spectrum analysis of respiratory sounds in exercising horses with experimentally induced laryngeal hemiplegia or dorsal displacement of the soft palate. *American Journal of Veterinary Research* 62:659–664.

Franklin SH, Naylor JR, Lane JG. 2002. Effect of dorsal displacement of the soft palate on ventilation and airflow during high-intensity exercise. *Equine Veterinary Journal Supplement* 34:379–383.

Franklin SH, Price C, Burn JF. 2004. The displaced equine soft palate as a source of abnormal respiratory noise during expiration. *Equine Veterinary Journal* 36:590–594.

Franklin SH, Naylor JR, Lane JG. 2006. Videoendoscopic evaluation of the upper respiratory tract in 93 sports horses during exercise testing on a high-speed treadmill. *Equine Veterinary Journal Supplement* 36:540–545.

Haynes PF. 1981. Persistent dorsal displacement of the soft palate associated with epiglottic shortening in two horses. *Journal of the American Veterinary Medical Association* 179:677–681.

Holcombe SJ, Ducharme NG. 2004. Abnormalities of the upper airway. In: Hinchcliff W, Kaneps AJ, Goer RJ, eds. *Equine Sports Medicine and Surgery.* (pp. 569–573). Philadelphia, PA: W.B. Saunders Company.

Holcombe SJ, Derksen FJ, Stick JA, Robinson NE. 1997. Effects of bilateral hypoglossal and glossopharyngeal nerve blocks on epiglottic and soft palate position in exercising horses. *American Journal of Veterinary Research* 58:1022–1026.

Holcombe SJ, Derksen FJ, Stick JA, Robinson NE. 1998. Bilateral nerve blockade of the pharyngeal branch of the vagus nerve produces persistent soft palate dysfunction in horses. *American Journal of Veterinary Research* 59:504–508.

Holcombe SJ, Cornelisse CJ, Berney C, Robinson NE. 2002. Electromyographic activity of the hyoepiglotticus muscle and control of epiglottis position in horses. *American Journal of Veterinary Research* 63:1617–1621.

Kannegieter NJ, Dore ML. 1995. Endoscopy of the upper respiratory tract during treadmill exercise: A clinical study of 100 horses. *Australian Veterinary Journal* 72:101–107.

Lane JG, Bladon B, Little DR, Naylor JR, Franklin SH. 2006a. Dynamic obstructions of the equine upper respiratory tract. Part 1: Observations during high-speed treadmill endoscopy of 600 Thoroughbred racehorses. *Equine Veterinary Journal* 38:393–399.

Lane JG, Bladon B, Little DR, Naylor JR, Franklin SH. 2006b. Dynamic obstructions of the equine upper respiratory tract. Part 2: Comparison of endoscopic findings at rest and during high-speed treadmill exercise of 600 Thoroughbred racehorses. *Equine Veterinary Journal* 38:401–408.

Martin BB, Reef VB, Parente EJ, Sage AD. 2000. Causes of poor performance of horses during racing, training, or showing: 348 cases (1992–1996). *Journal of the American Veterinary Medical Association* 216:554–558.

Morris EA, Seeherman HJ. 1990. Evaluation of upper respiratory tract function during strenuous exercise in racehorses. *Journal of the American Veterinary Association* 196:431–438.

Ortved KF, Cheetham J, Mitchell LM, Ducharme NG. 2010. Successful treatment of persistent dorsal displacement of the soft palate and evaluation of laryngohyoid position in 15 racehorses. *Equine Veterinary Journal* 42:23–29.

Parente EJ, Martin BB. 1995. Correlation between standing endoscopic examinations and those made during high-speed exercise in horses: 150 cases. In: *Proceedings of the 41st Annual Convention of the American Association of Equine Practitioners.* (pp. 170–171). Lexington, KY.

Parente EJ, Martin BB, Tulleners EP. 1998. Epiglottic retroversion as a cause of upper airway obstruction in two horses. *Equine Veterinary Journal* 30(3):270–272.

Parente EJ, Martin BB, Tulleners EP, Ross MW. 2002. Dorsal displacement of the soft palate in 92 horses during high-speed treadmill examination (1992–1998). *Veterinary Surgery* 31(6):507–512.

Rehder RS, Ducharme NG, Hackett RP, Neilan GJ. 1995. Measurement of upper airway pressures in exercising horses with dorsal displacement of the soft palate. *American Journal of Veterinary Research* 56:269–274.

Robertson JT. 1991. Pharynx and larynx. In: Beech J, ed. *Equine Respiratory Disorders.* (pp. 331–387). Philadelphia, PA: Lea and Febiger.

Tate LP, Sweeney CL, Bowman KF, Newman HC, Duckett WM. 1990. Transendoscopic Nd:YAG Laser surgery for treatment of epiglottal entrapment and dorsal displacement of the soft palate in the horse. *Veterinary Surgery* 19(5):356–363.

Van Erck E. 2011. Dynamic respiratory videoendoscopy in ridden sports horses: Effect of head flexion, riding and airway inflammation in 129 cases. *Equine Veterinary Journal Supplement* 43:18–24.

Woodie JB, Ducharme NG, Kanter P, Hackett RP, Erb HN. 2005. Surgical advancement of the larynx (laryngeal tie-forward) as a treatment for dorsal displacement of the soft palate in horses: a prospective study 2001–2004. *Equine Veterinary Journal* 37(5):418–423.

18 Ultrasonography of the Horse with Suspected Dorsal Displacement of the Soft Palate

Heather Chalmers

Introduction

Dorsal displacement of the soft palate (DDSP) is well recognized as an important performance-limiting condition of horses. Experimental models that induce DDSP include bilateral blockade of the pharyngeal branch of the vagus nerve (Holcombe et al. 1998), bilateral transection of the thyrohyoid muscles (Ducharme et al. 2003), and blockade of the hypoglossal nerve at the level of the thyrohyoid bones (Cheetham et al. 2009). The mechanisms by which these models induce DDSP are not clear; however, current understanding suggests that the actions of the intrinsic and extrinsic nasopharyngeal muscles and their effects on airway size and position may contribute to DDSP during exercise.

The use of ultrasound to characterize the laryngohyoid position in the resting horse with and without DDSP has been evaluated (Chalmers et al. 2009). This work tested the hypothesis that the spatial relationship of the basihyoid bone and the larynx is different in horses that are affected with DDSP compared to unaffected horses. This idea was developed via the observations that laryngeal tie-forward and myectomy procedures are consid-

ered effective in treating DDSP, and that these procedures alter upper airway conformation (Carter et al. 1993; Cheetham et al. 2008.; Llewellyn and Petrowitz 1997; Smith and Embertson 2005; Woodie et al. 2005). Accurate assessment of the anatomic position of upper airway structures is challenging and many of the structures are not readily visualized or palpated externally or measured endoscopically. Ultrasonography has been established as a complementary means of assessing nonluminal upper airway structures in horses (Chalmers et al. 2006). Therefore, the concept that upper airway conformation may be different in horses affected with DDSP compared to normal horses was assessed in the standing horse using ultrasound. This study was performed as a blinded cross-sectional study, in which 56 racing horses presenting for evaluation of poor performance were evaluated with ultrasound. The main finding from this study was that the position of the basihyoid bone at rest in the standing horse was found to be more superficial, or more ventral, in horses that exhibited DDSP at exercise compared to horses that did not exhibit DDSP at exercise (Chalmers et al. 2009).

Advances in Equine Upper Respiratory Surgery, First Edition. Edited by Jan Hawkins.
© 2015 ACVS Foundation. Published 2015 by John Wiley & Sons, Inc.

Ultrasonographic technique

The ultrasonographic approach to a horse suspected of having DDSP is identical to that described for horses suspected of having RLN and involves a previously described technique of laryngeal ultrasound examination (Chalmers et al. 2006). In summary, the examination is performed with the horse unsedated and the head in a neutral position. Ultrasonography is performed with an 8.5–12.5 MHz linear or curvilinear probe. Five measurements of the laryngohyoid structures are made in the horse with suspected DDSP: depth of the rostral lingual process, depth of the basihyoid bone at base of the lingual process, depth of the caudal aspect of the basihyoid bone, depth of the thyroid cartilage, and distance between the thyroid cartilage and basihyoid bone. The measurements are obtained using two windows: the rostroventral window in a transverse plane and in a longitudinal plane using the caudoventral window.

Using the rostroventral window, measurements are made in the transverse plane with an 8.5 MHz transducer from the depth of the rostral aspect of the lingual process and the depth of the base of the lingual process at the basihyoid bone by following the lingual process caudally in real time and obtaining an image at the junction of the lingual process and the base of the basihyoid bone. The next measurements are obtained in the longitudinal plane at the caudoventral window using a 12.5 MHz transducer from the depth of the caudal aspect of the basihyoid bone (measurement A), depth of the rostral aspect of the thyroid cartilage (measurement B), and distance from the caudal aspect of the basihyoid bone to the rostral aspect of the thyroid cartilage (measurement C).

In horses without any abnormalities in the ventral acoustic windows, careful measurements of the laryngohyoid position should be performed. Specifically, from the midventral acoustic window the depth of the base of the basihyoid bone should be measured (Figure 18.1) as detailed above. In horses with DDSP, there is a significant difference between the depths of the basihyoid bone at the base of the lingual process compared to horses without a diagnosis of DDSP (Chalmers et al. 2009). For horses with DDSP the mean measurement for the depth of the basihyoid bone at the base of the

lingual process was 1.18 cm and for horses without DDSP the mean measurement was 1.34 cm. The odds ratio for the measurement of the depth of the base of the basihyoid bone was found to be 16.95 (95% CI 1.3–128), indicating that the odds of a horse experiencing DDSP at exercise increased by approximately 17-fold with each 1-cm decrease in the depth of the basihyoid bone (Chalmers et al. 2009). It is unclear if this relationship is causative and is reflective of differing conformation of the upper airway, or if this finding is a consequence of having DDSP, such as due to muscle atrophy of the sternohyoideus or sternothyroideus muscles.

Discussion

The focus of the ultrasound examination when assessing for DDSP involves determining the location of the ventral structures of the larynx and hyoid apparatus. This includes a thorough assessment of structures of the ventral throat region including the lingual process and base of the basihyoid bone, the paired ceratohyoid bones, the paired thyrohyoid bones, the ventral and lateral aspects of the thyroid cartilage, and the vocal folds at the cricothyroid notch. Many of these structures are not visible with endoscopy, and therefore the use of ultrasound is considered highly complementary to the endoscopic examination. Abnormalities that can be observed in the ventral region during a routine examination include masses, abscesses, hyoid bone fractures, and lymphadenopathy. It is frequently possible to detect evidence of previous surgery, which may include the presence of tie-forward prosthesis suture or fibrosis of the soft tissues.

Importantly, it has been shown that head and neck positions affect the laryngohyoid position (McCluskie et al. 2008). As such, every effort should be made to standardize head and neck position in a neutral and repeatable location. This may include the use of a modified goniometer or other measurement device. The lack of standardization of head and neck position are important limitations of the radiographic (Cheetham et al. 2008.) and ultrasonographic (Chalmers et al. 2009) studies exploring the laryngohyoid position in DDSP and may limit the clinical utility of these techniques.

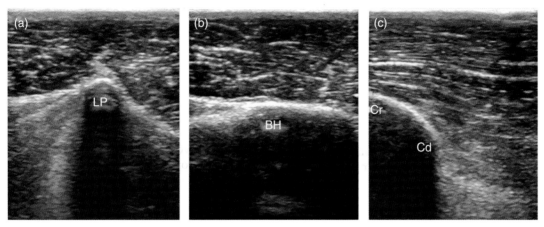

Figure 18.1   Composite ultrasound images of the rostroventral (a, b) and midventral (c) acoustic windows of the throat region of a 4-year-old Standardbred gelding presenting with and upper respiratory noise during exercise. Images (a) and (b) depict the bony landmarks used to locate the basihyoid bone, beginning cranially in the transverse plane the lingual process (LP) and the base of the basihyoid bone (BH). Both can be identified by the hyperechoic surface and the strong acoustic shadow. Image (c) is obtained in a cranial (Cr) to caudal (Cd) direction, and demonstrates the characteristic slope of the base of the basihyoid bone, such that the depth of the basihyoid bone is different cranially (Cr) than caudally (Cd). For this reason, to ensure standardization of findings, it is recommended to assess basihyoid depth at the cranial aspect of the basihyoid bone, as the lingual process is merged with the base of the bone, as depicted in (b).

The exact application of laryngeal ultrasound will depend on the clinical setting and the tools available. Because neither treadmill videoendoscopy, overground videoendoscopy, nor ultrasound are ideal diagnostic tests, it is strongly recommended to use these techniques together to increase the diagnostic accuracy for DDSP. The diagnosis of intermittent DDSP remains problematic and is generally not possible in the resting horse (Lane et al. 2006; Parente et al. 2002). High-speed treadmill examination has been criticized on the basis that treadmill protocols are inherently nonrepresentative of racing conditions, but the use of a treadmill allows the clinician to work the horse to a level of exertion that mimics that experienced in racing (Allen and Franklin 2010; Lane et al. 2006). Increasingly, the use of wireless overground endoscopy systems is forming the front line of diagnosis when upper airway problems are suspected. Yet, limitations of overground endoscopy compared to treadmill endoscopy have been reported for DDSP (Allen and Franklin 2010). Thus, even where exercising endoscopy is available, the diagnosis of DDSP remains problematic and may often be made presumptively. Because of these limitations and the intermittent nature of

DDSP, a new diagnostic approach such as laryngeal ultrasonography may address some of the outlined limitations of exercising endoscopic techniques. As an adjunct to exercising endoscopy, the initial data support the use of laryngeal ultrasound to aid in the diagnosis of DDSP (Chalmers et al. 2009). In situations where exercising endoscopy is not readily available, laryngeal ultrasound prior to referral for exercising endoscopy can increase the justification for recommending the exercising test to the client. In cases where the exercising test is available and was negative, the clinician may use the ultrasound findings in concert with other suggestive diagnostic criteria to provide further support for a clinical diagnosis of DDSP.

References

Allen KJ, Franklin SH. 2010. Comparisons of overground endoscopy and treadmill endoscopy in UK Thoroughbred racehorses. *Equine Veterinary Journal* 42(3):186–191.

Carter BG, Robertson JT, Beard WL, Moore RM. 1993. Sternothyroideus myectomy, tenectomy, and staphylectomy for treatment of dorsal displacement of the soft palate in horses. *Veterinary Surgery* 22(5):374.

Chalmers HJ, Cheetham J, Yeager AE, Ducharme NG. 2006. Ultrasonography of the equine larynx. *Veterinary Radiology and Ultrasound* 47(5):476–481.

Chalmers HJ, Yeager AE, Ducharme NG. 2009. Ultrasonographic assessment of laryngohyoid position as a predictor of dorsal displacement of the soft palate in horses. *Veterinary Radiology and Ultrasound* 50(1):91–96.

Cheetham J, Pigott JH, Thorson LM, Mohammed HO, Ducharme NG. 2008. Racing performance following the laryngeal tie-forward procedure: A case-controlled study. *Equine Veterinary Journal* 40:501–507.

Cheetham J, Pigott JH, Hermanson JW, Campoy L, Soderholm LV, Thorson LM, Ducharme NG. 2009. Role of the hypoglossal nerve in equine nasopharyngeal stability. *Journal of Applied Physiology* 107(2):471–477.

Ducharme NG, Hackett RP, Woodie JB, Dykes N, Erb HN, Mitchell LM, Soderholm LV. 2003. Investigations into the role of the thyrohyoid muscles in the pathogenesis of dorsal displacement of the soft palate in horses. *Equine Veterinary Journal* 35(3):258–263.

Holcombe SJ, Derksen FJ, Stick JA, Robinson NE. 1998. Bilateral nerve blockade of the pharyngeal branch of the vagus nerve produces persistent soft palate dysfunction in horses. *American Journal of Veterinary Research* 59(4):504–508.

Lane JG, Bladon B, Little DR, Naylor JR, Franklin SH. 2006. Dynamic obstructions of the equine upper respiratory tract. Part 1: Observations during high-speed treadmill endoscopy of 600 Thoroughbred racehorses. *Equine Veterinary Journal* 38(5):393–399.

Llewellyn HR, Petrowitz AB. 1997. Sternothyroideus myotomy for the treatment of dorsal displacement of the soft palate. *Proceedings of the American Association of Equine Practitioners* 43:237–238.

McCluskie LK, Franklin SH, Lane JG, Tremaine WH, Allen KJ. 2008. Effect of head position on radiographic assessment of laryngeal tie-forward procedure in horses. *Veterinary Surgery* 37(5):608–612.

Parente EJ, Martin BB, Tulleners EP, Ross MW. 2002. Dorsal displacement of the soft palate in 92 horses during high-speed treadmill examination (1993–1998). *Veterinary Surgery* 31(6):507–512.

Smith JJ, Embertson RM. 2005. Sternothyroideus myotomy, staphylectomy and oral caudal soft palate photothermoplasty for treatment of dorsal displacement of the soft palate in 102 Thoroughbred racehorses. *Veterinary Surgery* 34(1):5–10.

Woodie JB, Ducharme NG, Kanter P, Hackett RP, Erb HN. 2005. Surgical advancement of the larynx (laryngeal tie-forward) as a treatment for dorsal displacement of the soft palate in horses: A prospective study 2001–2004. *Equine Veterinary Journal* 37(5);418–423.

19 Sternothyroideus Myotenectomy and Staphylectomy

Jan Hawkins

Introduction

Sternothyroideus myotenectomy and/or staphylectomy have been used as treatment for DDSP for many years (Anderson et al. 1995; Barakzai et al. 2004; Harrison and Raker 1988; Shappell et al. 1989; Smith and Embertson 2005; Tate et al. 1990; Tulleners et al. 1997). Since the late 1990s sternothyroideus myotenectomy and staphylectomy has been used for surgical management of DDSP, particularly in the Standardbred racehorse. This procedure was first popularized by Llewellyn. In 1997, Llewellyn reported that sternothyroideus myotenectomy and staphylectomy resulted in 35 of 41 horses achieving either the same or a faster race time (Llewellyn and Petrowitz 1997). Results have also been reported for Thoroughbred racehorses (BonenClark et al. 1999). Until the advent of the laryngeal tie forward sternothyroideus myotenectomy and staphylectomy were preferred by many surgeons as the surgical treatment of choice for DDSP in racehorses. In some areas, it is still the first-line surgical procedure for horses with DDSP. This surgical procedure has the advantages of being performed under short-term general anesthesia,

requires a minimum of surgical equipment, does not require referral to a surgical facility, and short convalescent time.

Surgical technique

Prior to general anesthesia and surgery, the horse is administered prophylactic antimicrobials and anti-inflammatories. Inhalational anesthesia is not necessary for the completion of this surgical procedure. Short-term intravenous anesthesia is preferred, with xylazine, ketamine, and butorphanol most commonly used. If additional anesthetic time is required injectable anesthesia can be supplemented with guaifenesin administered to effect. If desired, the horse can be intubated. If intubation is elected, the endotracheal tube should be inserted nasotracheally. This avoids extubation of the horse during the surgical procedure as the soft palate will not be obstructed by the endotracheal tube. The procedure can be performed while recumbent in a recovery stall or the horse can be positioned on a surgical table. The horse is positioned in dorsal recumbency and the ventral aspect of the larynx is prepared for

Advances in Equine Upper Respiratory Surgery, First Edition. Edited by Jan Hawkins.
© 2015 ACVS Foundation. Published 2015 by John Wiley & Sons, Inc.

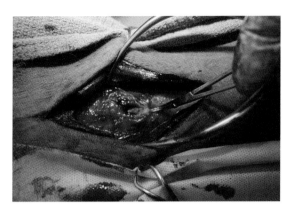

Figure 19.1   Ventral midline incision centered over the caudal aspect of the cricoid cartilage. The hemostat marks the cricoid cartilage. Rostral is toward the left and caudal is toward the right of the photograph.

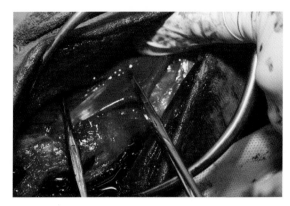

Figure 19.3   Gross postmortem photograph depicting clamping of the tendon of insertion of the sternothyroideus muscle and the muscle belly.

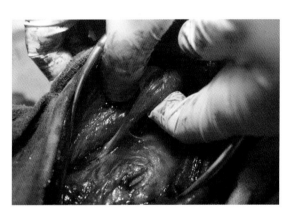

Figure 19.2   Gross postmortem photograph depicting isolation of the left sternothyroideus muscle. Note insertion of the sternothyroideus on the thyroid cartilage. Rostral is toward the left and caudal is toward the right of the photograph.

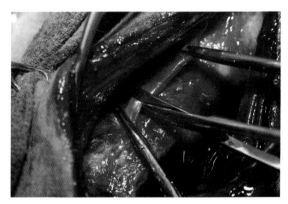

Figure 19.4   Gross postmortem photograph depicting transection of the tendon of insertion of the sternothyroideus muscle with Metzenbaum scissors.

aseptic surgery. An 8–10 cm incision is made centered over the cricoid cartilage (Figure 19.1). If the incision is positioned so that it begins at the level of the cricoid cartilage it increases the difficulty of accessing the tendon of insertion of the sternothyroideus muscle. A more caudal incision than that used for a standard laryngotomy approach to the larynx eliminates this complication. Following skin incision the sternothyroideus muscle bellies are split on the midline to access the ventral aspect of the larynx. Blunt digital dissection is used to isolate the tendon of insertion of the sternothyroideus muscle (Figure 19.2). Once isolated, the tendon is

clamped with a Carmalt hemostat (Figure 19.3). There is a small vein associated with the tendon of insertion and it should be avoided. As much of the muscle belly as possible is isolated and clamped with either an angiotribe or an additional Carmalt hemostat. The tendon of insertion is transected adjacent to the clamp site as is the sternothyroideus muscle belly (Figure 19.4). Occasionally small vessels are located within the muscle belly but typically they are controlled via clamping. It is important to remove a section of the muscle belly as some surgeons have reported fibrosis of the muscle belly to the larynx with the end result being recurrence of signs of soft palate displacement. Following transection and removal of the sternothyroideus

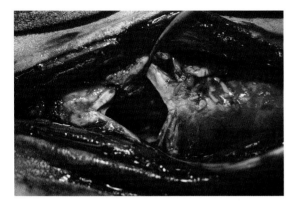

Figure 19.5   Gross postmortem photograph depicting a laryngotomy incision through the cricothyroid ligament. Gelpi retractors are being used to open the cricothyroid space. Rostral is toward the left and caudal is toward the right.

muscle the cricothyroid ligament is incised to enter the laryngeal lumen (Figure 19.5). A Gelpi or similar retractor is used to open the laryngeal lumen. A finger is inserted into the laryngeal lumen and the epiglottis is depressed to displace the soft palate. Following displacement the soft palate can be visualized (Figure 19.6). A straight sponge forceps is used to grasp the soft palate on the midline and using a pair of curved Metzenbaum or Satinsky scissors the sponge forceps is used as a template to trim the soft palate (Figure 19.7). When this is done this leaves two "tags" of tissue on each side of the soft palate (Figure 19.8). Each of these palate tags is also trimmed (Figure 19.9). This completes the staphylectomy (Figure 19.10). For obvious reasons it is important to be conservative when trimming the soft palate to avoid problems with dysphagia following the staphylectomy. The laryngotomy retractors are removed and the procedure is completed by removing a 4 × 8 cm section of the sternohyoideus muscle centered over the laryngotomy incision.

Complications associated with sternothyroideus myotenectomy and staphylectomy include hemorrhage associated with transection of the tendon or insertion of the sternothyroideus, muscle belly, or iatrogenic injury to adjacent vessels (e.g., linguo-facial vein), incisional infection, and dysphagia if an excessive amount of soft palate was resected. Overall, the complication rate of this procedure is low.

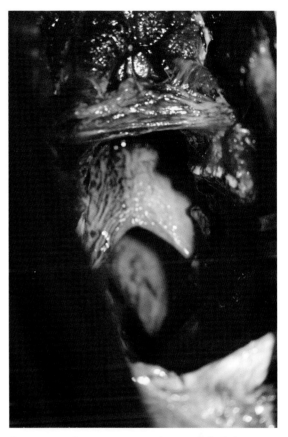

Figure 19.6   Gross postmortem photograph depicting exposure of the caudal aspect of the soft palate. The thyroid cartilage and rostral aspect of the larynx have been removed. Note the characteristic V shape of the soft palate.

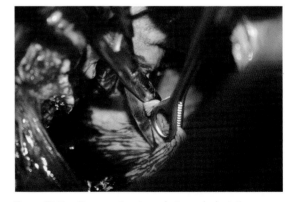

Figure 19.7   Gross postmortem photograph depicting grasping of the soft palate on the midline with straight sponge forceps and the incision of the soft palate on the left side with curved scissors.

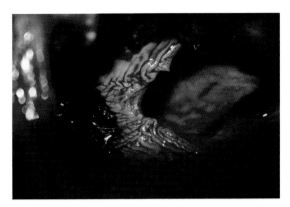

Figure 19.8   Gross postmortem photograph depicting the two "tags" left behind following excision of the soft palate in the clamp of the sponge forceps.

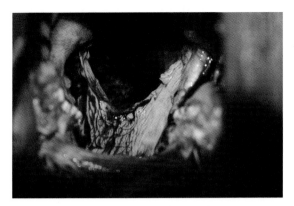

Figure 19.10   Gross postmortem photograph depicting completion of the staphylectomy procedure. Rostral is at the bottom of the photograph and caudal is toward the top of the photograph.

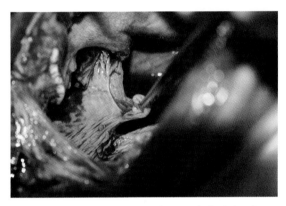

Figure 19.9   Gross postmortem photograph depicting the excision of one of the soft palate "tags." The tag is grasped with an Allis tissue forceps and is excised with scissors.

Aftercare

Antimicrobials are rarely needed after surgery. Anti-inflammatories are administered for 5–7 days following the surgical procedure. The laryngotomy incision is cleaned twice daily until healed which is typically within 2–3 weeks. The author prefers to withhold horses from exercise until the laryngotomy is healed although it is common practice for racehorses, particularly Standardbreds to return to training within days of the surgical procedure.

The reported success of sternothyroideus myotenectomy and staphylectomy has ranged from 60% to 70%. Horses that do not respond positively to this surgical technique are candidates for a laryn-geal tie forward but apparently have a decreased prognosis when compared to horses treated for DDSP with laryngeal tie forward as the initial surgical technique.

References

Anderson JD, Tulleners EP, Johnston JK, Reeves MJ. 1995. Sternothyrohyoideus myectomy or staphylectomy for treatment of intermittent dorsal displacement of the soft palate in racehorses: 209 cases (1098–1991). *Journal of the American Veterinary Medical Association* 206(12):1909–1912.

Barakzai SZ, Johnson VS, Baird DH, Bladon B, Lane JG. 2004. Assessment of the efficacy of composite surgery for the treatment of dorsal displacement of the soft palate in a group of 53 racing Thoroughbreds (1990–1996). *Equine Veterinary Journal* 36(2):175–179.

BonenClark G, Bryant J, Hernandez J, Ferrell EP, Colahan PT. 1999. Sternothyroideus tenectomy or sternothyroideus tenectomy with staphylectomy for the treatment of soft palate displacement. *Proceedings of the American Association of Equine Practitioners* 45: 85–86.

Harrison IW, Raker CW. 1988. Sternothyroideus myectomy in horses: 17 cases (1984–1985). *Journal of the American Veterinary Medical Association* 193(10):1299–1302.

Llewellyn HR, Petrowitz AB. 1997. Sternothyroideus myotomy for the treatment of dorsal displacement of the soft palate. *Proceedings of the American Association of Equine Practitioners* 43:239–243.

Shappell KK, Caron JP, Stick JA, Parks AJ. 1989. Staphylectomy for treatment of dorsal displacement of the soft palate in two foals. *Journal of the American Veterinary Medical Association* 195(10):1395–1398.

Smith JJ, Embertson RM. 2005. Sternothyroideus myotomy, staphylectomy, and oral caudal soft palate photothermoplasty for treatment of dorsal displacement of the soft palate in 102 Thoroughbred racehorses. *Veterinary Surgery* 34(1):5–10.

Tate LP, Sweeney CL, Bowman KF, Newman HC, Duckett WM. 1990. Transendoscopic Nd: YAG laser surgery for treatment of epiglottal entrapment and dorsal displacement of the soft palate in the horse. *Veterinary Surgery* 19(5):356–363.

Tulleners EP, Stick JA, Leitch M, Trumble TN, Wilkerson JP. 1997. Epiglottic augmentation for treatment of dorsal displacement of the soft palate in racehorses: 59 cases (1985–1994). *Journal of the American Veterinary Medical Association* 211(8):1022–1028.

20 Dorsal Displacement of the Soft Palate: Laryngeal Tie-Forward

Norm G. Ducharme

Introduction

The rationale of this treatment is that the action/dysfunction of muscles that affects the position of the basihyoid and laryngeal complex affects the stability (i.e., patency of the nasopharynx) of the nasopharynx. Surgical elevation and advancement of the larynx in horses termed "laryngeal tie-forward" was introduced in 2003 when it was discovered that resection of the thyrohyoideus (TH) muscle bilaterally resulted in dorsal displacement of the soft palate (DDSP) during exercise (Ducharme et al. 2003). Furthermore, this induced displacement could be resolved by placement of sutures or an external device (Ducharme et al. 2003; Woodie et al. 2005b). The occurrence of DDSP following removal of the TH muscles bilaterally provided the second experimental evidence that the position of the basihyoid/laryngeal complex influenced the stability of the upper airway of horses at exercise. Previously, transection of the sternothyroideus (ST) and sternohyoideus (SH) muscles bilaterally has been associated with increased upper airway pressures during exercise,

an indication that strap muscles affected the stability of the upper airway at exercise (Holcombe et al. 1994). Further support for the importance of muscles/nerves influencing the position of the basihyoid and larynx was obtained more recently when the application of local anesthetic solution around the hypoglossal nerves bilaterally at the level of the ceratohyoid bones also resulted in DDSP at exercise (Cheetham et al. 2009).

The laryngeal tie-forward procedure results in a rostral and dorsal movement of the larynx and a caudal and dorsal movement of the basihyoid bone (Cheetham et al. 2008). Although the optimal position or relationship of the larynx/hyoid apparatus to stabilize the upper airway at exercise is unknown, a more dorsal basihyoid and larynx was associated with a better prognosis (i.e., rate of return to racing). This is consistent with the finding that a more ventral position of the basihyoid based on ultrasonographic assessment (see Chapter 18) was associated with a higher likelihood of DDSP during exercise to those findings (Chalmers et al. 2009). The results of these two studies support the hypothesis that we should target a more dorsal

Advances in Equine Upper Respiratory Surgery, First Edition. Edited by Jan Hawkins.
© 2015 ACVS Foundation. Published 2015 by John Wiley & Sons, Inc.

position of the larynx and thus we have modified the positions of the sutures to emphasize a more dorsal movement of the larynx.

The following describes in detail the modifications of the technique since it was first introduced. These modifications are based on two objectives: (1) improving success (i.e., position of the larynx) and (2) minimizing complications. Indeed, as in any procedure, there are complications associated with the laryngeal tie-forward procedure. The emphasis of this chapter is on technical details that minimize the likelihood of these complications. The author's experience is based on over 600 operations with the majority of horses treated being racehorses. The procedure has been performed in sport horses with success but the pathophysiology of the disease in those horses as well as their response to treatment are far less known.

Surgical technique

After induction of general anesthesia, the horse is placed in dorsal recumbency and the ventral cervical area is prepared for aseptic surgery. A right-handed surgeon can perform this procedure without changing sides if standing on the left side of the horse (reverse for a left-handed surgeon). A ventral midline incision is made from 1 cm caudal to the cricoid cartilage extending cranially up to 1 cm rostral to the caudal border of the basihyoid bone (Figure 20.1). The paired SH muscles are bluntly separated on the midline and the larynx freed from the surrounding tissue so it can be mobilized. The left and right ST muscles/tendons are then elevated separately before placing the sutures in the caudal aspect of the wing of the left and right thyroid cartilages. Elevation of the ST muscles/tendons is done by placing a curved Crile hemostat immediately caudal to the cricoid cartilage; this prevents inadvertent damage to the cricothyroid (CT) muscles or its innervation from the external branch of the cranial laryngeal nerve. This step is done first prior to placement of sutures into the thyroid cartilages as inadvertent perforation of the caudal laryngeal vein/artery can result in bleeding that renders identification of the ST tendon more difficult. As a consequence, elevation of the ST tendon in a bloody field can lead to damage to the CT muscles, which have been shown or proposed to result in vocal cord

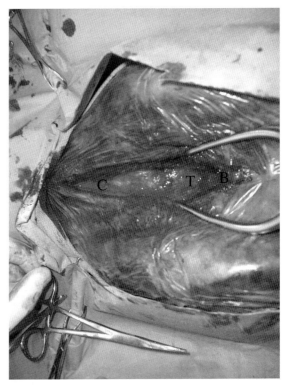

Figure 20.1   Intraoperative image showing the ventral aspect of the throatlatch area after skin incision and separation of the sternohyoideus muscle. C, cricoid cartilage; T, ventral aspect of the rostral aspect of the thyroid cartilage; B, basihyoid bone.

collapse (Dart 2006; Holcombe et al. 2006). The site of placement of the suture is the caudal aspect of the wing of the thyroid cartilage starting ~6 mm from its ventral border extending dorsally to the ventral border of the ST tendon attachment on the thyroid cartilage (Figure 20.2). Tearing of the suture in the cartilage has been observed occasionally, especially in 2-year-old horses. To minimize this complication, we originally reported to pass the suture twice in the thyroid cartilage. This is extrapolated from work for increased stability in the muscular process during prosthetic laryngoplasty (Kelly et al. 2008). To further minimize this complication and prevent lateral deviation of the larynx we pass the suture four times into the thyroid cartilage approximately 3–4 mm apart (Figures 20.2 and 20.3b). The ST muscle/tendon is then elevated and a 2–3 cm section removed. Removing a section of the tendon prevents reattachment of the ST onto the cricoid cartilage, thus re-establishing a caudal traction force on the larynx. The procedure is then repeated on the contralateral side.

The sutures are then passed around the basihyoid bone. This is a modification of the originally

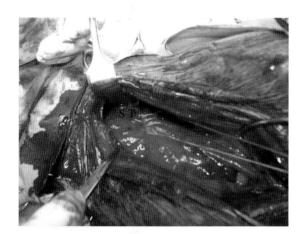

Figure 20.2   Intraoperative image showing the placement of the sutures into the thyroid cartilage ventral to the ST tendon. Four bites are placed to divide the forces between suture and cartilage and thus minimizing the likelihood of suture pull through.

described technique whereby a hole was drilled through the basihyoid bone (Ducharme et al. 2003; Woodie 2005). This was eliminated from the procedure because we and others have observed cases where the suture either breaks on the cut edge of the basihyoid bone or cuts through the basihyoid bone, thus fracturing the caudal aspect of the bone. Using a suture or wire passer placed immediately adjacent to the junction of the lingual process and basihyoid bone, the ipsilateral dorsal suture and contralateral ventral suture are retrieved together and tagged with separate hemostats (Figure 20.3a). It is important that the suture passer is placed immediately dorsal to the basihyoid bone and on its midline to avoid injuring a branch of the lingual artery/vein that is abaxial. The procedure is repeated on the contralateral side. (Note: If this vessel is inadvertently damaged, profuse bleeding can occur. Placement of a temporary tagged sponge can be used to control the hemorrhage until the sutures are tied.) In most instances, tying of the sutures leads to pressure by the rostral aspect of the thyroid cartilage on the bleeding vessels dorsal to the basihyoid bone and arrests the bleeding. A complication associated with suture breakage or the suture cutting through the thyroid cartilage is deviation of the larynx toward the intact suture (Figure 20.4). To

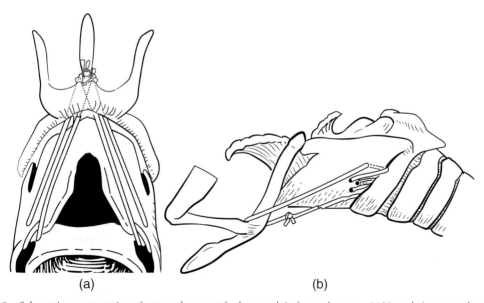

(a)   (b)

Figure 20.3   Schematic representation of suture placement for laryngeal tie-forward sutures. (a) Ventral view: note that the dorsal suture is placed ipsilateral while the ventral suture crosses to the contralateral side. (b) Lateral view: note that both sutures are placed dorsal to the basihyoid bone to enhance the dorsal mobilization of the larynx.

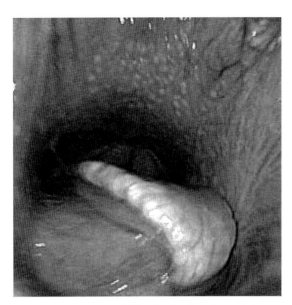

Figure 20.4   Two-year-old Standardbred racehorse 1 day postoperatively. Note deviation of the epiglottis to the left associated with suture pull through from the right thyroid cartilage.

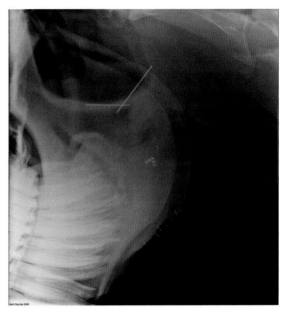

Figure 20.5   Radiograph of a 6-year-old Thoroughbred mare after laryngeal tie-forward using metal implants to reinforce the thyroid cartilage based on Rossignol's technique.

prevent this complication, the ventral sutures are first tied together. Because of the friction associated with the multiple passes in each side of the thyroid cartilage, the ventral sutures (one from each side) can be tied securely without applying any tension on the dorsal suture. The horse's nose is lifted by a nonsterile assistant so the head and neck are angled at ~90°. After the first throw on the ventral sutures, the surgeons verify that the ventral aspect of the thyroid cartilage is 1 cm dorsal to the basihyoid bone and ~1.5 cm rostral to its caudal edge. The dorsal sutures (one from each side) are then tied. The head is then returned to a semiextended position with the bridge of the nose supported by a wedge pad to prevent tension on the sutures.

An alternative method to prevent tearing of the suture in the thyroid cartilage is to place the sutures through a stainless steel button that adds stability to the thyroid cartilage (Figure 20.5). This has been introduced by Rossignol et al. (2012). The sutures are first passed through the metallic button (Arthrex® suture button) and each thread is then passed through the thyroid cartilage ventral to the ST tendon. Sutures are then placed around the basi-

hyoid as described above. Because of the lack of suture friction at the thyroid lamina, the ventral sutures cannot be tied together without the dorsal sutures. However, the ventral and dorsal sutures can be tied together.

A complication of the procedure is seroma formation surrounding the larynx. To prevent this complication, when reapposing the SH muscle with absorbable size 0 suture, the fascia on the ventral aspect of the larynx is incorporated in the muscle layer closure to minimize dead space.

Closure of the subcutaneous tissue and skin is routine with the incision protected with an impervious drape during the recovery period. The head should be supported when placing the horse in the recovery stall to avoid excessive tension on the prosthetic sutures. For the same reason, we avoid the use of head rope and assisted recovery with traction on the head. Return to training is recommended at 2 weeks following surgery. In the first 2 weeks postoperatively the horses are fed and watered at shoulder height. If 2-year olds are operated on between racing seasons, we do not recommend pasture turnout to minimize constant lowering of the head while grazing.

Results

It is worth noting that a recent meta-analysis (evidence-based level II) was performed to identify which procedure was the most effective treatment for DDSP in racehorses (Allen et al. 2012). In their review, major obstacles were identified in the pursuit of their analysis: the diagnosis was not always confirmed at exercise, controls were often missing, and when controls were present the disease status of the control was not established by exercising videoendoscopy. Their conclusion was that "it is currently not possible to determine which procedure is the most appropriate." This is also true for publications evaluating the laryngeal tie-forward. Originally, the procedure was reported without control in 116 horses (Woodie et al. 2005a) (evidence-based level IV) and was associated with a success rate of ~80%. Earnings and owners/trainer assessment was used as a surrogate for the disease status after surgery. Our second study was a case-control study (evidence-based level II; $n = 106$) where we documented that following surgery the performance/earnings of horses with DDSP were restored to that of matched control (Cheetham et al. 2008). This last data set was collected in racehorses only (<2400 m) and the results may or may not be extrapolated to other groups of horses.

Management of complications

Of 608 horses, our short-term complication rate was 7.2%. Specific short-term complications included 3.3% intraoperative bleeding, 1.8% intraoperative suture problems, 1.6% incisional (0.5% infection, 1.1% swelling/seromas), and 0.3% stylohyoid bone fracture. Of the horses operated 1.7% had previously been treated with a laryngeal tie-forward.

Suture failure may occur intra- or postoperatively. If the left or right sutures were tied separately and implant failure occurs, coughing is often observed and upon endoscopy the epiglottis is deviated to one side (Figure 20.5). When this complication develops, revision of the procedure is required. This is why it is preferable to have the left and right sutures tied together where failure would lead to caudal retraction of the larynx (see Chapter 23 on failed treatment of DDSP), rather than epiglottic deviation.

Incisional infection

Early incisional infection can be treated with appropriate drainage followed by lavage with sterile saline and broad-spectrum antibiotics. If the infection does not resolve and a draining tract develops, so that no abscess is formed, delaying suture removal for 60 days would allow for perilaryngeal fibrosis to occur, therefore preventing caudal retraction of the larynx after suture removal. If an abscess is present, it must be addressed to prevent compression of the larynx. Removal of the suture can be done standing with the horse sedated appropriately and infiltration with local anesthesia. The knots are identified with ultrasound and the incision is centered on the knots. If the knots cannot be identified on ultrasonography, the incision is centered on the aspect of the basihyoid bone where most surgeons place the knots. After the knot is grasped with a hemostat, the suture is cut and removed. We have not treated an incisional infection with the technique modification where each suture is passed four times in the thyroid cartilage nor if metallic implants have been placed. General anesthesia may be needed in those cases for a more detailed surgical exploration or manipulation. The incision is left to heal by second intention.

Recurrence

Horses that initially responded to treatment may experience recurrence (see Chapter 23 for further details).

Vocal cord collapse

Vocal cord collapse has been reported in one case following a laryngeal tie-forward (Dart 2006). The authors have proposed that the cause of vocal cord collapse is likely interference with the function of the cricothyroid muscle or its innervation. The authors have proposed that the cause of this complication is likely interference with the function of the CT muscle or its innervation either by surgical dissection or fibrosis after surgery. That is, why emphasis is placed on preserving this muscle during elevation of the ST tendon/muscle. Possible additional explanations for this type of complication are sutures that are inadvertently placed around the cricoid cartilage instead of the thyroid cartilage, thus interfering with the contraction of the CT muscle (see chapter 23 on revision of DDSP treatment). We have seen the latter in a few cases.

Other technical tips/concerns

- Do not place the sutures in the thyroid lamina too dorsally and rostrally as you may penetrate the ventricle that is most caudal in the dorsal location.
- Ventriculocordectomy performed at the same time as the laryngeal tie-forward should be done with caution as the sutures will lose the laryngeal mucosal barrier and be separated from contamination only by the cricoarytenoideus lateralis muscle. If bleeding is observed from the ventricle postoperatively you may want to consider continuing the antimicrobials a little longer as ventricle penetration has occurred.
- Swelling from one or more ventricles postoperatively is likely due to hematoma near the ventricle and is of no permanent consequence.

References

Allen KJ, Christley RM, Birchall MA, Franklin SH. 2012. A systematic review of the efficacy of interventions for dynamic intermittent dorsal displacement of the soft palate. *Equine Veterinary Journal* 44(3):259–266.

Chalmers HJ, Yeager AE, Ducharme NG. 2009. Ultrasonographic assessment of laryngohyoid position as a predictor of dorsal displacement of the soft palate in horses. *Veterinary Radiology* 50(1):91–96.

Cheetham J, Pigott JH, Thorson LM, Mohammed HO, Ducharme NG. 2008. Racing performance following the laryngeal tie-forward procedure: A case-controlled study. *Equine Veterinary Journal* 40(5):501–507

Cheetham J, Pigott JH, Hermanson JW, Campoy L, Soderholm LV, Thorson LM, Ducharme NG. 2009. Role of the hypoglossal nerve in equine nasopharyngeal stability. *Journal of Applied Physiology* 107(2):471–477.

Dart AJ. 2006. Vocal fold collapse after laryngeal tie forward correction of dorsal displacement of the soft palate in horses. *Veterinary Radiology Ultrasound* 50(1):584–585.

Ducharme NG, Hackett RP, Woodie JB, Dykes N, Erb HN, Mitchell LM, Soderholm LV. 2003. Investigations into the role of the thyrohyoid muscles in the pathogenesis of dorsal displacement of the soft palate in horses. *Equine Veterinary Journal* 35(3):258–263.

Holcombe SJ, Beard WL, Hinchcliff KW, Robertson JT. 1994. Effect of sternothyrohyoid myectomy on upper airway mechanics in normal horses. *Journal of Applied Physiology* 77(6):2812–2816.

Holcombe SJ, Rodriquez K, Lane J, Caron JP. 2006. Cricothyroid muscle function and vocal fold stability in exercising horses. *Veterinary Surgery* 35(6):495–500.

Kelly JR, Carmalt J, Hendrick S, Wilson DG, Shoemaker R. 2008. Biomechanical comparison of six suture configurations using a large diameter polyester prosthesis in the muscular process of the equine arytenoid cartilage. *Veterinary Surgery* 37(6):580–587.

Rossignol F, Ouachee E, Boening KJ. 2012. A modified laryngeal tie forward procedure using metallic implants for treatment of dorsal displacement of the soft palate in horses. *Veterinary Surgery* 41(6):685–688.

Woodie JB, Ducharme NG, Kanter P, Hackett RP, Erb HN. 2005a. Surgical advancement of the larynx (laryngeal tie forward) as a treatment for dorsal displacement of the soft palate in horses: A prospective study 2001–2004. *Equine Veterinary Journal* 37(5):418–423.

Woodie JB, Ducharme NG, Hackett RP, Erb HN, Mitchell LM, Soderholm LV. 2005b. Can an external device prevent dorsal displacement of the soft palate during strenuous exercise? *Equine Veterinary Journal* 37(5):425–429.

21 Laser Palatoplasty

Jan Hawkins

Introduction

Dorsal displacement of the soft palate (DDSP) is a common cause of exercise intolerance and upper respiratory tract noise in performance horses. Laser palatoplasty is one of many surgical procedures which have been described to manage DDSP (Alkabes et al. 2010; Hogan and Palmer 2002; Ortved et al. 2010; Smith and Embertson 2005; Tate et al. 1990). Laser palatoplasty has been used to stiffen the soft palate through laser-induced fibrosis. There have been three studies detailing the use of laser palatoplasty in the horse (Alkabes et al. 2010; Hogan and Palmer 2002; Smith and Embertson 2005). Two are clinically based and concentrated on racehorses and one details clinical, histologic, magnetic resonance imaging, and biomechanical findings associated with laser palatoplasty. Laser palatoplasty is frequently combined with other surgical procedures including sternothyroideus myotenectomy and laryngeal tie-forward.

Surgical technique

Laser palatoplasty can be performed with the horse standing or while under general anesthesia. Standing laser palatoplasty is performed with the horse restrained in stocks and sedated with detomidine hydrochloride (0.01–0.02 mg/kg, IV) and butorphanol tartrate (0.01–0.02 mg/kg, IV). The most important part of the standing procedure is to initiate DDSP. This can be accomplished by initiating a swallow and then topically desensitizing the soft palate with anesthetic solution (Cetacaine, Lidocaine, or Mepivacaine) under endoscopic guidance to maintain palate displacement or a mouth speculum can be used to facilitate manual displacement of the soft palate. Finally, if neither of these two techniques work the epiglottis can be retracted caudally using bronchoesophageal grasping forceps (Figure 21.1).

A diode laser is used for the procedure. The laser is set to 15 watts in continuous wave and delivered in 1 second on and 1 second off intervals. A 600-μm,contact-sculpted fiber is passed down the biopsy channel of the endoscope to contact the caudal free edge of the soft palate. The calculated power density for this procedure is $10417\ \text{W/cm}^2$. The procedure begins with the laser fiber contacting the soft palate on the midline of the soft palate ~2–3 mm from the caudal free edge. The laser fiber is then moved 2–4 mm and the laser

Advances in Equine Upper Respiratory Surgery, First Edition. Edited by Jan Hawkins.
© 2015 ACVS Foundation. Published 2015 by John Wiley & Sons, Inc.

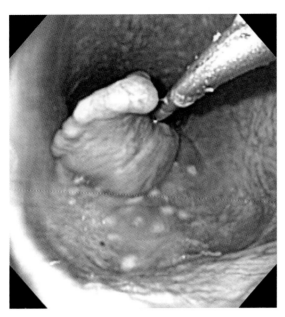

Figure 21.1   Endoscopic photograph depicting retraction of the esophagus with bronchoesophageal grasping forceps.

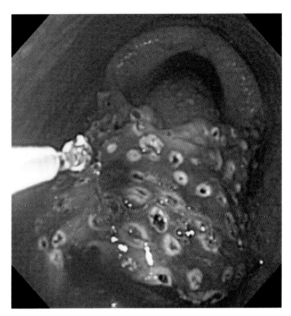

Figure 21.2   Intraoperative endoscopic photograph of diode laser palatoplasty under general anesthesia prior to laryngeal tie-forward.

is discharged. Typically laser contact points go beyond the tip of the epiglottis and extend to both sides of the soft palate adjacent to the epiglottis (see Figure 21.2). This procedure is repeated until a total of 2400 joules have been delivered to the soft palate (Figure 21.2). Based on a previous study (Alkabes et al. 2010), this number of joules consistently resulted in fibrosis and replacement of soft palate musculature with fibrous connective tissue and is what the author has done clinically without adverse effects.

Laser palatoplasty under general anesthesia

When performed under general anesthesia, the horse is orotracheally intubated and positioned in lateral recumbency (side does not matter). Because the laser can initiate airway fire in the presence of 100% oxygen, the horse should not be connected to anesthetic gases in the presence of an activated laser. With orotracheal intubation the soft palate is located dorsal to the epiglottis and greatly facilitates the surgical procedure. I commonly perform laser palatoplasty immediately prior to laryngeal tie-forward and certainly prefer to perform laser

palatoplasty under general anesthesia because it greatly shortens the time necessary to complete the procedure when compared to performing the procedure with the horse standing.

Aftercare

Prophylactic antimicrobials are not necessary for laser palatoplasty. Systemic and topical anti-inflammatory medication is recommended. The author typically administers phenylbutazone 2.2 mg/kg, PO, q12h; dexamethasone, IV (20 mg, q24h for 2 days; then 10 mg q24h for 2 days; then 10 mg q48h for two treatments); and topical pharyngeal spray (dimethyl sulfoxide, glycerin, prednisolone, and sterile water) 10 mL per transnasal catheter twice a day for 7–10 days. Horses have a variable amount of soft palate inflammation following the procedure and some horses do experience postoperative dysphagia associated with painful swallowing (Figure 21.3). These anti-inflammatories help minimize this complication. The author recommends 30 days of

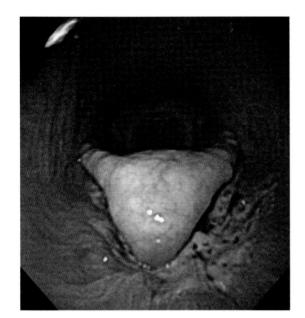

Figure 21.3   Standing endoscopic photograph 7 days post diode laser palatoplasty and laryngeal tie-forward.

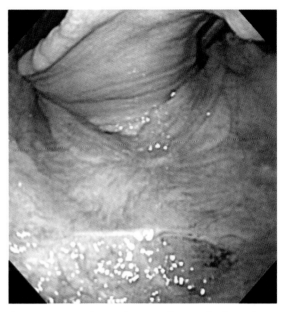

Figure 21.4   Standing endoscopic photograph of complete healing of the soft palate post diode laser palatoplasty. Note areas of fibrosis and contracture of the caudal free edge of the soft palate.

rest before returning to exercise to ensure healing of the soft palate (Figure 21.4).

Complications

Postoperative complications associated with laser palatoplasty include dysphagia and coughing, and soft palate granulation tissue masses occasionally develop (Figure 21.5). In most instances, these complications resolve with anti-inflammatory medication and within the first 7–14 days following the surgical procedure.

Discussion

Of the two studies reported, one reported improved racing performance in 63% of treated horses (Smith and Embertson 2005) and the other reported 50 of 52 returning to racing after surgery (Hogan and Palmer 2002). Other than these two studies, most of the evidence regarding the efficacy of laser palatoplasty is largely anecdotal. Owners elect for laser palatoplasty for two primary reasons: (1) the procedure can be performed standing on an outpatient basis and (2) as an ancillary procedure to

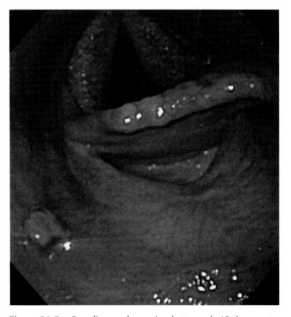

Figure 21.5   Standing endoscopic photograph 45 days post diode laser palatoplasty. Note granulation tissue mass on right aspect of the caudal soft palate.

laryngeal tie-forward. Laser palatoplasty can also be combined with sternothyroideus tenectomy as described by Hogan and Palmer. Unfortunately, the indications for laser palatoplasty over other surgical techniques for the management of DDSP are not very clear but are the author's subjective opinion that laser palatoplasty is a useful technique. I routinely recommend laser palatoplasty in combination with laryngeal tie-forward because I have had some treatment failures (recurrence of DDSP) when laryngeal tie-forward was performed alone. Subjectively, these treatment failures have been less when combined with laser palatoplasty. Finally, laser staphylectomy has been reported as an adjunctive treatment for persistent DDSP following laryngeal tie-forward (Ortved et al. 2010) (see Chapter 24). In that study, six of eight horses with continued persistent DDSP following laryngeal tie-forward were successfully treated with laser staphylectomy. Although the techniques of laser palatoplasty and laser staphylectomy differ, one can extrapolate that the outcome is similar. Laser palatoplasty results in contracture and fibrosis of the caudal aspect of the soft palate and thus alters its biomechanical properties. How laser palatoplasty alters the function of the soft palate is not well understood. In one study, biomechanical testing of the soft palate post laser palatoplasty failed to show an increase in elastic modulus (Alkabes et al. 2010). It actually resulted in a decrease in soft palate elastic modulus. Perhaps

any change in the biomechanical properties alters the change in function may lead to the desired outcome.

References

Alkabes KC, Hawkins JF, Miller MA, Nauman E, Widmer W, Dunco D, Kras J, Couetil L, Lescun TB, Gautam R. 2010. Evaluation of the effects of transendoscopic diode laser palatoplasty on clinical, histologic, magnetic resonance imaging, and biomechanical findings in horses. *American Journal of Veterinary Research* 71(5):575–582.
Hogan PM, Palmer SE. 2002. Transendoscopic laser cauterization of the soft palate as an adjunctive treatment for dorsal displacement in the racehorse. *Proceedings of the Annual Convention of the American Association of Equine Practitioners* 48:228–230.
Ortved KF, Cheetham J, Mitchell LM, Ducharme NG. 2010. Successful treatment of dorsal displacement of the soft palate and evaluation of laryngohyoid position in 15 racehorses. *Equine Veterinary Journal* 42(1):23–29.
Smith JJ, Embertson RM. 2005. Sternothyroideus myotomy, staphylectomy, and oral caudal soft palate photothermoplasty for treatment of dorsal displacement of the soft palate in 102 thoroughbred racehorses. *Veterinary Surgery* 34(1):5–10.
Tate LP, Sweeney CL, Bowman KF, Newman HC, Duckett WM. 1990. Transendoscopic Nd:YAG laser surgery for treatment of epiglottal entrapment and dorsal displacement of the soft palate in the horse. *Veterinary Surgery* 19(5):356–363.

22 Surgical Management of Dorsal Displacement of the Soft Palate in the Racehorse

Patricia Hogan

Introduction

Dorsal displacement of the soft palate (DDSP) is a common cause of expiratory upper respiratory noise and exercise intolerance in the racehorse. The challenge is in confirming the presumptive diagnosis of DDSP. The disease is frequently suspected based on poor racing performance and upper respiratory noise made during exercise and is often not definitively diagnosed prior to evaluation for surgery. It is also not unusual for DDSP to be confused with epiglottic entrapment as some trainers will refer to DDSP as "entrapping." For obvious reasons, the diseases differ in regard to definitive treatment. It is also critical for the clinician to consider the important underlying role that inflammatory airway disease plays in the transient expression of upper airway obstructions, particularly DDSP and dynamic pharyngeal collapse. This is a particularly important consideration in the young 2-year-old racehorse, and also in the older seasoned racehorse with normal airway anatomy and no previous history of an upper airway obstruction. Many of these horses are mistakenly diagnosed as surgi-

cal candidates and instead, respond very well to medical treatment of lower airway inflammation.

Evaluation of the racehorse suspected with DDSP should have a complete physical examination performed before standing endoscopic examination. It is not uncommon for horses to be referred for surgical treatment of DDSP and upon physical examination have been found to have other problems such as lower airway disease, cardiac arrhythmias (i.e., atrial fibrillation), and even lameness. In those situations, these abnormalities must be treated before considering surgical correction as some of these horses will have DDSP resolve with treatment of the initiating cause. Standing endoscopic examination for DDSP has been described previously in Chapter 17. Racehorses suspected of DDSP may have a normal endoscopic examination at rest, or subjectively, may have easily inducible DDSP at rest. An endoscopic finding that can be indicative of DDSP is ulceration of the caudal border of the soft palate (Figure 22.1). Standing endoscopic examination can also rule out recurrent laryngeal neuropathy (RLN), epiglottic entrapment, arytenoid chondritis, or other abnormalities

Advances in Equine Upper Respiratory Surgery, First Edition. Edited by Jan Hawkins.
© 2015 ACVS Foundation. Published 2015 by John Wiley & Sons, Inc.

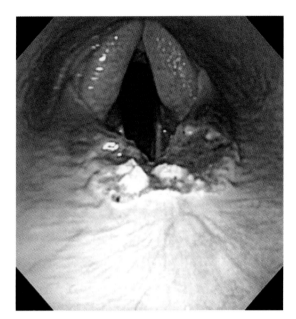

Figure 22.1   Standing endoscopic photograph of a Standardbred racehorse with ulceration of the caudal free edge of the soft palate in a horse with DDSP.

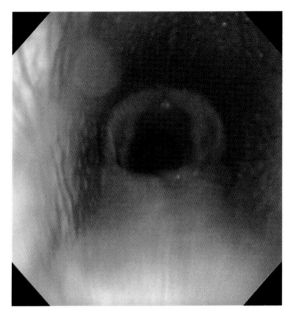

Figure 22.2   Endoscopic photograph of a Standardbred racehorse with DDSP during high-speed treadmill exercise.

which could potentially cause the same clinical signs of exercise intolerance and upper respiratory noise. It is very important that the endoscopic examination include the lumen of the trachea down to the bifurcation. Once the standing endoscopic examination has been performed, options should be discussed with the owner/trainer.

For all racehorses suspected of DDSP without confirmation of the disorder on resting endoscopic examination, the author recommends either high-speed treadmill (HSTM) or overground endoscopy to confirm the suspected diagnosis of DDSP before pursuing surgical treatment. However, some owners/trainers are convinced of the diagnosis based on their own clinical observations and experience, and prefer to pursue corrective surgery without treadmill or overground endoscopy.

The purpose of treadmill or overground endoscopy is to either confirm the diagnosis of DDSP or rule out other upper respiratory abnormalities which can only be diagnosed during exercising endoscopy. This includes, but is not limited to, axial deviation of the aryepiglottic folds, RLN, vocal cord collapse, or pharyngeal

collapse. Horses with these conditions require other treatments besides those used for DDSP. Horses with confirmed DDSP during exercising endoscopy (Figure 22.2) are candidates for surgical correction. It is not unusual for a racehorse to not exhibit DDSP during exercising endoscopy but have clinical signs compatible with the disease. The author typically recommends surgical correction for these horses.

Surgical correction

Most horses the author is asked to evaluate for DDSP have already had some form of conservative management. This typically includes figure 8 noseband, tongue tie, Cornell collar, or a Z-bit. Therefore, all horses with a diagnosis of DDSP, in spite of conservative treatment, are considered candidates for surgery. Three surgical options are discussed with the owner/trainer: laryngeal tie-forward, laser palatoplasty, and sternothyroideus myotenectomy. The author believes that the laryngeal tie-forward provides the best prognosis for the racehorse in confirmed cases of DDSP and is recommended to the owner as the ideal treatment choice. Laser palatoplasty can be recommended as a standalone procedure or in combination with laryngeal tie-forward or sternothyroideus myotenectomy, particularly if soft palate ulceration is present. Laser palatoplasty is appealing to some trainers because it can be performed standing and on an outpatient basis. Finally, sternothyroideus myotenectomy, without *staphylectomy*, is preferred by many Standardbred trainers and can be performed in the field (see Chapter 19). In the author's experience, when surgical options are discussed with the owner/trainer, laryngeal tie-forward is most frequently chosen, unless financial limitations are a concern. For those cases, laser palatoplasty or sternothyroideus myotenectomy is elected.

Laryngeal tie-forward

With the recent advent and economic availability of the portable dynamic endoscopic units, many more horses are being diagnosed definitively with DDSP at the racetrack. Largely due to the perceived success of an external laryngeal device, the Cornell Collar (Woodie et al. 2005b), a surgical procedure was developed in the 1990s to permanently mimic the actions of the collar. The premise of the laryngeal tie-forward is to surgically position the larynx dorsal to the basihyoid bone during exercise (Ducharme et al. 2003; Cheetham et al. 2008; Woodie 2005a, 2005b).

The current technique of laryngeal tie-forward is described in Chapter 20. Surgeon differences with this procedure are detailed here. There are two methods described for securing the suture to the basihyoid bone: (1) suture insertion through a hole drilled through the basihyoid bone and (2) suture placement around the basihyoid bone on each side of the lingual process. Drilling through the basihyoid bone has largely been omitted from the surgical procedure because of the rare possibility of a fracture of the basihyoid through the drill hole and loss of the desired laryngeal position. The alternate and most recently described method requires passing the suture around the basihyoid bone, rather than drilling a hole through it. This technique, utilizes two strands of No. 5 suture material. Both Fiberwire (Arthrex) and Mer-

silene are acceptable suture materials, with Fiberwire being preferred by most surgeons. Therefore, instead of drilling through the basihyoid bone, an ASIF wire passer is placed on one side of the lingual process and directed dorsal to the basihyoid bone, so that it exits at the caudal aspect of the basihyoid bone. This is then repeated on the other side. Once the wire passer is positioned under the basihyoid bone, the suture needle is placed inside the end of the wire passer and the suture is pulled under the bone. Once the suture is secured through or around the basihyoid bone, each free end containing the needle is directed through each respective side of the thyroid cartilage. If not already transected from a prior surgery, the tendon of insertion of the sternothyroideus muscle is elevated and transected before making the pass with the needle. The needle is then passed through the thyroid lamina using the remnant of the tendon as a landmark for needle placement. The initial pass is just ventral to the tendon of insertion, extends approximately 1.5 cm and exits rostrally. The second pass is placed then just dorsal to the tendon of insertion and is angled in the same direction. These two passes thus serve to form a loop in the thyroid lamina. The needle is then cut from the end of the suture and the two free ends held together with a hemostat while the procedure is repeated on the other side of the larynx. Once both sutures are securely in position, a triple throw is placed in the suture on one side of the larynx, a nonsterile assistant elevates the nose of the horse into flexion, and the suture is gathered until the larynx is pulled forward enough that the ventral aspect of the thyroid cartilage is just even with or slightly rostral to the caudal aspect of the basihyoid bone. It is helpful to have a sterile assistant place the tip of a ground-down needle holder on the first knot to secure the degree of tension and prevent slippage until the second throw is thrown and secured. The author uses a small fly-fishing forceps that is smooth and will not fray or crush the suture when applied. Multiple knots (at least —five to six) are applied and then the nose of the horse is gently lowered back to the neutral position. The entire process is then repeated on the other side of the larynx. If the larynx is secured properly into place, the previously palpable ventral space between the cricoid cartilage and the basihyoid bone is no longer present, and the small muscles alongside this area will be visibly "bunched up." The objective is to place the larynx in such a position that the rostral edge of the thyroid cartilage is just ahead of the caudal aspect of the basihyoid bone.

Closure is very simple and consists of an opposing sternohyoideus musculature using 0 polydioxanone (PDS), taking care to occasionally tack down to the ventral fascia of the larynx. Incorporating the ventral fascia into the closure will limit seroma formation in the postoperative period. The author places just two centrally located simple interrupted subcutaneous sutures to oppose the skin edges and then staples are used to close the skin. There is no tension in this area at all once the horse is standing and therefore a complete subcutaneous closure is not required. A rolled gauze stent is sutured over the incision line with No. 1 polypropylene to protect the site and provide incisional compression for the first 5 days. It is very important when removing the horse from the operating table and placing it into the recovery stall, that the head is supported in a ventroflexed position so as not to place undue tension on the surgically secured larynx. A lead rope attached to the chin ring of the halter and run through the rings of the leg hobbles in the hoist is held by an assistant and maintains the head in a flexed position until the horse is secured in lateral recumbency.

Horses are provided stall rest with daily hand walking for 2 weeks prior to a return to training. Antibiotics are not routinely used postoperatively but oral phenylbutazone administration (4 mg/kg, PO) is recommended for 5–7 days. Occasionally a horse will develop a seroma at the incision site 10–14 days postoperatively, but this can usually be resolved with the administration of anti-inflammatories (phenylbutazone and Naquasone) and rarely requires surgical drainage. Horses are recommended to be fed and watered at shoulder level whenever possible in order to lessen tension on the laryngeal fixation.

Laser cautery of the soft palate (palatoplasty)

Transendoscopic diode or Nd:YAG laser cautery of the pharyngeal surface of the soft palate was initially reported as an adjunctive treatment for DDSP by the author in 2002 (Hogan 2002). The procedure was recommended in conjunction with a sternothy-roideus tenectomy and was designed to replace the staphylectomy. At the time of publication, a staphylectomy through a ventral laryngotomy was a very common surgical procedure for DDSP in horses. The purpose of staphylectomy is to remove a central portion of the free edge of the palate, resulting in fibrosis or scarring, and thus theoretically, a tighter seal between the soft palate and the epiglottis.

The hypothesis for laser cautery of the soft palate was borrowed from human medicine where people with persistent issues with snoring were thought to have excessive flaccidity of the soft palate. Surgical procedures, including thermal cautery, were designed to create fibrosis of this tissue, thus reducing the incidence of airway stridor during sleep. It was thought that cauterizing the free edge of the soft palate in horses would achieve the desired fibrosis or "stiffening" of the palate, be less invasive than a staphylectomy, and thus requires a reduced lay-up period. Recent research has raised questions as to whether transendoscopic laser cautery actually creates enough fibrosis to result in an appreciable "stiffening" of the soft palate (Alkabes et al. 2010), but the procedure is still popular.

Horses are restrained with a nose twitch or lip chain and lightly sedated with xylazine or detomidine hydrochloride only; butorphanol is not recommended due to the subtle side effects of facial tremors or head movement. The soft palate is locally anesthetized with mepivacaine and swallowing is induced to maintain the soft palate in a displaced position. A 600-µm bare diode laser fiber is passed through the biopsy channel of the endoscope and using contact technique, is applied for 1–2 seconds at 2-mm intervals along the free edge of the soft palate under 15 watts of power. The zone of application should extend approximately 1.5 cm rostrally and extend around most of the rim of the palate. If an ulcer is present, it is fully cauterized (Figure 22.3).

Antibiotics are not required but horses are treated perioperatively with intravenous phenylbutazone (4 mg/kg) and tetanus toxoid. Postoperatively phenylbutazone is continued orally for 5–7 days, pharyngeal spray for 14 days, and a decreasing regimen of oral prednisolone is prescribed for 21 days. Horses are allowed hand walking for 3 days and then may return to light training. The laser site is

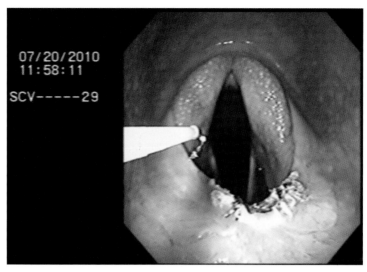

Figure 22.3   Endoscopic photograph of diode laser palatoplasty of an ulcer on the caudal free margin of the soft palate in a racehorse with DDSP.

evaluated endoscopically at 7 days, and if no excessive swelling is noted, horses may return to full training.

Sternothyroideus myotenectomy with/without staphylectomy (Llewellyn procedure)

The Llewellyn procedure is still preferred by some trainers/owners and veterinary practitioners (Llewellyn and Petrowitz 1997). This procedure does not require specialized equipment and can be performed in the field. It is not unusual to have this procedure performed prior to referral to a surgical center and owners/trainers should be asked if the procedure has been performed. It is the least expensive of the surgical techniques used for the management of DDSP in the racehorse. Refer Chapter 19 for further details regarding this surgical technique.

In summary, management of DDSP in the racehorse centers on the confirmation of the correct diagnosis preferably with exercising endoscopy and a frank discussion with the owner/trainer about the available surgical options and the prognosis for each. Each of the described procedures has its pros and cons. However, mounting clinical evidence suggests that the laryngeal tie-forward plus or minus being combined with laser palatoplasty

is the treatment of choice for the management of DDSP in the racehorse.

References

Alkabes KC, Hawkins JF, Miller MA, Nauman E, Widmer W, Dunco D, Kras J, Couetil L, Lescun TB, Gautam R. 2010. Evaluation of the effects of transendoscopic diode laser palatoplasty on clinical, histologic, magnetic resonance imaging, and biomechanical findings in horses. *American Journal of Veterinary Research* 71(5):575–582.

Cheetham J, Pigott JH, Thorson LM, Mohammed HO, Ducharme NG. 2008. Racing performance following the laryngeal tie-forward procedure: A case-controlled study. *Equine Veterinary Journal* 40(5):501–507.

Ducharme NG, Hackett RP, Woodie JB, Dykes N, Erb HN, Mitchell LM, Soderholm LV. 2003. Investigations into the role of the thyrohyoid muscles in the pathogenesis of dorsal displacement of the soft palate in horses. *Equine Veterinary Journal* 35(3):258–263.

Hogan PM, Palmer SE. 2002. Transendoscopic laser cauterization of the soft palate as an adjunctive treatment for dorsal displacement in the racehorse. *Proceedings of the Annual Convention of the American Association of Equine Practitioners* 48:228–230.

Llewellyn HR, Petrowitz AB. 1997. Sternothyroideus myotomy for the treatment of dorsal displacement of the soft palate. *Proceedings of the Annual Convention of the American Association of Equine Practitioners* 43:239–243.

Woodie JB, Ducharme NG, Kanter P, Hackett RP, Erb HN. 2005a. Surgical advancement of the larynx (laryngeal tie forward) as a treatment for dorsal displacement of the soft palate in horses: A prospective study 2001–2004. *Equine Veterinary Journal* 37(5):418–423.

Woodie JB, Ducharme NG, Hackett RP, Erb HN, Mitchell LM, Soderholm LV. 2005b. Can an external device prevent dorsal displacement of the soft palate during strenuous exercise? *Equine Veterinary Journal* 37(5): 425–429.

23

Dorsal Displacement of the Soft Palate: Evaluation of the Horse with Poor Performance Following Attempted Surgical Correction

Norm G. Ducharme

Introduction

Horses that have failed to respond to prior surgical treatment for intermittent displacement of the soft palate should be examined carefully to ensure the actual diagnosis and the cause of failure. Indeed a dynamic exercising, endoscopic examination should follow a failed surgical treatment to ensure that the original diagnosis was correct. In addition, one should consider that given that complex diagnosis (meaning more than one cause of obstruction) has been reported in 24–69.7% of horses at exercise (Strand and Skjerve 2011; Witte et al. 2011) the potential exists that the cause of the current obstruction may not be secondary to dorsal displacement of the soft palate (DDSP). Therefore, the horse may have responded to treatment for DDSP but the comorbid cause of obstruction persists. Treatment should then be focused on the proven cause of obstruction, not a speculative diagnosis. If inflammation is still present after the prior surgical treatment and results in an inflammatory epiglottic or subepiglottic process, this must be addressed before proceeding with additional diagnostics. Ongoing epiglottic and subepiglottic

inflammation can certainly predispose to the induction of DDSP.

As a surgical principle, it is unwise to repeat a surgical procedure for which the animal has never responded to the original treatment unless the surgical procedure can be documented to have been performed suboptimally or has technically failed (i.e., broken or loose tie-forward suture). Furthermore, the morbidity associated with certain procedures makes their repetition risky. For example, if DDSP is seen after laser-assisted or sclerotic agent treatment of the soft palate, repeating the procedure is not indicated. Indeed, given the lack of positive change in the biomechanical property of the soft palate after "stiffening" procedures (Alkabes et al. 2010; Munoz et al. 2008) and the risk of damage to the palatinus muscle by the procedure, recurrence of DDSP should be treated with an alternative mode of therapy. Likewise given the morbidity associated with staphylectomy, mainly oronasal contamination, repeating the staphylectomy would increase the likelihood of nasopharyngeal contamination to an unwise level.

Horses that originally responded to sternothyrohyoideus muscle resection or laryngeal

Advances in Equine Upper Respiratory Surgery, First Edition. Edited by Jan Hawkins.
© 2015 ACVS Foundation. Published 2015 by John Wiley & Sons, Inc.

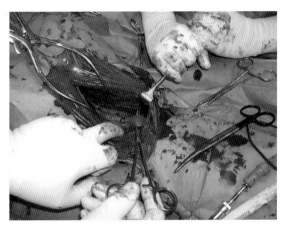

Figure 23.1   Intraoperative images of a failed tie-forward. A Crile hemostat is placed under the left ST muscle that has healed to the cricoid cartilage, re-establishing a caudal force on the larynx.

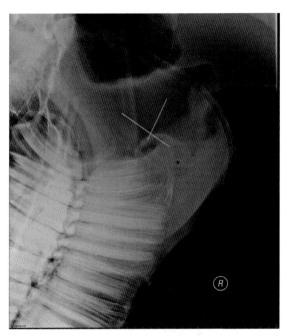

Figure 23.2   Radiograph of a horse with failed tie-forward. Note the ossification at the base of the thyroid cartilage (*) is caudal to the thyrohyoid bone.

tie-forward can be revised without significant increase in patient morbidity. Recurrence after sternothyroideus myotenectomy has been hypothesized to be due to fibrosis of the larynx to the surrounding tissue (Llewellyn, personal communication) or reattachment of the muscle(s) to the larynx (Figure 23.1). In those horses, surgical revision is aimed at lysis of the adhesions surrounding the larynx and transection of the reattachment of the sternothyroideus tendons/muscles.

Horses that initially responded to laryngeal tie-forward may experience recurrence (Witte et al. 2011; Woodie et al. 2005a). Failures are usually acute (i.e., from one race to another). Laryngeal tie-forward revision is indicated if the horse had an initial positive response to surgery and then experiences recurrence of soft palate displacement. A second reason for tie-forward revision is that one can document the diagnosis at exercise and document a technical failure of the surgical procedure. In both cases, a dynamic assessment is obtained by training/racing the horse with an external device that temporarily repositions the larynx more dorsally and forward (Woodie et al. 2005b). Positive response to the device would indicate the need for revision surgery. Alternatively, the horse may be managed by use of the external device.

Evidence of technical failure of the procedure is seen if the sutures have failed to maintain the intraoperative position of the larynx. This can be

assessed radiographically by identifying a caudal position of the ossification at the base of the thyroid cartilage in relation to the thyrohyoid bone (Figure 23.2). One should be careful of the angle of the neck while obtaining those radiographs and the best assessment is obtained with the head in an extended position (Allen et al. 2011; McCluskie et al. 2008) and comparing with pre- and immediate post-operative radiographs. The latter is easier if metal implants have been used (see Chapter 20). Alternatively, the detection of a loose tie-forward suture upon head extension with ultrasound would indicate technical failure (Figure 23.3). Finally, ultrasonographic detection of a suture through the cricoid cartilage instead of the thyroid cartilage would also be indicative of suboptimal surgical procedure (Figure 23.4).

Revision of the laryngeal tie-forward

Revision of the laryngeal tie-forward procedure should take 10–15 minutes longer than the standard procedure if done as follows. One should be aware

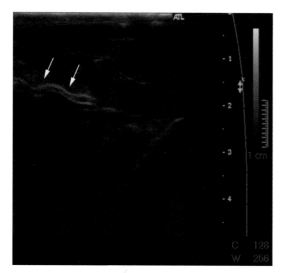

Figure 23.3   Ultrasound image obtained with an 8.5-MHz semiconvex probe showing a loose tie forward suture upon head extension in a 3-year-old Thoroughbred filly.

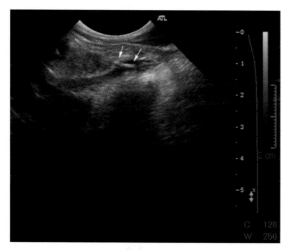

Figure 23.4   Ultrasonographic image obtained with an 8.5-mHz semiconvex probe showing a suture in the cricoid cartilage after laryngeal tie-forward in a 3-year-old Thoroughbred filly.

that endotracheal intubation is more difficult after laryngeal tie-forward either because of narrowing of the nasopharynx or because of the change in angulation between the larynx and oropharynx associated with elevation of the larynx, which tends to result in a more dorsal approach to the larynx. Regarding the actual surgical procedure, the skin

incision is done using the same surgical landmarks as before (1 cm caudal to cricoid cartilage extending rostrally to the base of the lingual process). Blunt separation of the sternohyoideus muscles is done. Using a mixture of blunt and sharp dissection, the adhesions surrounding the ventral and lateral aspects of the larynx are lysed to free the larynx from the surrounding adhesions. The adhesions between the thyroid and basihyoid bone are then released using a curved mayo scissors placed immediately dorsal to the basihyoid. Any remnant of fibrous adhesion between the sternothyroideus tendon/muscle and cricoid or thyroid cartilage is sharply incised. Previous sutures are left in place and new sutures are passed as described in Chapter 20. At this point in the procedure it is important to identify the caudal edge of the thyroid cartilage and not inadvertently place the sutures in the cricoid cartilage. With adhesions the differentiation of caudal edge of the cricoid cartilage and thyroid cartilage are not as evident. Closure is routine although given the amount of dissection needed, the surgical incision is more likely to become more swollen when compared to the initial surgical procedure. Incisional seroma formation is more likely following surgical revision.

References

Alkabes KC, Hawkins JF, Miller MA, Nauman E, Widmer W, Dunco D, Kras J, Couetil LL, Lescun TB, Gautam R. 2010. Evaluation of the effects of transendoscopic diode laser palatoplasty on clinical, histologic, magnetic resonance imaging, and biomechanical findings in horses. *American Journal Veterinary Research* 71(5):575–582.

Allen KJ, Christley RM, Birchall MA, Franklin SH. 2011. A systematic review of the efficacy of interventions for dynamic intermittent dorsal displacement of the soft palate. *Equine Veterinary Journal* 44(3):259–266.

McCluskie LK, Franklin SH, Lane JG, Tremaine WH, Allen KJ. 2008. Effect of head position on radiographic assessment of laryngeal tie-forward procedure in horses. *Veterinary Surgery* 37(7):608–612.

Munoz JA, Marcoux M, Picandet V, Theoret CL, Perron MF, Lepage OM. 2008. Histological and biomechanical effects of palatal sclerotherapy in the horse using sodium tetradecyl sulfate. *The Veterinary Journal* 183(3):316–321.

Strand E, Skjerve E. 2011. Complex dynamic upper airway collapse: Associations between abnormalities in

99 harness racehorses with one or more dynamic disorders. *Equine Veterinary Journal* 44(5):524–528.

Witte SH, Witte TH, Harriss F, Kelly G, Pollock P. 2011. Association of owner-reported noise with findings during dynamic respiratory endoscopy in Thoroughbred racehorses. *Equine Veterinary Journal* 43(1):9–17.

Woodie JB, Ducharme NG, Kanter P, Hackett RP, Erb HN. 2005a. Surgical advancement of the larynx (laryngeal tie-forward) as a treatment for dorsal displacement of the soft palate in horses: A prospective study 2001–2004. *Equine Veterinary Journal* 37(5):418–423.

Woodie JB, Ducharme NG, Hackett RP, Erb HN, Mitchell LM, Soderholm LV. 2005b. Can an external device prevent dorsal displacement of the soft palate during strenuous exercise? *Equine Veterinary Journal* 37(5): 425–429.

24 Treatment of Persistent Dorsal Displacement of the Soft Palate

Norm G. Ducharme

Introduction

Persistent dorsal displacement of the soft palate (DDSP) is easy to recognize endoscopically at rest as the soft palate is permanently positioned dorsal to the epiglottic cartilage. One should ensure that the permanent DDSP observed is real by its persistence despite multiple swallowing attempts and after removal of the twitch to ensure that the lack of replacement of the soft palate is not due to anxiety. Persistent DDSP is associated with respiratory deficit, dysphagia, or both. The emphasis here is "associated with" not necessarily a causal relationship as persistent DDSP may be the cause or the result of the swallowing deficit leading to feed material at the nose and tracheal aspiration. Although rare, we do see horses that are persistently displaced at rest yet during dynamic endoscopy (treadmill or overground) no displacement is present. Therefore one should ensure that there are clinical signs consistent with DDSP during exercise. The old adage of "treating the horse not the radiographs" also applies to endoscopic images. If true persistent displacement is present, the horse should have signs of respi-

ratory abnormality (i.e., gurgling noise and/or decreased performance). Affected horses may also exhibit clinical signs associated with swallowing (i.e., dysphagia, nasopharyngeal, and/or tracheal contamination with food material).

Pathogenesis

There are multiple causes for persistent DDSP. Neuromuscular dysfunction of the soft palate muscles, specifically palatinus and palatopharyngeus muscles or its innervation (pharyngeal branch of the vagus nerves), leads to persistent displacement of the soft palate with dysphagia (Holcombe et al. 1998). Muscular damage is seen in animals with vitamin E/selenium deficiency. Neural deficit can be seen with inflammation surrounding the nerve usually as it courses in the guttural pouches. This represents an efferent neuromuscular failure but a sensory failure may also lead to DDSP presumably because of failure of recruitment of, at least, the palatinus and palatopharyngeal muscles (Holcombe et al. 2001). We believe that an intense sensory stimulation may also lead

Advances in Equine Upper Respiratory Surgery, First Edition. Edited by Jan Hawkins.
© 2015 ACVS Foundation. Published 2015 by John Wiley & Sons, Inc.

to laryngeal descent causing the epiglottic cartilage to become ventral to the soft palate. This may be confirmed following application of local anesthesia to the nasopharynx and correction of persistent DDSP. Sources of enhanced sensory input causing laryngeal descent and persistent DDSP include soft palate and subepiglottic ulceration, and tracheal irritation (causes by tracheal aspiration, ulceration, tracheal catheter, etc.). They are also secondary causes for permanent displacements associated with epiglottic cartilage abnormalities (Ortved et al. 2010). It is presumed that a deformed epiglottic cartilage interferes with a normal laryngopalatal seal creating an unstable palate.

Historical complaints

Horses with persistent DDSP are reported to make a "gurgling" or "snoring" noise at rest and early during exercise. This differs from horses with intermittent DDSP where noise is reported near the end of the exercise event. Coughing is reported more often in horses with persistent DDSP then intermittent DDSP. Horse performance is also diminished with persistent DDSP because the latter interferes with exhalation due to resistive breathing associated DDSP (Holcombe et al. 1998). If dysphagia is present the owner or caretaker will report food and/or water at the nose after eating. We hypothesize that failure of elevation of the larynx during swallowing is also a cause of DDSP with dysphagia. Those are observed following perilaryngeal surgery where postoperative fibrosis limits the laryngeal movement. Likewise hypoglossal nerve disease interferes with contraction of the thyrohyoid muscles whose main function is to elevate the larynx during swallowing. Finally pain associated with temporohyoid disease has been suspected to prevent laryngeal elevation.

Clinical signs and examination

Evidence of dysphagia and/or coughing includes food at the nose and water exiting the nose immediately after drinking. Evidence of coughing is observed either while eating or by detecting feed deposits on the wall of the stall. Endoscopic confirmation of DDSP is seen by observing the position

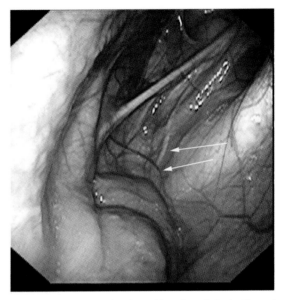

Figure 24.1   Horse with enlarged lymph node in the floor of the medial compartment of the guttural pouch near the pharyngeal branch of the vagus (white arrows).

of the soft palate dorsal to the epiglottic cartilage throughout the exam despite multiple swallows. The goal is to identify the cause of permanent DDSP after its identification. Careful endoscopic exam at rest should identify if persistent displacement is an efferent neurological deficit by evaluating the interior of the guttural pouch. Guttural pouch abnormalities which could affect soft palate function include enlargement of retropharyngeal lymph nodes on the floor of the medial compartment of the guttural pouch (Figure 24.1 or fungal lesion) over the bundle of IX, X, XI, and XII near the internal carotid artery (Figure 24.2). Epiglottic abnormalities can also contribute to persistent DDSP. The latter can be suspected by examining if the soft palate is either flat (Figure 24.3) or has an epiglottic bulge visible through the surface of the soft palate (Figure 24.4). The exam should then continue to detect evidence of dysphagia in the nasopharynx, nasal cavity, and trachea. At that time local anesthesia is applied to the nasopharynx in preparation for manipulation with a laryngeal forceps to explore the epiglottic cartilage and subepiglottic tissues. If DDSP is corrected after application of local anesthesia, this would be evidence that the cause of the DDSP is an appropriate response to

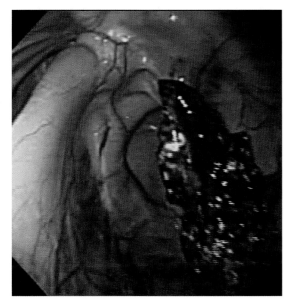

Figure 24.2   Fungal lesions over internal carotid artery in close proximity to cranial nerves IX, X, XI, XII.

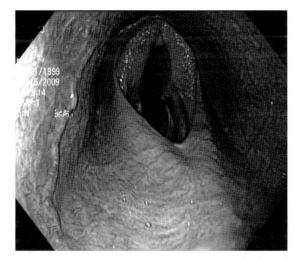

Figure 24.3   Horse with persistent DDSP; notice that the soft palate is flat with no evidence of an epiglottic bulge or mass on its oral surface. This is typically seen in horses with intermittent displacement as well.

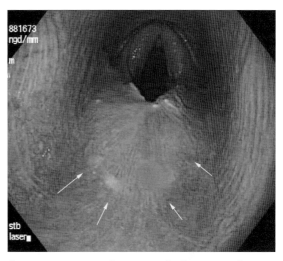

Figure 24.4   Horse with persistent displacement and an epiglottic bulge (white arrows) on its oral surface suggesting that the epiglottic cartilage is enlarged or deformed.

examination may also be beneficial in identifying potential causes of dysphagia or neural disease.

Management

Treatment is directed toward the cause when identified. If guttural pouch disease is present, surgical or pharmacological intervention aims at reducing or eliminating compression and/or inflammation surrounding specifically the vagal, glossopharyngeal, and hypoglossal nerves should be the focus of treatment.

Most cases are associated with deformity of the epiglottic cartilage. Typically an insult to the epiglottic cartilage has resulted in reduction in the size of the epiglottic cartilage and a change in its shape. The consequence of this is that the subepiglottic membrane is now relatively longer and entraps one or both sides of the epiglottic cartilage. Treatment is aimed at first removing the excessive subepiglottic membranes and elevating the larynx surgically using the laryngeal tie-forward (Ortved et al. 2010). This corrects the problem in 40–50% of horses. If the laryngeal tie-forward is not successful, and during endoscopic or radiographic exam, one can see an epiglottic bulge through the soft palate, a staphylectomy is indicated. Typically one can observe after laryngeal elevation, that the

sensory stimuli. The epiglottic cartilage is then elevated and the subepiglottic tissue examined for evidence of granulomas, deformity, chondritis, abscess, and excessive scarring. CT and/or MRI

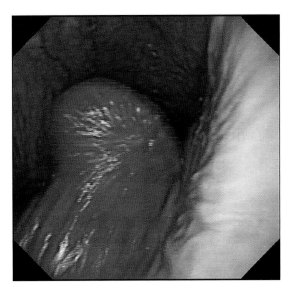

Figure 24.5 Horse with persistent displacement of the soft palate during a swallow after a laryngeal tie-forward. Note the epiglottic bulge underneath the soft palate.

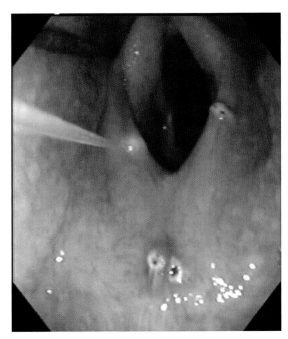

Figure 24.6 Horse with persistent DDSP after laryngeal tie-forward. The horse is being prepared for a laser staphylectomy. Note the three "dots" placed on the soft palate prior to resection with the diode laser. These "dots" serve as a guide for the soft palate resection. The bronchoesophageal grasping forceps are in the upper left of the photograph and the diode laser fiber is contacting the soft palate.

epiglottic bulge is enhanced causing a marked elevation of the soft palate (Figure 24.5). The goal of the staphylectomy is to allow the epiglottic cartilage during swallowing to reach its highest point and open the caudal edge of the soft palate. The enlarged opening allows for the epiglottic cartilage to access the dorsal aspect of the soft palate and stay over the soft palate during swallowing. It must be emphasized that staphylectomy has the potential for allowing feed from the oropharynx to reach the nasopharynx. Clients should be warned of this potential complication. Because of the prior laryngeal tie-forward staphylectomy via laryngotomy is not recommended because of increased risk for exposure and potential infection of the tie-forward prosthetic suture material. Therefore, laser-assisted staphylectomy is preferable as the risk of suture exposure is eliminated and the extent of the staphylectomy can be performed with the horse standing. To prevent excessive resection of the soft palate, the outline of the intended line of resection is first done with the diode laser (Figure 24.6). The soft palate is resected along the reference points placed on the soft palate. A contact, diode laser is used (15–20 watts, 1–3 seconds on and 1 second off). Bronchoesophageal forceps are used

to grasp the cut edge of the soft palate and are useful in completing the staphylectomy.

If tracheal aspiration is observed treatment should be directed toward resolution of this problem. Most commonly the problem is after laryngoplasty with or without ventriculocordectomy. The goal is to rebuild the laryngeal barrier provided by adduction of the vocal cord. This can be achieved by removing the laryngoplasty suture and adducting the arytenoid cartilage or 3–4 mL injection of a bulking agent in the remnant of the vocal fold (Radiesse® Voice, South Mateo, CA).

Rarely have we identified a painful soft palate ulcer that appears to induce the displacement. Most soft palate ulcers do not appear to be painful, however the occasional one is. Those are resected surgically via laryngotomy to resolve the DDSP.

In some cases no causes for persistent DDSP are found. On the hypothesis that this is a result of failure of laryngeal elevation, a laryngeal tie-forward is done empirically.

References

Holcombe SJ, Derksen FJ, Stick JA, Robinson NE. 1998. Effect of bilateral blockade of the pharyngeal branch of the vagus nerve on soft palate function in horses. *American Journal of Veterinary Research* 59(4):504–508.

Holcombe SJ, Derksen FJ, Berney C, Becker AC, Homer NT. 2001. Effect of topical anesthesia of the laryngeal mucosa on upper airway mechanics in exercising horses. *American Journal of Veterinary Research* 62(11):1706–1710.

Ortved KF, Cheetham J, Mitchell LM, Ducharme NG. 2010. Successful treatment of persistent dorsal displacement of the soft palate and evaluation of laryngohyoid position in 15 racehorses. *Equine Veterinary Journal* 42(1):23–29.

Section III

Surgery of the Head

25 Nasal Septum Removal

David E. Freeman

Introduction

Diseases of the nasal septum are rare in horses and a challenge to treat. In particular, the challenge in a performance horse is restoring airflow to the point that the horse can achieve its full athletic potential. Most nasal septal diseases that result in permanent deformity and nasal occlusion require almost complete resection of the nasal septum to improve airflow.

Congenital deformities, cystic degeneration, abscessation, traumatic injury, amyloidosis, fungal infection, and neoplasia of the nasal septum narrow the nasal passages and reduce airflow (Doyle and Freeman 2005; Garrett et al. 2010; Sharma et al. 2010; Shoemaker et al. 2005; Tulleners and Raker 1983). Typical traumatic diseases that require nasal septum resection include septal thickening, malformation, and deviation, because the cartilage in the septum responds to trauma in an exaggerated manner and heals without restoring the normal shape and contour. An important component of traumatic injury is damage to the overlying nasal bones that depress them into the nasal passages,

thereby creating nasal passage compression and partial occlusion that persist after septum removal. Occasionally, when the septal damage is caused by facial trauma, nasal bone deformity might not be evident, or may not correlate with the severity of septal deformity, largely because of the abnormal response of the septal cartilage to trauma. Nasal septum resection is also an important component of surgical correction of wry nose (see Chapter 26) (Schumacher et al. 2008).

Clinical signs of nasal septum disease

Clinical signs of nasal septum disease include abnormal respiratory noise, which can be evident at rest in many horses but is exacerbated by exercise. Exercise tolerance is markedly reduced. Head trauma is assumed and not witnessed in some cases caused by direct nasal injury, but definitive diagnosis can be made in all cases by combinations of palpation, visual inspection, endoscopy, dorsoventral skull radiographs, or computed tomography. The latter is particularly useful in defining the extent

Advances in Equine Upper Respiratory Surgery, First Edition. Edited by Jan Hawkins.
© 2015 ACVS Foundation. Published 2015 by John Wiley & Sons, Inc.

of injury from rostral to caudal, which is critical in defining the condition of the remaining septum after resection.

Surgery

Resection of the nasal septum of horses was first described in English by Bemis in 1916. The original technique used a wide guarded chisel, to make the ventral and dorsal cuts through the septum, and a vertical cut through the caudal part of the septum was made with an osteotome. The guarded chisel is not readily available but can be custom made. The vertical cut is made through a trephine hole placed on the dorsal midline of the face, immediately rostral to the frontal sinus at the point of divergence of the nasal bones. This cut is directed along the most rostral edge of a Doyen forceps inserted through the trephine hole and applied across the septum to clamp it at the proposed line of transection (Tulleners and Raker 1983). The forceps also acts as a stop to halt progression of the chisel during the dorsal and ventral cuts.

Section of the nasal septum in a vertical plane with the original method places the caudal septal stump very close to the ventral conchae, where subsequent granulation, swelling, or fibrosis could impinge on or produce adhesions to the conchae (Figure 25.1; Tulleners and Raker 1983). Such an effect in a narrow segment of nasal passage could cause continued airway occlusion (Tulleners and Raker 1983). To avoid this problem, Tulleners and Raker described a technique that involved making the caudal cut at a 60° angle with an osteotome so that the caudal remnant of the septum was in a wider part of the nasal passage (Figure 25.1) and a larger portion of the diseased septum could be removed (Tulleners and Raker 1983). One problem with this technique is the difficulty in cutting the septum through the vomer bone at the end of the nasal passage, because the floor of the nasal passage has a slightly ventral incline at this point (Figure 25.2), which would require a corresponding curve in the chisel or a deliberate redirection of the chisel to follow that curve. Tulleners and Raker described using obstetrical wire in one horse to create the ventral and dorsal cuts in the nasal septum, and proposed that this method would elim-

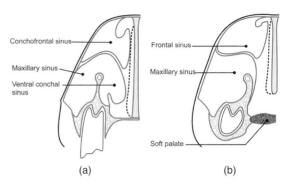

(a)   (b)

Figure 25.1 A vertical cut through the caudal part of the septum directly below the trephine places the septal stump where swelling from edema, granulation tissue, and fibrosis (broken line) could occlude the nasal passage by impinging on the adjacent conchae (a). If the caudal cut is directed as far caudally as possible on the septum (b), then the swelling in the septal stump (broken line) will be in a wide part of the nasal passage and will not impinge on adjacent structures.

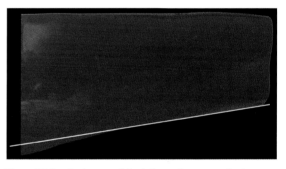

Figure 25.2 Resin cast of the left nasal passage of a horse between the septum and the bony components of the nasal passages showing the septal surface. Note that the caudal part of the floor of the nasal passage declines ventrally at the caudal end (below white line).

inate trauma to the adjacent conchae and allow complete resection. Preplaced wires should allow for more precise, cleaner, and faster cuts than the chisel, because the wires would closely follow the dorsal and ventral attachments of the septum throughout the length of the nasal passage. By comparison, trauma from the chisel could be considerable if the abnormal septum were severely thickened or deviated and required multiple cuts. Wire cuts could be made simultaneously and therefore more rapidly than with the chisel method, which could reduce the time for blood loss before intranasal packing could be placed.

Three-wire method of septal resection

The three-wire method is an extension of the method originally described by Tulleners and Raker and has been modified to include a caudal cut with a preplaced wire (Doyle and Freeman 2005). Theoretical advantages of this technique are that it would allow almost complete resection of the septum, be technically easier to perform than previously described techniques, minimize trauma to the adjacent conchae, and be fast enough to minimize hemorrhage.

Surgical preparation

Preoperative cross matches are required to identify possible blood donors in case of intraoperative or postoperative hemorrhage, which places the patient at risk of hemorrhagic shock. Preoperative antibiotics and anti-inflammatory medications are administered. The horse is anesthetized in lateral recumbency, a speculum is placed in the mouth, and the trachea is intubated with a cuffed tube, which is removed when necessary to pass wires. An area on the midline of the head corresponding to the surgical field for the trephine hole is clipped and prepared for aseptic surgery, all long hairs on the nostrils and muzzle are clipped, and the nostrils are cleaned and rinsed with a dilute chlorhexidine solution. An area of skin centered at the junction of the upper and middle third of the ventral midline of the neck is clipped and prepared for a tracheotomy. Tracheotomy is required because both nasal passages will be packed with gauze following removal of the nasal septum.

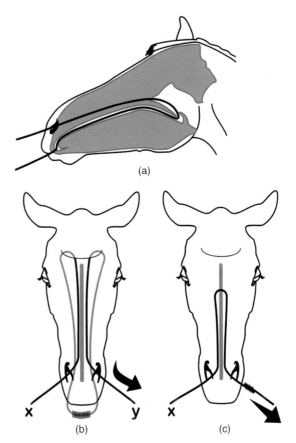

Figure 25.3   Introduction of wire x through one nasal passage and exiting through the mouth (a,b) after manual retrieval around the soft palate. Wire y is introduced the same way through the contralateral nostril and the two ends outside the mouth are spliced together with adhesive tape (c). The nasal portion of each wire is black and the oral portion is gray in (b). Wire y is pulled in the direction of the arrow (c) to bring the splice and the other end of wire x out of the nasal passage so that wire x is positioned for the ventral cut.

Ventral wire

An approximately 100 cm length of obstetrical wire (Jorgensen Laboratories, Inc., Loveland, CO), inserted into a Chamber's mare catheter (Jorgensen Laboratories, Inc., Loveland, CO) or insemination pipette, is passed along the lower ventral meatus until it can be retrieved around the free border of the soft palate with a hand passed orally (Doyle and Freeman 2005; McIlwraith and Robertson 1998). Once grasped, the end of the wire is withdrawn until it exits the oral cavity, taking care to simulta-

neously feed the other end into the catheter so that the wire can make the sharp turn into the oropharynx (Figure 25.3). The tip of the catheter or pipette can be directed caudal to the soft palate so that the wire does not drag over and traumatize its caudal border. A second obstetrical wire, approximately 100 cm long, is passed through the upper nasal passage and is retrieved from the mouth in a similar manner as the first wire. The wire ends exiting the mouth are spliced together by tying them in a knot or by wrapping adhesive tape around them and covering the cut ends (Figure 25.3). A hand in the caudal part of the oropharynx guides the spliced end around the free edge of the soft palate and the wire exiting from one nostril is withdrawn until the spliced section exits the nostril. This maneuver places a single wire through one nostril, along the length of the septum, around its caudoventral edge to exit through the opposite nostril (Figure 25.3). The splice is undone to remove the extra wire. The end protruding from each nostril is grasped and kept taut along the floor of the ventral meatus to eliminate any slack or gap between the wire and septum, and thereby prevent inadvertent looping of subsequent wires around this wire.

Dorsal wire

A trephine hole at least 1.5 cm in diameter is made through the nasal bones immediately caudal to a point on the face where these bones diverge toward the eyes (Figure 25.4) to expose the dorsal edge of the nasal septum. Bleeding from the trephine hole can be substantial, and so this step should be delayed until needed for placement of the caudal and dorsal wires. Mucosa is incised to allow entry into the nasal passages, which might be narrower than normal if the septum is thickened to that level. A Chambers mare catheter is passed through the downside dorsal meatus until the tip exits through the trephine hole. Approximately 100 cm length of obstetrical wire is passed through the catheter, and the catheter is withdrawn from the nose so that one wire end exits from the lower nostril and the other through the trephine hole (Figure 25.4). The catheter is passed through the up side and out of the trephine hole. The wire coming through the down side of the trephine hole is inserted into the catheter on the up side and is drawn through the up nostril, to encircle the septum at the rostral edge of the trephine hole (Figure 25.4). The wire ends are grasped and pulled rostrally and dorsally to ensure a snug fit and avoid any loops that could ensnare the third or caudal wire.

Caudal wire

A Chamber's catheter is inserted through the trephine hole toward the free border of the soft palate (Figure 25.5). Approximately 100 cm length

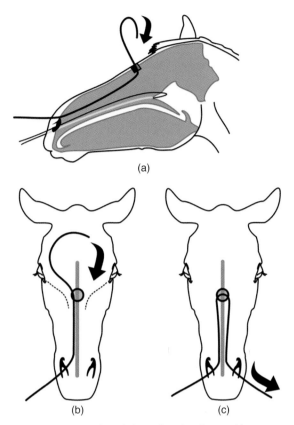

(a)

(b)   (c)

Figure 25.4   A trephine hole is placed in the nasal bones at the point of divergence to the eyes (broken lines) and a wire is passed through a Chamber's catheter, up one nostril, to exit through the trephine hole (a, b). The same wire is then passed through a Chamber's catheter (not shown) to exit the opposite nostril (along arrows in b, c). This wire is then seated around the septum at the rostral edge of the trephine hole (c) for the dorsal cut. An alternative is to pass both wire ends down each nasal passage through the trephine hole.

of obstetrical wire is passed through this catheter into the oral cavity to be grasped by a hand inserted through the mouth and that wire is then drawn orally to exit the mouth (Figure 25.5). This procedure is repeated with another wire on the opposite side of the septum. The two wire ends exiting the mouth are spliced together and one wire end exiting the trephine hole is withdrawn until the splice is pulled into the pharynx and then exits the trephine hole. The splice is undone so the two ends of one wire exit the trephine hole at each side of the septum and this wire encircles the ventral edge of the vomer bone (Figure 25.5).

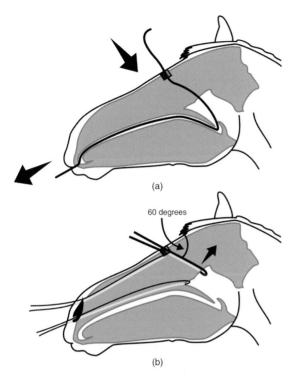

(a)

60 degrees

(b)

Figure 25.5   The third wire is threaded through the trephine hole, retrieved around the caudal edge of the soft palate, and brought through the mouth (direction of arrows in (a)). Another wire is placed in similar fashion through the contralateral nasal passage, and the ends are spliced together outside the mouth (not shown). Traction on one wire draws the spliced end of the other wire out of the trephine hole. The remaining wire is then directed by a Chamber's catheter (as described in the text) to direct the wire as far caudally as possible around the vomer bone to form a 60° angle with the nasal bones (b). In (b), all three wires are shown in the desired locations in preparation for septal resection.

Nasal septum resection by three-wire method

The ends of wires are secured in special handles or with pliers and septal cuts are made in the following sequence. The most rostral cut is made with a scalpel as far caudally as the lesion will allow, leaving at least a 5-cm strut of septum rostrally to support the nostrils and alar folds. This cut is started on the floor of the ventral meatus and curved dorsally and caudally to leave more intact septum dorsally for alar fold support. The convex edge of the cut should be directed rostrally to obtain as much opening at the nares as possible. Although the lateral alae of the nares can be incised to improve access for the rostral cut in some cases (McIlwraith and Robertson 1998), this step is rarely needed and can prolong surgery because the incision requires careful closure.

To produce a caudal cut at 60° in the nasal septum (Figure 25.5), a Chamber's mare catheter is threaded along the caudal wire on one side of the septum through the trephine hole and is used to direct the wire as far caudally as possible around the vomer bone. The caudal limit to this line of angled transection is the perpendicular plate of the ethmoid bone (Hare 1975). Once satisfied with the seating of the wire, an initial cut is started in the vomer bone and the catheter is then withdrawn. In this way, the wire engages the vomer bone as far caudally as possible so that the remainder of the cut can be made at the desired 60° angle.

The septum is cut with back and forth sawing motions synchronized to complete all wire cuts as rapidly as possible. The ventral and dorsal cuts are made simultaneously, and as soon as the caudal cut has started. Great care is taken to pull each wire as far as possible toward the edge of the septum that it must cut, ventrally for the ventral cut and dorsally for the dorsal cut. As the wires approach the nostrils, the rate of cutting is slowed, and the fingers are placed dorsally and ventrally in the rostral cut in the path of each wire to prevent it from cutting the rostral strut of the intact septum.

When the septum is free, the rostral edge of the resected piece is grasped with Ochsner forceps, Vulsellum forceps (Sklar Instruments, West Chester, PA), or a robust set of pliers and is extracted through one nostril. After removal, the resected septum must be examined to ensure that the cuts are clean, and that the entire septum was removed, including the entire lesion, and to assess the nature of the injury (Figure 25.6). The angle formed by the caudovertical cut with the ventral cut should range from 52° to 62° (Figure 25.6). Evidence of a satisfactory angle is an intact mucosal covering for 3–4 cm caudally, over the free edge of the vomer bone (Figure 25.6). The nasal cavity is palpated digitally to determine if the palatine process of the incisive bone, which forms a groove for the ventral edge of the septum (Hare 1975), has become detached to lie free in the nasal passage (Doyle and Freeman 2005). If so, it must be removed.

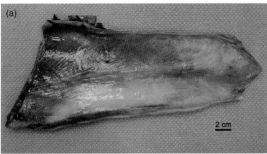

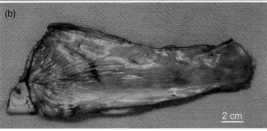

Figure 25.6 Two specimens of diseased septum removed by the three-wire method. Specimen (a) is close to normal shape because the septal thickening was not associated with nasal bone depression. The concave dorsal edge in (b) and the compressed profile at the rostral edge was caused by nasal bone fracture and depression across the bridge of the nose in this horse. Horse (b) would be at risk of continued airflow restriction at the rostral end of the nasal passage.

To control hemorrhage, a 3-inch stockinet (Johnson & Johnson, New Brunswick, NJ), knotted at one end and then inverted, is partly filled with a saline-soaked laparotomy sponge (Johnson & Johnson, New Brunswick, NJ) and is packed into the nasal passage (Doyle and Freeman 2005). To do this, a Chamber's catheter is inserted into the stockinet and pushed against the sponge to impact it against the cut end of the septum, as determined through the trephine hole. The stockinet is packed with additional saline-soaked laparotomy sponges tied together and to the trailing edge of the first sponge, until the rostral end of the stockinet expands to fill the nasal passage. The rostral end of this nasal tampon is then sutured to the false nostril by a mattress suture of size 2 nylon or similar material that passes through a 3 cm × 3 cm pledget of gauze on the external roof of the false nostril. This is preferred to suture closure of the nostrils, which is excessively traumatic and unnecessary. The trephine hole can be left open to heal by second intention or the skin can be sutured

over it. If skin closure is desired, the initial skin incision for the trephine should be curved so that a skin flap can be elevated and then replaced intact over the boney defect.

Although a tracheotomy can be performed while the horse is anesthetized and the trachea can be intubated through it for delivery of inhalant anesthetic, the author prefers to perform the tracheotomy after the surgery is completed, either before or shortly after the horse has been placed in the recovery stall. The tracheotomy required for an endotracheal tube can be considerably larger than what is needed for a tracheotomy tube after surgery. In the author's experience, there is a greater risk of web occlusion of a tracheotomy if the transverse incision between tracheal rings approaches half the diameter of the trachea; this size opening might be required for large endotracheal tubes or could inadvertently develop during the intubation procedure.

Variations in wire placement

Wire placement with manual retrieval of ends in the pharynx requires an individual with a hand small enough to be passed orally to that level, which would be impossible in a horse with a small head. In such cases, the wires can be placed in one nasal passage and then retrieved with an endoscopic biopsy instrument on the opposite side (McIlwraith and Robertson 1998) or with bronchoesophageal forceps (Richard Wolf Medical Instrument Corp., Vernon Hills, Illinois, USA) under endoscopic guidance (Figure 25.7). In one description of placing the caudal wire around the septum, the wire was passed through the trephine hole to pass beneath the vomer bone to be retrieved on the opposite side (McIlwraith and Robertson 1998). Although specific details were not provided on how the end was retrieved, blind retrieval with a long Ochsner forceps or sponge forceps would seem feasible. For endoscopic retrieval of wires, it is easier to grasp a length of size 2 nylon with the biopsy instrument of the endoscope than to grasp the thicker and more rigid obstetrical wire. This suture is introduced through a Chamber's mare catheter or similar so that 3 cm protrudes beyond the catheter to be grasped by the endoscopic biopsy instrument passed up the opposite nostril (Figure 25.8). The suture is drawn back through the nostril to be used

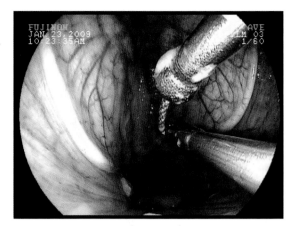

Figure 25.7 Method of using a bronchoesophageal forceps (bottom) under endoscopic guidance to grasp the obstetrical wire introduced into the contralateral nasal passage through a Chamber's catheter (top).

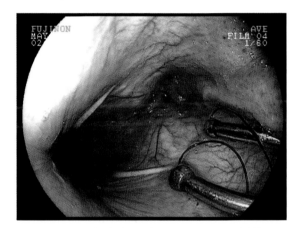

Figure 25.8 Method of introducing two sutures of different colors through two Chamber's catheters in the same nostril to prevent intertwining of sutures or wires. The ventral suture will be retrieved with the biopsy instrument introduced through the contralateral nostril and will be used to draw the ventral wire around the back of the septum. The dorsal suture will be retrieved in the same way but will be maintained dorsal to the first suture and will be used to make the caudal vertical cut.

as a leader by tying one end to the wire, which is folded at the tie so the cut end of the wire trails during traction through the nasal passages. The suture can then draw the wire through the nasal passages around the vomer bone and out of the opposite nostril, taking care to advance the wire simultaneously to facilitate the sharp turn around

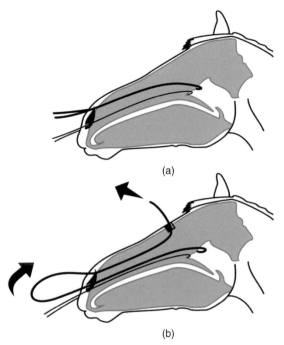

(a)

(b)

Figure 25.9 Method for placing the wire introduced by the endoscope for the caudal vertical cut. After the ventral wire (thin line) and caudal wire (thick line) are placed (a), a trephine hole is cut as described (b). A Chamber's catheter (not shown for clarity) is inserted through the trephine hole and directed out of the nostril, and the wire is fed through this so that it exits the trephine hole. This is repeated on the other side so that the wire is placed for the caudal cut (Figure 25.5b).

the ventral edge of the septum. The author has used endoscopic placement of two wires in this way so that one can be used for the ventral cut and one for the caudal cut (Figure 25.9). It is critical to prevent crossing of these wires by keeping the first wire constantly snugged against the floor of the ventral meatus as the second one is inserted. Alternatively, the two wires can be inserted by using two Chamber's catheters simultaneously in the same nasal passage to place different colored sutures (black nylon, blue polypropylene) as color-coded leaders for ventral and caudal wires (Figure 25.8), but again taking care not to cross sutures or wires.

Once the wire for the caudal cut is placed along the ventral meatus, its nasal ends must be redirected through the trephine hole, which is made after both wires have been placed to prevent obscuring the endoscopic procedures with blood

(Figure 25.9). Once these steps are completed, a Chamber's mare catheter is introduced through the trephine hole and then out of one nasal passage so the ends of one preplaced caudal wire can be fed into the tip. The catheter and wire end can then be drawn retrograde to exit through the trephine hole (Figure 25.9). This is repeated on the other side of the septum, so that this wire now passes through the trephine hole and around the vomer bones (Figures 25.5 and 25.9). The Chamber's catheter is used as described above to direct the caudal cut at an angle with this wire (Figure 25.5). The wire for the dorsal cut is then placed as described above through the trephine opening (Doyle and Freeman 2005).

In all the preceding descriptions, dorsal and ventral cuts are made from the caudal to cranial, which risks extending the cuts into the rostral septal strut. This can be avoided by bringing the dorsal and ventral wire ends through the edges of the rostral incision instead of relying on digital guidance to arrest their progress into the rostral strut (McIlwraith and Robertson 1998). For the dorsal wire, after the wire has been inserted through the nostril and out of the trephine hole on one side, the nasal end is then redirected through a Chamber's catheter that is introduced on the opposite side through the trephine hole, through the rostral cut (McIlwraith and Robertson 1998), and out of the same nostril as used for initial insertion (Figure 25.10). In this way, the dorsal wire is placed around the septum at the dorsal end of the rostral cut, rather than at the trephine, and can be sawed from cranial to caudal through the trephine hole without the risk of cutting the rostral strut. In a similar fashion, one end of the preplaced wire for the ventral cut can be redirected to emerge through the ventral edge of the rostral cut (McIlwraith and Robertson 1998) so that it emerges through the same nostril as the other end of that wire (Figure 25.10). This placement will prevent the ventral wire from proceeding into the rostral strut, provided the sawing motion is directed away from the strut as much as possible.

Approach via laryngotomy

Another wire method involves a laryngotomy that is used for insertion of a Doyen forceps through the

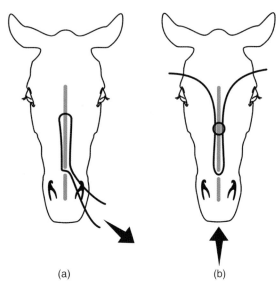

(a)   (b)

Figure 25.10   Method of placing the wires so as to minimize the risk of cutting into the rostral cartilaginous strut. (a) For the ventral wire, one end passes through the rostral incision and then exits the nares on the same side as it was introduced. (b) For the dorsal wire, the wire is inserted so that it passes around the septum at the rostral cut and exits through the trephine hole. The direction of cutting is indicated by the arrow in (b). Special care must be taken with the ventral wire to ensure that the end passing through the rostral incision does not engage on the edge of the rostral strut or it will cut and weaken it.

pharynx to grasp the caudal end of the septum at a 60° angle to the dorsal midline of the head (Loinaz et al. 2012). A wire is passed through the ventral meatus until it can be grasped in the pharynx or as it emerges from the laryngotomy. The same wire can then be passed from the laryngotomy, in front of the Doyen forceps, and then through a catheter in the opposite nasal passage to emerge from the opposite nostril. This wire can be used for the ventral cut. Another wire is placed in the same way except that it is brought behind the Doyen forceps. This wire will be used to make the caudal cut, which will follow the jaws of the forceps until the wire reaches the tips of the instrument at the attachment of the septum to the nasal bones. At that point, it will pass over the tips and continue along the dorsal edge of the septum, thereby making the dorsal cut. The rostral cut is made as for other methods. This procedure has all the advantages of the above described wire methods but requires one less wire and has the added advantage that it replaces the trephine hole

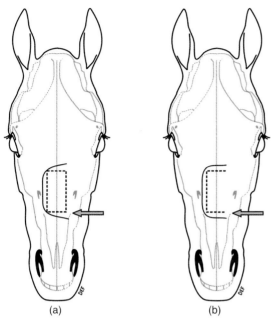

Figure 25.11   (a) Dorsal bone flap approach with temporary bone removal and (b) an attached bone flap (broken lines). Solid lines are soft tissue incisions. Gray arrow indicates the nasoincisive notch that is used to identify the rostral limit of the bone flap.

with a laryngotomy, which is easier to make, heals rapidly, and eliminates the risk of a bony blemish with the trephine hole. Also, this approach would eliminate any possible trephine-induced changes in the growth of nasal bones in young horses.

Bone flap method

A dorsal approach to the nasal bones has been described for nasal septum resection and offers some advantages under certain conditions (Shoemaker et al. 2005). With the horse anesthetized in left lateral recumbency and the dorsum of the head turned 45° from the horizontal, a three-sided curvilinear skin incision is made over the nasal bones to span the septal abnormality, the proposed length of septum to be removed, and the full width of the bridge of the nose (Figure 25.11). The skin, underlying fascia, and periosteum are reflected along three sides to form a soft tissue flap with the long side parallel to the midline (Figure 25.11). An oscillat-

ing bone saw (Stryker® bone saw, Stryker Instruments, Kalamazoo, MI) is used to cut a rectangular segment of bone (4–5 cm wide and 6–10 cm long). The most rostral limit of the flap must end at a point that leaves at least 1 cm of solid bone caudal to the nasoincisive notch, or the rostral extremities of the nasal bones will fracture and weaken nasal support (Figure 25.11). Once the bone flap is freed from the parent bone, the cartilaginous attachment of the nasal septum to the nasal bones is severed with an osteotome. The detached bone flap is then wrapped in gauze sponges soaked with saline (0.9% NaCl) solution. Eight-inch Rochester–Pean surgical clamps (Pilling Weck Inc., Markham, ON, Canada) are positioned across the nasal septum at the rostral and caudal ends and are angled as needed to include as much caudal septum as possible, leaving at least 4 cm of the rostral end. Mayo scissors are used to transect the septum between the clamps. The nasal mucosa is sharply incised along the ventral attachment of the septum. The septum is grasped with Rochester Ochsner forceps rostrally and caudally, and is removed by traction and rocking motion to detach it from the hard palate and vomer bone. Any palpable septal remnants or any remaining diseased portions of septum are removed by rongeurs. The nasal passages are packed with a stockinet and rolled gauze tampon from caudal to rostral as described (Doyle and Freeman 2005). The bone flap is replaced and secured with 0 polydioxanone (PDS) interrupted sutures (Ethicon, Novartis Animal Health Inc.) through predrilled holes. The periosteum is apposed with 0 PDS in a simple interrupted pattern, followed by subcutaneous and skin closures.

Although the original report described removing the nasal bone segment and replacing it after septal resection (Shoemaker et al. 2005), the author prefers to create a bone flap with all layers attached (Freeman et al. 1990; Figure 25.11). The argument against retaining bone flap attachments is possible fracture of the nasal bones as they are elevated off any residual septal attachments, and this can cause an unsatisfactory cosmetic repair (Shoemaker et al. 2005). Although cuts for the attached bone flap can be beveled toward the inner surface of the flap to allow proper seating against the parent bone, this is not necessary if an attached bone flap is raised (Doyle and Freeman 2005).

Nasal septoplasty

A septoplasty technique that preserves the nasal support from the septum has been described as a successful alternative to septum resection for correction of septal deviation in a foal (Yarbrough et al. 1997). This procedure would seem to be better suited to lesions in the most rostral part of the septum, as in the case reported (Yarbrough et al. 1997). It would also be of most benefit to foals, because they are so dependent on septal support to prevent facial deformity and nostril collapse, but presumably could be used in a horse of any age. This procedure involves mucosal elevation followed by parasagittal incisions in the cartilage. The incised segments of cartilage can be mobilized into positions that correct the deformity and confer stability to the repair through strategic angles of incisions and overlapping of edges (Yarbrough et al. 1997). Hemorrhage can be reduced by submucosal infiltration with 25 mg ephedrine diluted in 10 mL of normal saline. The procedure was completed by closure of the membrane and apposition of overlapped cartilage edges with absorbable suture.

Postoperative care

Postoperative care involves stall rest and antibiotics and anti-inflammatory medication for 72–96 hours. At 24–72 hours postoperatively, the inner gauze part of the nasal tampon is removed, followed by the stockinet. Tampon removal is followed by some mild-to-moderate epistaxis for approximately 15 minutes, but allows unobstructed airflow and hence removal of the tracheotomy tube. The nasal passages can be gently lavaged with warm water or physiologic solution through the trephine hole after the packing is removed to remove blood clots and mucus from the nasal passages. Owners are asked to return the horse 4–6 weeks after discharge for endoscopic evaluation of the surgical site and again at the same interval for a final examination.

Complications

Complications during or after surgery are usually minor and transient. Most horses develop transient fever in the postoperative period. It is not unusual for edema to develop over the nasal bones below the trephine site and this can persist for weeks after surgery, along with a persistent mucopurulent nasal discharge. Some horses can have an abnormal odor from the nares for several weeks after the surgery, as remnants of blood and tissue debris continue to decay in the cut edges. A bony thickening can persist for weeks at the trephine site but usually resolves with time. The gauze packing can enter the nasopharynx and be swallowed, but this can be prevented by placing it in stockinet (Doyle and Freeman 2005). Regardless of the method used, blood loss can be disconcerting but is rarely sufficient to require blood transfusion. Failure to remove all of the lesion is unusual with the resection methods described, but this risk is greatest if the most rostral extent of the septum is involved, regardless of disease process.

Prognosis

At 4–6 weeks after surgery, all surgical sites should be healing well, but some inflammation and granulation tissue will be evident along the lines of septal resection and on the nasal side of the trephine hole. Another 3–6 weeks will be required for incised septal edges to be free of thickening and granulation tissue on endoscopy (Figure 25.12), for nasal discharge to resolve, and to start exercise. Facial contour will remain unchanged and some horses will continue to make a respiratory noise. Noise will be evident mostly at a walk and slow gaits, but should disappear at high speeds. Any degree of persistent respiratory noise can be attributed to altered airflow dynamics and turbulence in the enlarged nasal cavity, conchal encroachment, turbulent airflow around the rostral remnant, or any remaining disease, deviation, or thickening in the rostral remnant.

Most horses return to their intended function at long-term follow-up, including racing (Thoroughbred and Standardbred), although some might fail to reach full athletic potential. An important determinant of outcome, especially with racehorses, is any residual nasal occlusion following surgery. Facial abnormalities after nasal septal resection include rostral flattening of the bridge of the nose, extreme convexity of the nose, and upper airway

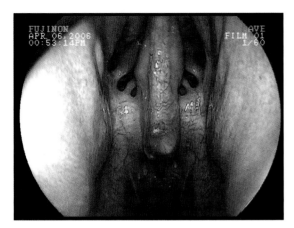

Figure 25.12 Endoscopic appearance of the dorsal and ventral conchae and the stump of the nasal septum at 10 weeks after surgery. Note the lack of reaction and thickening along the cut edges. Despite the favorable appearance of the surgery site, this horse had an abnormal nasal odor that resolved shortly afterward.

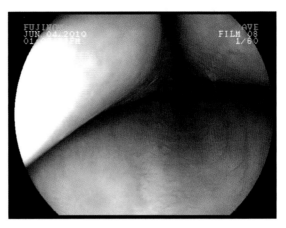

Figure 25.13 Endoscopic view of the rostral end of the nasal passage showing the ventral conchae are almost in contact as they encroach toward the floor of the nasal passage. This is likely to restrict airflow.

obstruction caused by loss of nostril support (Tulleners and Raker 1983). If any of these changes were evident before surgery, they could contribute to persistent airway obstruction after an otherwise successful septum resection.

Conchal encroachment would seem the most likely reason for failure of septum resection in horses with pre-existing deviation and deformity in the nasal bones from a compression fracture or wry nose (Doyle and Freeman 2005). In such cases, conchae from both sides seem to move axially to fill the void between them after septum removal in these horses and this can occlude the airway ventrally and rostrally (Figure 25.13). Presumably, the conchae were forced into contact with the nasal septum before surgery by depression of the injured nasal bones from the original injury. Removal of the nasal septum simply allows the conchae to continue this downward and axial displacement (Figure 25.13). Some of these horses might benefit from alar fold resection at the time of the original surgery or later, but the effects of this might be disappointing.

Ventral conchal encroachment cannot be alleviated by resecting the ventral and dorsal conchae through a large frontonasal bone flap, largely because this approach does not allow sufficient rostral access, where nasal passage encroachment is most severe (Doyle and Freeman 2005). The dorsal

bone flap method might be particularly useful to remove the encroaching conchae, and it also allows other cosmetic procedures, such as elevation of depressed nasal bones, reconstruction of concurrent nasal deformities, and application of a bone plate if needed to restore a defect in the nasal bones (Shoemaker et al. 2005). It also allows a more direct approach to hemostasis and packing placement, which can be critical after such procedures (Shoemaker et al. 2005).

In any horse younger than 1 year old, nasal septum resection is usually followed by loss of rostral support to the nostrils, presumably because the nares and the head in general outgrow any rostral cartilaginous strut that remains after resection. Although this can be partly relieved by resection of the alar folds, the prospects for recovery of airway function is poor. Also, it is not unusual for young horses to display some impaired growth of the upper jaw after nasal septum resection, possibly secondary to an effect of the trephination procedure or removal of the septum on nasal bone growth. Consequently, these animals will develop an underbite that is largely of cosmetic importance. In foals with a rostral lesion, nasal septoplasty might decrease airway obstruction while allowing normal development of the facial contour (Yarbrough et al. 1997). Owners probably should be advised to wait until the horse is 2 years old before it has resection of the nasal septum.

Although not tested in a large number of high-performance horses, nasal septum resection offers suitable candidates the best option for elimination of airway obstruction. Although all horses in recent reports did not take part in a strenuous athletic activity, horses have raced after nasal septum resection (Schumacher et al. 2008); however, prognosis for achieving full racing potential should be guarded. Any residual noise after surgery does not always indicate career-limiting obstruction.

Author comments

Horses receive intravenous fluids in sufficient volumes under general anesthesia to offset inhalant induced vasodilatation and associated low tissue perfusion, even in the face of intraoperative blood loss with nasal septum resection. Volume loading with intravenous fluids is not recommended because this can exacerbate hemorrhage when cardiovascular status is normal. Insemination pipettes are suitable alternatives for a Chamber's catheter, and they both greatly facilitate wire passage though tight passageways (McIlwraith and Robertson 1998); however, the rigidity of the steel catheter can be an advantage. The hub end of the catheter can be cut off to facilitate insertion of wire or suture through it.

All methods described above have produced comparable outcomes, although they have only been tested on a small numbers of cases. A two- or three-wire method severs the most caudal extent of the septum in a cleaner and less traumatic fashion than could be accomplished with an osteotome (Figure 25.6). The prerequisites for success with wire methods are adherence to the correct order for each step, prevention of wires intertwining, and synchronizing the cutting steps so that they are completed as quickly and smoothly as possible. This approach will keep hemorrhage and trauma to a minimum. Although the dorsal bone flap approach is more invasive than the wire methods, it allows excellent exposure to the nasal passages and allows reconstruction of deformed nasal bones if necessary. The author has found it to be useful for large lesions that might not be amenable to removal through the nares; however, such lesions are rare. Another positive claim for the dorsal flap is that it permits more targeted removal of focal lesions. However, limited resection of such lesions might run the risk of leaving a transected end of septum in a narrow portion of the nasal passages, which could cause airway obstruction if these ends heal with considerable thickening. The major limitation of the dorsal bone flap is restricted access to rostral lesions because the rostral limit of the flap is limited by the need to retain an intact nasoincisive notch (Figure 25.11).

Although, near total septum removal with the three-wire methods might seem excessive for a horse with a focal lesion in the middle of the septum, it does place the transected caudal stump in a position where thickening along its cut edge would do less harm than in a narrow portion of the nasal passages, where focal resection could place it (Figure 25.1). Also, failure to remove all diseased septum is not a problem with the three-wire method, except in those horses with very rostral involvement. If there is extensive involvement of the most rostral segment of septum by the disease process, leaving some diseased cartilage in place is preferable to resecting too much and removing rostral support. Any remaining disease process could be addressed later by debridement, septoplasty, or topical or medical treatment, depending on the nature of the primary disease.

References

Bemis HE. 1916. Removal of the nasal septum. *Journal of the American Veterinary Medical Association* 49:397–399.

Doyle AJ, Freeman DE. 2005. Extensive nasal septum resection in horses using a 3-wire method. *Veterinary Surgery* 34:167–173.

Freeman DE, Orsini PG, Ross MW, Madison JB. 1990. A large frontonasal bone flap for sinus surgery in the horse. *Veterinary Surgery* 19:122–130.

Garrett KS, Woodie JB, Cook JL, Williams NM. 2010. Imaging diagnosis–nasal septal and laryngeal cyst-like malformations in a Thoroughbred weanling colt diagnosed using ultrasonography and magnetic resonance imaging. *Veterinary Radiology and Ultrasound* 51:504–507.

Hare WCD. 1975. Equine respiratory system. In: Sisson S, Grossman JD, Getty R, eds. *Sisson and Grossman's the Anatomy of the Domestic Animals* (pp. 498–453). Philadelphia, PA: W.B. Saunders Company.

Loinaz RJ, Boutros CP, Rakestraw PC, Taylor TS. 2012. Evaluation of a laryngotomy approach for near-total resection of the nasal septum in the horse. *Veterinary Surgery* 41(5):643–648.

McIlwraith CW, Robertson JT. 1998. Nasal septum resection. In: McIlwraith CW, Robertson JT, eds. *McIlwraith and Turner's Equine Surgery Advanced Techniques*, 2nd ed. (pp. 264–269). Baltimore, MD: Williams and Wilkins.

Schumacher J, Brink P, Easley J, Pollock P. 2008. Surgical correction of wry nose in four horses. *Veterinary Surgery* 37:142–148.

Sharma A, Thompson MS, Schnabel LV, Mete A, Hackett RP. 2010. Imaging diagnosis-equine nasal septal thickening due to chronic chondritis. *Veterinary Radiology and Ultrasound* 51:65–68.

Shoemaker RW, Wilson DG, Fretz PB. 2005. A dorsal approach for the removal of the nasal septum in the horse. *Veterinary Surgery* 34:668–673.

Tulleners EP, Raker CW. 1983. Nasal septum resection in the horse. *Veterinary Surgery* 12:41–47.

Yarbrough TB, Carr EA, Snyder JR, Hornof WJ. 1997. Nasal septoplasty for correction of septal deviation in a foal. *Veterinary Surgery* 26:340–345.

26 Surgical Treatment of Horses with Wry Nose

Jim Schumacher

Introduction

Wry nose, or *campylorrhinus lateralis*, is a congenital facial malformation of horses characterized by slight-to-severe lateral deviation of the maxillae, premaxillae, nasal septum, and nasal bones (Baker 1999). The malformation occurs at or close to the junction of the premaxillae and maxillae. The premaxillae and maxillae are sometimes shorter than the mandible, and the deviated nasal bones and hard palate are sometimes arched. The malformation can be accompanied by other anomalies, such as cleft palate (palatoschisis), but only rarely.

Some investigators believe wry nose to be hereditary because it seems to occur most frequently in Arabians and miniature horses (Baker 1998; Mitz and Allen 2003), but the frequency with which it occurs in various breeds has not been investigated scientifically. Failure of the uterus, especially that of a primiparous mare, to expand to accommodate growth of the fetus has been postulated to account for the anomaly (Vandeplassche et al. 1984). This may account for malformations in which both the upper and lower jaws are deviated but fails to account for the more common malformation characterized by deviation of only the upper jaw.

Wry nose is easily diagnosed by the affected horse's facial appearance (Figure 26.1), but the degree of deviation is determined most accurately by examining a dorsoventral radiographic projection of the head. All or some of the premaxillary incisors fail to occlude with the mandibular incisors, and the tongue may protrude on the convex side of the malformation. Although most affected foals suckle effectively, some severely affected foals are unable to suckle well enough to survive (McKellar and Collins 1993). Horses with severe malformation have difficulty prehending grass, and the cheek teeth may wear abnormally because lateral excursion of the mandible is usually confined to the convex side of the malformation. Deviation of the septum results in obstruction of the nasal cavities, especially the nasal cavity on the convex side of the malformation, and severely affected horses may have respiratory stridor even while resting (Cousty et al. 2010; Puchol et al. 2004; Schumacher et al. 2008). The alar folds and alar cartilages may collapse into the nasal cavities.

Advances in Equine Upper Respiratory Surgery, First Edition. Edited by Jan Hawkins.
© 2015 ACVS Foundation. Published 2015 by John Wiley & Sons, Inc.

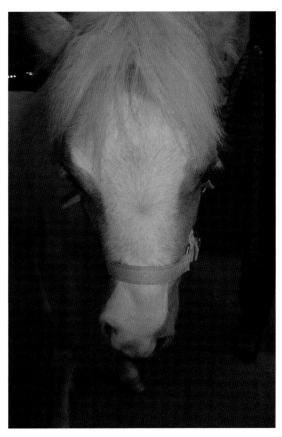

Figure 26.1   Horse affected with wry nose.

Most horses affected with wry nose require little or no special care to survive, but those exhibiting dyspnea while at rest because of severe deviation of the nasal septum may require a tracheostomy or insertion of an endotracheal tube into the nasal cavity on the convex side of the malformation to relieve dyspnea. Foals unable to suckle may be able to survive by drinking a milk replacer from a bucket. A mildly or moderately malformed face may straighten as the foal grows (Vandeplassche et al. 1984), but horses with a severe malformation require permanent tracheostomy or removal of the nasal septum to resolve dyspnea caused by obstruction of the nasal cavities. More radical surgery is required to improve prehension and mastication of feed and cosmesis. Reported surgical treatments to relieve respiratory impairment, improve mastication and prehension, and enhance cosmesis include: (1) distraction osteogenesis after bilat-

eral, partial osteotomy of the premaxillae/maxillae (Puchol et al. 2004); (2) bilateral osteotomy of the premaxillae/maxillae and external fixation of the transected bones (Cousty et al. 2010); and (3) bilateral osteotomy of the premaxillae/maxillae and the nasal bones, internal fixation of the transected bones, and excision of the nasal septum (Schumacher et al. 2008; Valdez et al. 1978).

Bilateral partial osteotomy of the maxillae/premaxillae and distraction osteogenesis

Using the technique of distraction osteogenesis, the right and left premaxillae/maxillae of a yearling horse were partly transected, using an oscillating saw, with the horse anesthetized, at their point of maximum curvature (Puchol et al. 2004). Each osteotomy was performed through a 4-cm long, longitudinal, cutaneous incision that extended through the periosteum at the midpoint between the dorsal and ventral aspects of the premaxillae/maxillae at the point of greatest curvature. A double bar was attached on the convex side of the malformation to four, 4-mm diameter Steinmann pins inserted through both premaxillae, rostral to the osteotomy, and to four similar pins inserted through both maxillae caudal to the osteotomy. A monolateral distraction external skeletal fixator was applied to the pins on the concave side of the malformation. By distracting the rostral and caudal pins on the concave side of the malformation by 1 mm daily for 55 days, growth of the concave side of the deformity was lengthened 5.5 cm, bringing the premaxillary and mandibular incisors into occlusion. Every 2 days, the clamps attaching the pins with the double connecting bar on the convex side of the malformation were slackened and retightened to accommodate the pressure generated by the distraction of bone on the concave side of the malformation. Although only the premaxillae/maxillae were distracted, the deviated nasal septum apparently also straightened. The authors failed to describe changes, if any, produced in the position of the nasal bones.

The technique of distraction osteogenesis to treat horses affected with wry nose is most appropriate for horses that have been weaned because, when placed on a suckling foal, the fixator may disturb or injure the dam when the foal suckles. Using this technique, the horse must be hospitalized for a lengthy period so that the external skeletal fixator can be adjusted daily to maintain a distractive force.

Bilateral osteotomy of the premaxillae/maxillae and external fixation

To treat a yearling horse for wry nose, the horse's premaxillae/maxillae were completely transected, straightened, and fixed by using an external skeletal fixator (Cousty et al. 2010). To perform the surgery, the horse was anesthetized and positioned in dorsal recumbency with its head in a lateral position with the concave side of the malformation upper most. The right and left maxillae/premaxillae and hard palate were transected with an oscillating saw through a 5-cm long, longitudinal, cutaneous incision exposing the concave side of the malformed premaxillae/maxillae. After suturing this incision, the head was positioned dorsally, and two, 20-cm long, 3-mm diameter, Steinmann pins were inserted in a transverse plane, through both premaxillae, rostral to the osteotomy, and two similar pins were inserted in a transverse plane, through both maxillae caudal to the osteotomy. The pins on each side of the osteotomy were incorporated into an external skeletal fixator with connecting bars placed as close as possible to the skin, after ensuring that the premaxillary and mandibular incisors were aligned properly. Two, unilateral, 10-cm long, 3-mm diameter, Steinmann pins were inserted into the ipsilateral maxilla, caudal to the osteotomy site, and secured to the external fixator, but these pins bent after the first week and were removed. The repair, however, remained stable. The nasal bones were not transected.

With this method of correction, the malformation is corrected at the time of surgery, and periodic distraction of the fixator is not required. Stabilization of transected bone is fragile, however, and disruption of repair could occur while the horse recovers from general anesthesia and during convalescence. When placed on a suckling foal, the fixator may disturb or injure the dam when the foal suckles. Care must be taken to ensure that the external fixator is adequately padded, that the connecting bars are applied close to the face, and that the pins situated cranial to the osteotomy do not interfere with the function of the lips.

Bilateral osteotomy of the premaxillae/maxillae and nasal bones and internal fixation

The surgical procedure most commonly used to correct wry nose consists of transecting the premaxillae/maxillae and nasal bones and stabilizing these transected bones in a more normal position and removing the nasal portion of the nasal septum (Schumacher et al. 2008; Valdez et al. 1978). These procedures can be staged several months apart (Valdez et al. 1978), but correcting the malformation during one anesthetic period decreases the time of convalescence and the cost of treatment (Schumacher et al. 2008).

Presurgical treatment

The horse should be evaluated, before surgery, for the presence of other congenital defects, such as cleft palate, and the cheek teeth should be rasped, if necessary, to establish normal occlusal angles between teeth in the mandibular and maxillary arcades. Hair should be clipped from the face, ventral portion of the neck, and the caudal half of one side of the thorax. Food is withheld for 12 hours before the horse is anesthetized, but foals are allowed to suckle until the time of surgery. The horse should be administered antimicrobial therapy and a nonsteroidal anti-inflammatory drug (NSAID) within an hour before surgery. The horse should receive a temporary tracheostomy, either before surgery, while sedated, or after general anesthesia is induced.

Anesthesia

Inhalation anesthesia is delivered through a cuffed endotracheal tube inserted into the trachea through the tracheostomy, either before or after the horse is anesthetized. Desensitizing the rostral region of the face by anesthetizing the infraorbital nerves with a long-acting anesthetic solution injected into the infraorbital canals allows the surgery to be performed with the horse in lighter plane of anesthesia than would otherwise be required. The horse should be administered a balanced electrolyte solution intravenously during surgery, but administration of blood is unlikely to be required, even though blood loss can be considerable.

Surgery

The malformation is corrected during one anesthetic period by performing the following procedures: transecting, straightening, and stabilizing the premaxillae/maxillae; procuring a portion of the rib for grafting at the site of the premaxillary/maxillary osteotomy; transecting, straightening, and stabilizing the nasal bones; and excising the nasal portion of the nasal septum. A laryngotomy is performed to assist in placing obstetrical wires for excising the nasal septum if the horse's oral cavity is so small that a hand cannot be inserted into the oropharynx. The order in which the procedures are performed is not crucial, but the bone graft should be procured first so that it can be procured aseptically.

Harvesting the bone graft

The section of the rib to be grafted at the site of maxillary/premaxillary osteotomy is procured with the horse in lateral or dorsal recumbency. The graft is harvested with the horse in dorsal recumbency if transecting, straightening, and stabilizing the premaxillae/maxillae are to be performed next. The graft is procured with the horse in lateral recumbency if excision of the nasal septum and transection, straightening, and stabilizing of the nasal bones are the procedures to be performed next.

The graft is harvested most easily from the distal aspect of a rib located in the caudal half of the rib cage. After preparing a site for aseptic surgery, an 8–12 cm long, cutaneous incision is created over the chosen rib. The incision begins slightly ventral to the costochondral junction of the rib and extends dorsally, through the skin, subcutaneous tissue, cutaneous trunci and external oblique muscles, and periosteum, along the longitudinal axis of the rib. The periosteum is elevated circumferen-

tially from the rib using a periosteal elevator, and the rib is transected 4–5 cm dorsal to its costochondral junction by using an oscillating bone saw or a loop of obstetrical wire. Care should be taken to avoid penetrating the pleura with the blade of the oscillating saw. The transected section of the rib is removed by cutting its ventral end at the costochondral junction with a scalpel blade. The section of rib is wrapped in gauze sponges soaked in blood or isotonic saline solution.

A long-acting local anesthetic solution, such as bupivacaine, is injected at the caudal border of the rib, proximal to the site at which the rib was transected, to provide analgesia to the surgical site. The periosteum, musculature, and subcutaneous tissue are each sutured separately with 2-0 (3.0 metric), absorbable, synthetic suture placed in a simple continuous pattern, and the cutaneous incision is sutured or stapled. A stent bandage is placed over the sutured incision.

Excising the nasal portion of the nasal septum

The nasal portion of the nasal septum is excised using previously published techniques (Bemis 1916; Doyle and Freeman 2005; Tulleners and Raker 1983) and is described in Chapter 25. The ventral, dorsal, and caudal borders of the septum can be incised most easily using three, 1-meter long loops of obstetrical wire. The rostral border is incised with a scalpel. Each end of the loop of wire is covered by a piece of tubing, such as a male dog urinary catheter, before it is inserted, to protect the respiratory mucosa from the sharp ends of the wire. To set the caudal and the dorsal loops, the dorsocaudal aspect of the nasal septum is exposed through a trephine hole created in the nasal bones just rostral to the conchofrontal sinuses.

The ventral wire can be positioned before the bridge of the nose is prepared for trephination. To position the ventral wire, one end of a piece of obstetrical wire is inserted through the right ventral nasal meatus, and the other end is inserted through the left ventral meatus. The ends of the wire can be grasped dorsal to the caudal edge of the soft palate, with the fingers of a hand inserted orally, and pulled out of the mouth. If the horse is so small that a hand cannot be introduced into the mouth, both ends of the wire are advanced caudally until they can be palpated with a finger inserted into the nasopharynx through a previously created laryngotomy, and the ends of the wire are guided through the larynx and out the laryngotomy with the finger. The two ends of the loop are tied to each other, the knot is covered with tape to prevent the frayed ends of the wire from damaging the respiratory mucosa, and the knot is pulled into the nasopharynx and through the right or left nasal cavity until it is exteriorized. Tension on both arms of the wire sets the loop around the caudoventral border of the septum.

In preparation for positioning the dorsal and caudal loops of wire, the horse is positioned in lateral recumbency with the concave side of the head uppermost (Figure 26.2), the dorsal aspect of its head elevated about 45° with a wedge or sand bag, and the bridge of the nose is prepared for surgery. The caudal aspect of the nasal bones is exposed through a semi-circular, cutaneous incision created just rostral to the conchofrontal sinuses, which is

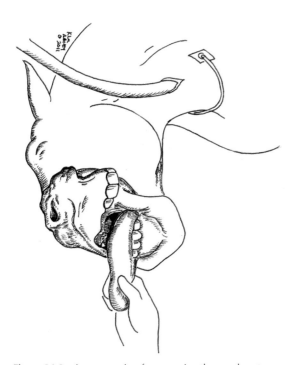

Figure 26.2   In preparation for removing the nasal septum or straightening the nasal bones, the horse is positioned in lateral recumbency, with the concave side of the malformation uppermost. Illustration by Kim Abney.

located close to where the nasal bones begin to widen, on a transverse plane half-way between medial canthus of the eye and the infraorbital foramen. A lateral radiographic projection of the skull, obtained with markers placed on the dorsal midline in the region of the rostral aspect of the conchofrontal sinuses helps to determine the exact site at which to expose the dorsocaudal aspect of the nasal portion of the nasal septum. The incision is extended through the periosteum, and the flap of skin and periosteum is reflected to expose the nasal bones.

A circular section of the nasal bones is excised from the dorsal midline rostral to the sinuses by using a 15–25 mm diameter Galt trephine, to expose a circular section of parietal cartilage of the septum, which is either excised with a scalpel or incised parallel to the long axis of the head on each side of the septum to expose the right and left nasal cavities. Hemorrhage is minimized by incising, rather than excising, the parietal cartilage. Exposing the right and left nasal cavities in this region provides access to the caudal and dorsal aspects of the septum.

To position the wire to incise the dorsal border of the septum, one end of a loop of obstetrical wire is inserted through the right incision into the right dorsal meatus, and the other end is inserted through the left incision into the left dorsal meatus. The ends of the loop are directed rostrally until they can be grasped at the external nares. Tension on both arms of the wire sets the loop around the dorsal border of the septum.

To position the wire for the caudal septal incision, one sheathed end of a piece of obstetrical wire is inserted through the incision in the parietal cartilage on the right side of the septum, and the other sheathed end of the wire is inserted through the incision in the parietal cartilage on the left side of the septum. The ends are directed into the nasopharynx until the ends of the wire can be palpated with fingers of a hand inserted through the mouth to the caudal border of the soft palate or with a finger inserted through a laryngotomy into the nasopharynx. The ends of the wires are grasped between two fingers and pulled out of the mouth or guided through the larynx and out the laryngotomy. The ends of the wire are tied together, and the knot is covered with tape to protect the respiratory mucosa. The knotted loop of wire is pulled back into the nasopharynx, and by pulling the loop in one direction, the knot is exteriorized at the trephine hole.

The caudal cut through the septum should be made at a 120–130° angle to the nasal bones, so that the caudal cut edge of the remaining portion of the septum, which inevitably thickens after surgery, resides within the nasopharynx, rather than between the nasal conchae. To position the caudal loop of wire so that it cuts at this angle, the jaws of a straight Doyen intestinal forceps are inserted through the trephine hole so that they span the septum and are directed caudoventrally, at a 120–130° angle to the nasal bones, until the ends of the jaws contact the soft palate. As the loop of wire is pulled from the oropharynx or the laryngotomy into the nasopharynx, the loop becomes positioned caudal to the jaws of the forceps, situating it to cut the septum along the angled jaws of the forceps.

When the three loops of wire are in position, the dorsal, ventral, and caudal aspects of the septum are cut simultaneously by the surgeon and two assistants, each making a cut with one of the loops of wire. More force is required initially to make the caudal cut because the loop of wire must cut through the vomer bone. When the dorsal and ventral borders of the septum have been cut to within 2 cm of the rostral end of the septum, a rostrally curved incision is made in the rostral end of the septum with a scalpel to connect the dorsal and ventral cuts. The nasal septum is grasped through one nostril with a large Vulsellum forceps and removed. The nasal chamber is packed tightly with rolled gauze to control hemorrhage, the nares are closed with a large mattress suture to retain the packing, and the cutaneous incision created over the bridge of the nose is closed with sutures or skin staples.

Straightening the nasal bones

In preparation for straightening the nasal bones, the horse is positioned in lateral recumbency, with the concave side of the malformation uppermost (Figure 26.3). If removal of the nasal septum preceded this procedure, the horse need not be moved. The dorsal aspect of the head is tilted 45° with a wedge or a sand bag, and the bridge of the nose is prepared for aseptic surgery.

A curved, 7–10 cm long, longitudinal, cutaneous incision, centered at the point of maximum curva-

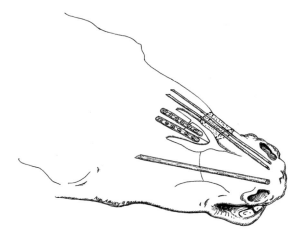

Figure 26.3   The nasal bones are transected at their point of maximum curvature, and the gap created on the concave side of the deformity when the bones are aligned along the longitudinal axis of the head is eliminated by performing a wedge osteotomy at the convex side of the nasal bones at the site of transection. The transected segment of each nasal bone is transfixed to its parent bone with a 2.7-mm reconstruction plate or a 2.7-mm dynamic compression plate, using 2.7-mm cortical bone screws, 6–8 mm long. Even though the transected nasal bones are attached to each other by a ligament, both should be fixed to its parent nasal bone in case one plate fails to provide fixation. To transfix the transected segment of the upper jaw, a 4–6 mm diameter Steinmann pin is inserted between the reserve crowns of the central and intermediate incisors on the convex side of the malformation, and driven through the transected segment of the upper jaw into the medullary cavity of the ipsilateral maxilla. Two or three, 2-mm diameter, Kirschner wires are inserted in similar fashion on the concave side of the jaw. These Kirschner wires penetrate and anchor a bone graft, harvested from a rib. Illustration by Kim Abney.

ture of the nasal bones, is made between the right and left nasal bones, being careful to avoid incising the narrow ligament connecting the nasal bones. The nasal bones and the periosteum covering them are exposed using a self-retaining retractor, and the periosteum over the center of each bone is incised longitudinally, and its edges reflected. The nasal bones are transected at their point of maximum curvature, with an oscillating bone saw, being careful to avoid penetrating the underlying parietal cartilage of the nasal septum. The bones are rotated into proper alignment, and the gap created on the concave side of the deformity is eliminated by performing a wedge osteotomy at the convex side of the nasal bones, with an oscillating saw, at the site of transection.

The transected segment of each nasal bone is transfixed to its parent bone with a 6–12 hole, 2.7-mm, reconstruction plate or a 2.7-mm, dynamic compression plate, using 2.7-mm, cortical bone screws, 6–8 mm long (Figure 26.3). Tapping the drill holes is unnecessary. A reconstruction plate is easier to conform to the surface of a deformed nasal bone than is a dynamic compression plate because it can be easily bent in various planes. Because the nasal bones are fixed firmly to each other by a ligament, fixing only one nasal bone to its parent bone with a plate stabilizes both nasal bones, but loss of stability provided by a single plate from loosening of the screws may result in collapse of both nasal bones into the airway. Transfixing each transected portion of the nasal bone to its parent bone decreases the likelihood of collapse of the nasal bones.

The subcutaneous tissue is closed with 2-0 (3.0 metric), absorbable, synthetic suture using a simple continuous pattern, the cutaneous incision is sutured or stapled, and a stent bandage is placed over the sutured incision.

Straightening the premaxillae/maxillae

In preparation for straightening the premaxillae/maxillae, the horse is positioned in dorsal recumbency, and its upper lip is retracted and fixed to the bridge of the nose with several towel clamps to expose the gingiva dorsal to the incisors. The mouth is held open using a narrow, triangular piece of wood or a dental wedge inserted between the maxillary and mandibular arcades of one side of the head. The rostral aspect of the mouth is cleansed with an antiseptic soap and rinsed with water.

A 3–5 cm long, longitudinal gingival incision, extending through the periosteum and centered at the point of greatest curvature, is created at each interdental space on the ventral border of the premaxillae/maxillae (Figure 26.4). The gingiva and periosteum are elevated from the medial and lateral surfaces of the bone using a periosteal elevator and are retracted with handheld retractors. The premaxillae/maxillae and palatine processes are transected though the incisions using an oscillating saw. If the bone is difficult to completely transect using the saw, the most dorsal portions of the

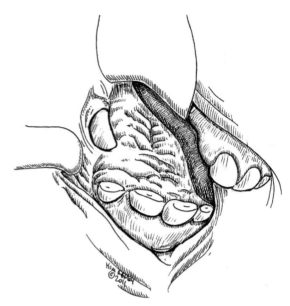

Figure 26.4 The ventral aspect of each premaxilla/maxilla is exposed through a longitudinal mucosal incision centered at the point of greatest curvature at the interdental space. After transecting the premaxillae/maxillae at the point of greatest curvature, a section of rib is inserted through the mucosal incision into the gap created on the concave side of the deformity when the bones are aligned along the longitudinal axis of the head. Illustration by Kim Abney.

premaxillae/maxillae can be transected by using a sharp osteotome and a mallet. The transected segment of the upper jaw is shifted toward the sagittal plane of the head until the mandibular and premaxillary incisors are aligned. Removing a small portion of bone on the convex side of the deformity with the saw may be necessary if the soft tissues on the concave side of the deformity restrict alignment of the transected portion of the jaw. A bone graft, usually 1.5–3 cm long, corresponding in length to the gap in the bone created on the concave side of the jaw when the maxillae/premaxillae are straightened, is removed from the harvested section of rib graft using an oscillating saw, and this bone is wedged firmly into the gap using a mallet and a dental punch (Figure 26.4).

To transfix the transected segment of the upper jaw, the tip of a 4–6 mm diameter Steinmann pin is inserted through a gingival incision, created between the reserve crowns of the central and intermediate incisors on the convex side of the malformation, and driven, using a high-speed drill, through the transected segment of the upper jaw into the medullary cavity of the ipsilateral maxilla. After being inserted firmly into the transected portion of the jaw, this pin can be used as a lever to help properly align the incisors before it is driven into the maxillae. A Steinmann pin of similar size or two or three, 2-mm diameter Kirschner wires are inserted in a similar fashion on the concave side of the jaw. The Steinmann pin or Kirschner wires penetrate and anchor the bone graft. Using two or more small Kirschner wires, rather than one Steinmann pin, prevents the graft from rotating. Inadvertent entry of the end of a pin or wire into the nasal cavity is not uncommon and seems to cause no adverse effects. The pins and wires are cut close to the gingiva by using a pin cutter or hack saw and are driven below the gingiva with a mallet and a punch.

.   The gingival incisions created for inserting the pins and wires can be sutured or left unsutured to heal by second intention. The gingival incisions at the interdental spaces are closed with 0 (3.5 metric), absorbable, synthetic suture using a simple interrupted, simple continuous, or cruciate pattern.

Postoperative care

The endotracheal tube is removed and replaced with a tracheostomy tube before or after the horse recovers from anesthesia. Anesthetizing the infraorbital nerves with a long-acting local anesthetic solution at the end of surgery provides temporary analgesia. Most horses are bright and alert after recovery from general anesthesia, and so, providing more potent analgesia than that which can be attained with an NSAID is seldom necessary. A horse that displays signs of more than mild discomfort, however, can be administered an opioid, such as butorphanol tartrate (0.02–0.05 mg/kg, IV), methadone (0.1 mg/kg, IV), or morphine (0.15 mg/kg, IV), on one or more occasions. The horse should be administered an $\alpha2$ agonist before it is administered an opioid to avoid opioid-induced dysphoria. Antimicrobial and nonsteroidal, anti-inflammatory therapy should be continued for 5 or more days.

The tracheostomy tube and nasal gauze packing are removed the day after surgery. The packing may be difficult to remove if it becomes impaled on the

point of a pin or wire that inadvertently entered a nasal cavity. The stent bandage over the incision on the bridge of the nose and that over the incision on the thorax are removed at 4 or 5 days, and skin staples or sutures are removed at 12–14 days. Horses can be discharged from the hospital at 4 or 5 days after surgery if no complications develop.

Steinmann pins and Kirschner wires used to stabilize the premaxillae/maxillae are removed at 4–6 weeks, but most loosen and are shed spontaneously at about this time. Failure to remove the Steinmann pins and Kirschner wires from a rapidly growing horse could result in retarded growth of one or both sides of the upper jaw. Plates used to transfix the transected nasal bones are not removed.

The time of anesthesia varies from 2.5–4 hours and is related directly to the number of surgeons assisting with the procedures. Having one surgeon and an assistant procure the bone graft while another surgeon and an assistant perform another procedure speeds the surgery. Positioning the loops of wire to remove the nasal septum from a horse affected with wry nose is often difficult because the curvature of the septum complicates passage of the wires, and so, if difficulty in positioning the wires is encountered, the surgeons should be prepared to remove the septum using other means, such as with a guarded chisel (Tulleners and Raker 1983).

The age of the horse at which surgery is performed does not seem to affect outcome, but surgery is more easily performed on horses 6 months old or older. By this age, the nasal bones are firmer than those of younger horses, making fixation of the transected nasal bones with plates and screws more stable.

Postoperative complications experienced by horses after correction of wry nose include failure of fixation of the transected nasal bones leading to their collapse into the airway; infection of tissue surrounding a plate on a nasal bone, necessitating removal of the plate after the nasal bones have healed; sequestration of the bone graft, necessitating removal of the graft; retardation and uneven growth of the premaxillae/maxillae resulting in brachygnathism and deviation of the premaxillae/maxillae; abnormal respiratory noise at exercise caused by collapse of the alar folds and cartilages, especially the fold and cartilage on the concave side of the deformity; and difficulty in removing the nasal pack caused by penetration of

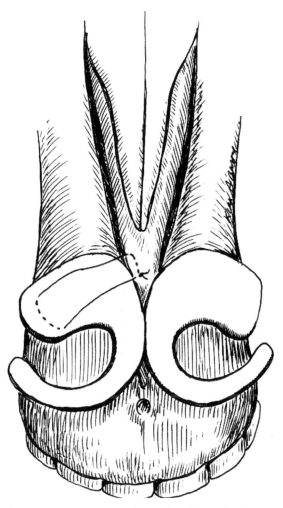

Figure 26.5   To prevent an alar cartilage from collapsing into the airway, the lateral edge of the alar cartilage can be anchored to nasal cartilage rostral to the nasal bones with a monofilament, nonabsorbable suture. Tightening and tying the suture permanently elevates the alar cartilage out of the airway. Illustration by Kim Abney.

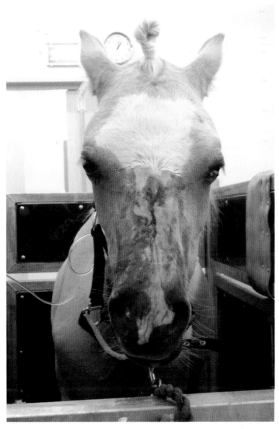

Figure 26.6   Postoperative appearance of the horse in Figure 26.1.

the end of one or more Steinmann pins or Kirschner wires into the nasal chamber (Schumacher et al. 2008).

Abnormal noise caused by collapse of the alar folds can be alleviated permanently by excising both alar folds. Collapse of an alar cartilage into the airway can be prevented by anchoring the alar cartilage to the conjoined tendons of the levator labii superioris muscles rostral to the nasal cartilages with a monofilament, nonabsorbable suture (Figure 26.5). The suture is inserted into the alar cartilage, close to the lateral edge of the cartilage, which is exposed through a 1.5-cm long, longitudinal incision, and the swaged on suture needle and end of the suture are passed subcutaneously to a similar incision created on the midline of the nose slightly caudal to the lateral incision. The needle is inserted through the conjoined tendons of the levator labii superioris muscles on the midline, creating a mattress suture, which when tightened and tied, permanently elevates the alar cartilage out of the airway.

The various procedures performed to correct wry nose can be performed in any sequence, but if the nasal septum is removed before the maxillae/premaxillae and the nasal bones are straightened, less force is required to properly align these bones. If the nasal septum is excised after the premaxillae/maxillae are straightened, loops of wire used to excise the septum can become ensnared on pins or wires inserted inadvertently into the nasal cavity.

The client should be informed before surgery that even though the horse's appearance after surgery is likely to be greatly improved, its appearance will remain abnormal (Figure 26.6). The owner should also be advised that more surgery, such as removal of the alar folds or elevation of the alar cartilages, may be necessary to eliminate abnormal respiratory noise and to improve respiratory capacity. The owner should be advised of all the other possible complications associated with the surgery.

References

Baker GJ. 1998. Problems involving the mouth. In: Reed S and Bayly W, eds. *Equine Internal Medicine* (pp. 605). Philadelphia, PA: W.B. Saunders Company.

Baker GJ. 1999. Abnormalities of development and eruption. In: Baker G and Easley J, eds. *Equine Dentistry* (pp. 49–59). Philadelphia, PA: W.B. Saunders Company.

Bemis H. 1916. Removal of the nasal septum. *Journal of the American Veterinary Medical Association* 2:397–399.

Cousty M, Haudiquet P, Geffroy O. 2010. Use of an external fixator for the correction of a wry nose in a mare. *Equine Veterinary Education* 22:458–451.

Doyle AJ, Freeman DE. 2005. Extensive nasal septum resection in horses using a 3-wire method. *Veterinary Surgery* 34:167–173.

McKellar GM, Collins AP. 1993. The surgical correction of a deviated anterior maxilla in a horse. *Australian Veterinary Journal* 70:112–114.

Mitz Carl, Allen Tom. 2003. Dentistry in miniature horses. In: Allen T. ed. *Manual of Equine Dentistry* (pp. 175–192). St Louis, MO: Mosby.

Puchol JL, Herrán R, Durall I, López J, Díaz-Bertrana C. 2004. Use of distraction osteogenesis for the correction of deviated nasal septum and premaxilla in a horse. *Journal of the American Veterinary Medical Association* 224:1147–1150.

Schumacher J, Brink P, Easley J, Pollock P. 2008. Surgical correction of wry nose in four horses. *Veterinary Surgery* 37:142–148.

Tulleners EP, Raker CW. 1983. Nasal septum resection in the horse. *Veterinary Surgery* 12:41–47.

Valdez H, McMullan WC, Hobson HP, Hanselka DV. 1978 Surgical correction of deviated nasal septum and premaxilla in a colt. *Journal of the American Veterinary Medical Association* 173:1001–1004.

Vandeplassche M, Simoens P, Bouters R, De Vos N, Verschooten F. 1984. Aetiology and pathogenesis of congenital torticollis and head scoliosis in the equine foetus. *Equine Veterinary Journal* 16(5):419–424.

27 Choanal Atresia

Jan Hawkins

Introduction

Choanal atresia is a congenital abnormality resulting in unilateral or bilateral obstruction of the choanae. Choanal atresia is caused by failure of the bucconasal membrane to rupture. The obstruction can be membranous or fibrocartilaginous. Choanal atresia results from failure of the bucconasal membrane to separate from the primitive buccal or oral cavity from the nasal pits during embryologic development. This membrane can be complete, consisting of bone or fibrocartilage or membranous. In horses, the majority of affected cases are membranous (Aylor et al. 1984; Crouch and Morgan 1983; Goring et al. 1984; Hogan et al. 1995; James et al. 2006; Richardson et al. 1994; Sprinkle et al. 1984). Bilateral choanal atresia results in dyspnea at birth and can result in death if an emergency tracheotomy is not performed. Unilateral choanal atresia is typically not diagnosed until the horse is placed into training and is not life threatening (Hogan et al. 1995).

There is no known breed or sex predilection, although most of the reported cases have been in Standardbreds. Bilateral choanal atresia is readily diagnosed because affected foals are unable to breath at birth and will die unless an emergency tracheotomy is performed. Placement of hands over the nares reveals no air movement. An additional abnormality is failure to pass a nasogastric tube on the affected side(s). Unilateral choanal atresia may not be clinically evident till the horse is placed into training. Affected horses make a respiratory noise and develop exercise intolerance.

Diagnosis of choanal atresia

The diagnosis of choanal atresia is suspected based on clinical signs of nasal obstruction or severe dyspnea in foals at birth. Evaluation of airflow from the nares reveals no air movement from the affected side(s). Endoscopy is the best method to confirm choanal atresia. Endoscopic findings compatible with choanal atresia include failure to pass the endoscope into the nasopharynx and the presence of a sheet of tissue at the caudal aspect of the nasopharynx (Figure 27.1).

Radiography can also be performed to confirm a diagnosis of choanal atresia. Contrast medium can be placed into the nasal passage and lateral, dorsoventral, and oblique skull radiographic views

Advances in Equine Upper Respiratory Surgery, First Edition. Edited by Jan Hawkins.
© 2015 ACVS Foundation. Published 2015 by John Wiley & Sons, Inc.

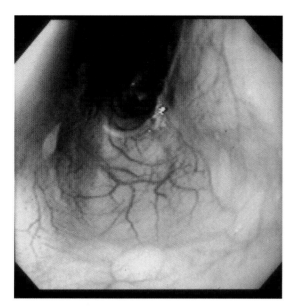

Figure 27.1   Endoscopic photograph of right-sided unilateral choanal atresia in a Standardbred race horse. Note the inability to view the nasopharynx because of the obstructing membrane.

are obtained. The contrast medium will outline the obstructing membrane.

Surgical management

Foals with bilateral choanal atresia must have an emergency tracheotomy as soon as possible after birth. Following the tracheotomy treatment options can be discussed with the owner. Few cases of choanal atresia have been reported in the veterinary literature. This makes treatment recommendations difficult because of the lack of experience with the condition. Nonetheless, there are basically two methods of surgical management: resection of the membrane through unilateral or bilateral nasal osteoplastic flaps and surgical ablation using a non-contact or contact diode or Nd:YAG laser (Aylor et al. 1984; Goring et al. 1984; Hogan et al. 1995; James et al. 2006).

Resection of the membrane through nasal osteoplastic flaps

Resection of the membrane through unilateral or bilateral nasal osteoplastic flaps has been described.

This technique was described before the widespread use of the surgical lasers. This technique should be considered when a diode or Nd:YAG or diode laser is not available, following failed attempts at laser resection of the membrane, or when the obstructing tissue contains fibrocartilage and is not membranous. A unilateral osteoplastic flap is required for unilateral atresia and bilateral flaps are required for bilateral atresia. A frontonasal osteoplastic flap is created centered over the choanae. This can be aided with intraoperative endoscopy. The endoscope is inserted to the level of the membrane and a measurement is taken from the endoscope. The endoscope is then removed and placed at the same level on the side of the face. Once the flap has been created the floor of the caudal maxillary sinus is removed to access the membrane. The membrane is resected by sharp dissection. To increase the size of the choanae it is recommended to remove the caudal aspect of the nasal septum as postoperative stricture to some degree is expected. To minimize the chances for postoperative stricture a shortened nasotracheal tube is placed to stent the newly created opening. The stent is sutured to the nares and gauze packing is placed to minimize postoperative hemorrhage. The packing can be positioned to exit the nares or through one corner of the osteoplastic flap(s). For obvious reasons the tracheotomy tube is maintained until the nasal packing is removed 2–3 days following surgery. It is imperative that the stent(s) be maintained for 4–6 weeks to minimize the risks for stricture of the choanae. In one of the few reported case reports detailing this technique, stenting for 6 weeks resulted in a successful outcome.

Laser ablation of the choanae

Laser ablation of the choanae was first described in 1995 (Hogan et al. 1995); however, the author has been associated with unreported cases of choanal atresia that have been treated with either the Nd:YAG or diode laser. Laser ablation can be performed standing or with the horse under general anesthesia. It is preferable to anesthetize foals with choanal atresia because of the risk for intraoperative hemorrhage requiring pressure and suction and to facilitate endoscopic examination and laser fenestration of the choanae (James et al. 2006).

Foals diagnosed with choanal atresia typically have bilateral choanal atresia thus requiring prompt surgical treatment. Horses with unilateral choanal atresia are usually diagnosed as yearlings or following introduction to training and therefore may be amenable to standing laser surgery.

If the procedure is performed standing, the horse is sedated and the membrane is topically desensitized with Cetacaine. Having performed both contact and noncontact laser incision/ablation of the membrane, the author prefers noncontact laser ablation of the membrane. This is preferred because it is associated with less hemorrhage and the delayed thermal necrosis associated with noncontact techniques can be used to the surgeon's advantage. Contact techniques are good for direct tissue incision but are not very successful for control of hemorrhage. Hemorrhage makes visualization difficult and can be severe enough to require suction or direct pressure with gauze packing. For noncontact surgery the diode laser is set to a minimum of 50 watts and the laser is delivered 3 seconds on and 1 second off. Contact surgery requires a laser setting of 15–20 watts and the delivery time is the same. Noncontact laser ablation begins by deployment of the laser in the center of the membrane. If hemorrhage is mild the entire circumference of the membrane is ablated with the laser. In some instances the surgery must be done in stages if hemorrhage prevents adequate visualization. In these situations if an opening can be created but complete ablation of the membrane cannot be accomplished at the initial surgery the opening is stented with a shortened, appropriately sized endotracheal tube. Endotracheal tubes used as stents are prone to obstructive with upper respiratory tract secretions and may require frequent cleaning. The membrane should be ablated so that it is level with the walls of the nasal passage (Figure 27.2). This is aided with delayed thermal necrosis associated with noncontact laser techniques. Once an acceptable lumen size has been achieved, it is imperative to stent the new opening. Of the few reported cases stricture of the new opening is common. The opening should be stented for a minimum of 4–6 weeks. In one instance, multiple laser procedures and bougienage were required to maintain and achieve an acceptable choanal opening (James et al. 2006). Horses with extreme narrowing of the choanal or nasal passage may require partial nasal septum resection. To accomplish this, a frontonasal bone flap will be required

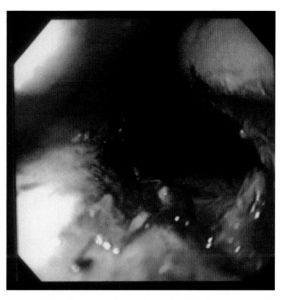

Figure 27.2   Postoperative radiograph of the horse pictured in Figure 27.1. The obstructing membrane was incised with a contact Nd:YAG laser fiber. With the membrane removed the nasopharynx and soft palate can be visualized.

to resect the caudal aspect of the nasal septum (see Chapter 25).

Complications

The most common intraoperative complication is hemorrhage. The amount of hemorrhage is difficult to predict. Subjectively, I feel the amount of hemorrhage is less when noncontact laser techniques are used. This does require the use of a diode or Nd:YAG laser capable of at least 50 watts of laser energy. In some instances higher wattages are helpful in minimizing hemorrhage. Hemorrhage can be managed with suction, lavage, and gauze packing. This can be greatly aided with general anesthesia because it ensures complete patient compliance. As stated previously it may be necessary to perform the procedure in stages until an acceptable opening has been achieved.

Another less common complication is fibrocartilage within the membrane. This may be difficult to assess with endoscopy only. Probing of the obstructing tissue with an instrument passed through the biopsy channel of the endoscope may be useful to help determine the nature of the membrane. Laser ablation may not be successful if the membrane is not completely membranous. These cases will most likely require osteoplastic bone flaps to access the tissue.

The most common postoperative complication is stricture of the new opening. Multiple authors have reported problems with stricture. The consensus is that stricture will occur to some degree but can be minimized with either chronic stenting of the opening or partial resection of the caudal aspect of the nasal septum. Sequential radial cuts with the diode laser or bougienage may also be helpful if postoperative stenosis occurs.

The prognosis following surgical correction of choanal atresia has to be guarded because of the potential of postoperative stricture. However, there are anecdotal reports of horses returning to race training. Since the majority of reported cases have been Standardbreds, obviously the desired end point is racing. If an acceptable airway diameter can be achieved with surgery then horses should be able to return to training and eventually racing.

References

Aylor MK, Campbell ML, Goring RL, Hillidge CJ. 1984. Congenital bilateral choanal atresia in a Standardbred foal. *Equine Veterinary Journal* 16:396–398.

Crouch GM, Morgan SJ. 1983. Bilateral choanal atresia in a foal. *Compendium on Continuing Education for the Practicing Veterinarian* 5:S206–S211.

Goring RL, Campbell M, Hillidge CJ. 1984. Surgical correction of congenital bilateral choanal atresia in a foal. *Veterinary Surgery* 13:211–216.

Hogan PM, Embertson RM, Hunt RJ. 1995. Unilateral choanal atresia in a foal. *Journal of the American Veterinary Medical Association* 207:471–473.

James FM, Parente EJ, Palmer JE. 2006. Management of bilateral choanal atresia in a foal. *Journal of the American Veterinary Medical Association* 229:1784–1789.

Richardson JL, Lane JG, Day MJ. 1994. Congenital choanal restriction in 3 horses. *Equine Veterinary Journal* 26:162–165.

Sprinkle FP, Crowe MW, Swerczek TW. 1984. Choanal atresia in foals. *Modern Veterinary Practice* 65:306.

28 Frontonasal and Maxillary Sinusotomy Performed with the Horse Standing

Jim Schumacher and Justin Perkins

Introduction

The paranasal sinuses can be explored endoscopically through one or more trephine holes to determine the cause of clinical signs associated with disease of the paranasal sinuses, and occasionally, the disease process can be resolved endoscopically through these holes. But when examination or treatment for a paranasal sinus disease through one or more trephine holes is difficult or impossible, access to the paranasal sinuses to diagnose or resolve disease is provided by a frontonasal or maxillary osteoplastic flap.

The frontonasal flap is created more commonly than the maxillary flap because it is easier to create and provides access to more sinus compartments. Creating a maxillary flap is more difficult because the site is partially covered with the levator labii superioris muscle, the angularis oculi artery and vein cross this site, and the attachment of the maxillary septum to maxillary bone sometimes makes elevating the flap difficult. The maxillary flap, however, provides better access to the cheek teeth than the frontonasal flap and so is used to access the apex or alveolus of the first (109, 209) or second (110, 210) maxillary molars. The apex or alveolus of the third (111, 211) maxillary molar is sometimes best accessed through a frontonasal flap.

Exposing a maxillary molar or its alveolus through a maxillary flap, rather than through a trephine hole, permits a larger portion of the sinuses to be examined visually and allows easier manipulation of instruments within the sinuses. The most common indications for creating an osteoplastic maxillary flap are tooth repulsion and removal of dental or osseous alveolar sequestra.

Although inspissated exudate within the ventral conchal sinus is best removed through a frontonasal flap, it can be removed through a maxillary flap. To remove inspissated exudate from the ventral conchal sinus through a maxillary flap, a portion of the sagittal bony plate beneath the infraorbital canal and a portion of the lateral wall of the ventral conchal sinus are removed using a small trephine or a bone rongeur. The reserve crowns of the first (109, 209) and second (110, 210) maxillary molars of horses less than 7 years old obscure this site for penetration, but the ventral conchal sinus can be examined through a maxillary flap, if the horse is less than 7 years old, by deforming the conchomaxillary aperture, located medial to the infraorbital canal, with a finger.

Advances in Equine Upper Respiratory Surgery, First Edition. Edited by Jan Hawkins.
© 2015 ACVS Foundation. Published 2015 by John Wiley & Sons, Inc.

Although surgery of the paranasal sinuses through an osteoplastic, frontonasal, or maxillary flap is usually performed with the horse anesthetized and recumbent, it can be performed with the horse standing, thereby eliminating the risks and expense of general anesthesia. When surgery of the sinuses is performed with the horse standing, structures within the sinuses are oriented in their normal position, and hemorrhage is less than if the same procedure were to be performed with the horse recumbent (Schumacher et al. 2000).

Local and regional anesthesia for sinusotomy performed with the horse standing

Surgery of the paranasal sinuses performed with the horse standing is most conveniently accomplished with the horse restrained in stocks, but can be performed safely without stocks. The horse is sedated with Xylazine HCl (0.3–1.0 mg/kg, IV or 0.6–2.0 mg/kg, IM) or detomidine HCl (0.005–0.01 mg/kg, IV or 0.03–0.04 mg/kg, IM) and an opioid, such as butorphanol tartrate (0.02–0.05 mg/kg, IV) or morphine (0.15 mg/kg, IV) (Doherty and Valverde 2006).

When administered intramuscularly, Xylazine and detomidine should be administered at least 15 minutes before surgery. Sedation is repeated just prior to surgery to minimize movement, if necessary, with Xylazine (0.25–0.5 mg/kg, IV) or detomidine (0.001–0.002 mg/kg, IV). Alternatively, a combination of detomidine (0.02 mg/kg/h) and butorphanol (0.01 mg/kg/h) can be administered by intravenous continuous rate infusion after first administering a loading dose of detomidine (0.005–0.01 mg/kg, IV) and butorphanol (0.02 mg/kg, IV) (Doherty and Valverde 2006). A constant state of sedation can also be maintained by using morphine (0.15 mg/kg/h), rather than butorphanol, after first administering a loading dose of morphine (0.15 mg/kg, IV).

The proposed site of incision is desensitized with local anesthetic solution instilled subcutaneously, and the paranasal sinuses are desensitized by instilling 30–50 mL of local anesthetic solution through a small hole created in the frontal bone with a 3-mm-diameter Steinmann pin or preferably, by anesthetizing the maxillary nerve at the pterygopalatine fossa where it enters the infraorbital

canal through the maxillary foramen. One technique of anesthetizing the maxillary nerve at the pterygopalatine fossa is to insert a 20–22 gauge, 8.9-cm (3.5 inch) spinal needle just ventral to the ventral border of the zygomatic process of the temporal bone at the narrowest point of the zygomatic arch. The needle is directed rostromedially and ventrally in the direction of the third molar (111 or 211) of the contralateral maxillary dental arcade (Bardell et al. 2010). Ten to 15 mL of local anesthetic solution is injected. Structures innervated by the maxillary nerve, such as the ipsilateral paranasal sinuses, nasal cavity, and teeth, are usually desensitized within 15 minutes. Another technique of anesthetizing the maxillary nerve at the pterygopalatine fossa is to insert a 20-gauge, 8.9-cm (3.5 inch) spinal needle ventral to the zygomatic process of the malar bone and dorsal to the transverse facial vessels on an imaginary line drawn perpendicular to the long axis of the head through the lateral canthus of the eye, until the needle strikes bone, usually at a depth of about 5.0–6.5 cm (2–2.5 inches) (Fletcher 2004). The horse may jerk its head if the needle contacts the nerve. When inserting the needle into the pterygopalatine fossa, the needle may inadvertently penetrate a large vessel close to the maxillary nerve causing extravasation of blood, which can result in enlargement of the horse's retrobulbar region, slight protrusion of the eye, and ineffectual blinking, which can, in turn, result in a corneal ulcer.

To avoid complications associated with the maxillary nerve block, the needle can be inserted only 4.5–5.0 cm ($1\frac{3}{4}$ to 2 inches) into the extraperiorbital fat body in which the maxillary nerve resides (i.e., the extraperiorbital fat body insertion technique) (Staszyk et al. 2008). Using this technique, the tip of the needle is inserted through the masseter muscle (about 3.0–3.5 cm) into the extraperiorbital fat body. A change in resistance to insertion is appreciated when the tip of the needle passes through the masseter muscle and enters the extraperiorbital fat body. The needle is then advanced about 15–20 mm, and 10–15 mL of local anesthetic solution is deposited at this site.

Creating an osteoplastic frontonasal or maxillary flap

The surgical site is prepared for surgery after the horse's paranasal sinuses and skin at the proposed site of incision have been desensitized. The horse's head should be supported on a stand so that the head is elevated above the heart and at a comfortable level for the surgeon to perform the sinusotomy. The surgical site is best left undraped so that the horse's reactions to surgery can be more closely monitored.

To create a medially hinged, osteoplastic, frontonasal flap, an incision that extends through the skin, subcutis, and periosteum is created along the caudal, lateral, and rostral confines of the frontal and dorsal conchal sinuses (i.e., the conchofrontal sinus) (Freeman et al. 1990). The caudal portion of this incision extends perpendicular to the long axis of the head, from a point on the dorsal midline anywhere between an imaginary line through the supraorbital foramina and point midway between that line and the medial canthi of the eyes, to a point about 1.5–2 cm medial to the most medial aspect of the rim of the orbit (Figure 28.1). The rostral portion of the incision extends perpendicular to the long axis of the head, from a point on the dorsal midline 1–2 cm caudal to the rostral limit of the conchofrontal sinus, which is located at the level of an imaginary line perpendicular to the long axis of the head, halfway between the infraorbital foramen and the medial canthus of the eye, to an imaginary line extending from the medial canthus of the eye to the nasoincisive incisure (Figure 28.1). The rostral limit of the conchofrontal sinus can also be located by passing a thumb and index finger caudally along

the nasal bones. The site at which the digits begin to deviate from each other marks the rostral extent of the conchofrontal sinuses.

The lateral portion of the incision connects the lateral extent of the caudal incision to the lateral extent of the rostral incision (Figure 28.1). The lateral portion of the incision should not cross the nasolacrimal duct, which is located on a line between the medial canthus of the eye and a point midway between the infraorbital foramen and the nasoincisive notch. The rostral aspect of the lateral portion of the incision can be angled medially, if necessary, so that the incision does not cross the duct (Freeman et al. 1990).

To create a dorsally hinged, osteoplastic, maxillary flap, an incision that extends through the skin, subcutis, and periosteum is created along the caudal, ventral, and rostral confines of the rostral and caudal maxillary sinuses. The incision begins at a point about 1 cm rostral to and slightly ventral to the medial canthus of the eye and extends ventrally, perpendicular to the facial crest, to a point about 1 cm dorsal to the facial crest. The incision is continued rostrally, parallel to the facial crest, to a point about 1 cm caudal to the rostral end of the facial crest, where it is redirected dorsally and extended to a point about 1 cm caudal to the infraorbital foramen. The rostral portion of the incision transects a portion of the levator labii superioris muscle and, usually, the angularis oculi artery and vein.

Before incising the bone to create the frontonasal or maxillary flap, the periosteum is reflected several millimeters from the underlying bone on either side of the incision. The incision is extended through bone by using an oscillating bone saw, a motorized cast cutter with a sharp, sterile blade, or a mallet and osteotome (Figure 28.2). Incising the bone in a straight line using an osteotome and mallet is difficult, and some horses react adversely to the concussive forces created when the mallet strikes the osteotome. To maintain sterility when using a cast cutter, the cast cutter can be wrapped with sterile, cohesive tape (Figure 28.2).

A twitch should be applied to the horse's upper lip to prevent the horse from moving while the bone is being incised. The bone is incised at a 45° angle so that the bone's external lamina is slightly larger than the bone's internal lamina. The blade of the saw should be lubricated with sterile, isotonic saline solution to prevent the bone from

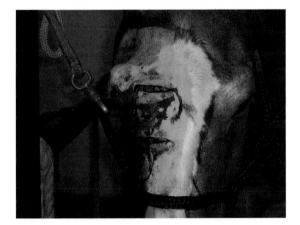

Figure 28.1   To create the flap, a three-sided, rectangular, cutaneous incision, extending through the periosteum, is created over the conchofrontal sinus.

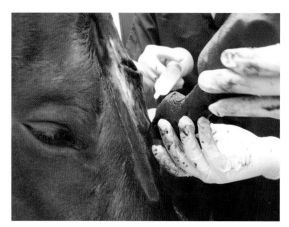

Figure 28.2   Bone exposed by the cutaneous incision is incised using an oscillating bone saw, a motorized cast cutter with a sharp, sterile blade, or a mallet and osteotome. This figure shows the osteotomy being created with a cast cutter. To maintain sterility when using a cast cutter, the cast cutter is wrapped with sterile, cohesive tape.

overheating. When creating the rostral portion of the bony incision over the conchofrontal sinus with an oscillating saw, care should be taken to avoid lacerating the floor of the dorsal conchal sinus with the blade of the saw. When creating the rostral portion of the maxillary sinusotomy, care should be taken to avoid damaging the infraorbital canal and nerve.

The osteoplastic flap is elevated slightly using a chisel or osteotome, fingers are introduced beneath the flap, and the flap is fractured at its base (Figure 28.3). When elevating a maxillary flap, the septal attachments between the rostral and caudal maxillary sinus may require division with an osteotome. The flap remains attached to the skull by skin, subcutaneous tissue, and periosteum. The twitch can usually be removed after the flap is fractured.

The paranasal sinuses can also be exposed, with the horse standing, by creating a hole in the bone of the forehead using a 5-cm (2 inch) diameter trephine (Quinn et al. 2005) (Figure 28.4). Exposing the sinuses through a large trephine hole, rather than through an osteoplastic flap, simplifies surgery, while still providing adequate exposure for removal of diseased tissue, but removing the large section of bone often results in a deep, disfiguring concavity on the horse's forehead.

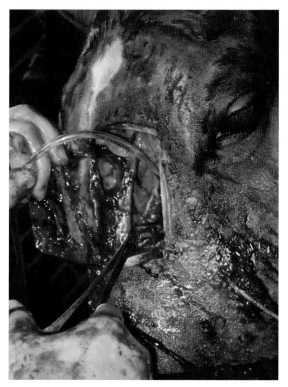

Figure 28.3   The osteoplastic flap, which is fractured at its base. The flap remains attached to the skull by skin, subcutaneous tissue, and periosteum.

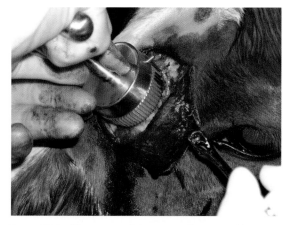

Figure 28.4   The paranasal sinuses can be exposed by creating a hole in the bone of the forehead using a 5-cm (2 inch) diameter trephine. Photograph courtesy of Henry Tremaine, University of Bristol, Bristol, UK.

Elevating an osteoplastic, frontonasal flap or removing a disc of bone with a large trephine exposes the conchofrontal sinus, which communicates ventrally with the caudal maxillary sinus through the large frontomaxillary aperture. The ethmoidal turbinates are seen occupying the caudomedial aspect of the frontal and caudal maxillary sinuses. Within the caudal maxillary sinus lies the infraorbital canal and the apices of the second (110, 210) and third (111, 211) molars. The maxillary septum, the bony septum separating the rostral and caudal maxillary sinuses, usually spans the apex of the second maxillary molar (110, 210). The entrance to the sphenopalatine sinus is seen medial to the infraorbital canal at the caudal aspect of the caudal maxillary sinus.

The bulla of the ventral conchal sinus, which forms the medial portion of the maxillary septum, is usually seen protruding into the caudal maxillary sinus beneath the rostral margin of the frontomaxillary aperture, provided that the compartments of the sinuses are not distorted by disease. Uncommonly, the bulla may lie rostral to the rostral margin of the frontomaxillary aperture making it difficult to visualize. A portion of the bulla is excised to expose the rostral maxillary sinus, which is seen lateral to the infraorbital canal, and the ventral conchal sinus, which is seen medial to the infraorbital canal. The infraorbital canal is supported by a thin plate of bone. These two compartments communicate with each other dorsal to the infraorbital canal through the conchomaxillary aperture. To better expose the ventral conchal and rostral maxillary sinuses, the rostrolateral portion of the floor of the conchofrontal sinus and the closely associated dorsolateral portion of the ventral conchal bone can be removed. The rostral and caudal maxillary sinuses communicate with the middle nasal meatus through the shared, slit-like nasomaxillary aperture, the caudal opening of which is located at the rostral aspect of the frontomaxillary aperture and which lies between the floor of the dorsal conchal sinus and the roof of the ventral conchal sinus.

A portion of the medial wall of the dorsal or ventral concha is sometimes excised through the frontonasal flap to establish a portal for drainage of fluid from the paranasal sinuses into the nasal cavity, and creating this portal is accompanied by substantial hemorrhage. Establishing this portal is usually not necessary because the nasomaxillary aperture is rarely obstructed. Establishing a new portal may be necessary, however, if the mucosa of the sinuses is so grossly thickened that mucociliary transport of fluid to the nasomaxillary aperture is likely to be functioning poorly. When this occurs the establishment of a new portal should be done at the end of the surgical procedure so that the opening can immediately be packed to prevent hemorrhage. Direct endoscopic access to the paranasal sinuses through the ipsilateral nasal cavity should be established if subsequent endoscopic examination of the sinuses is anticipated, such as for examining the sinuses for recurrence of a progressive ethmoid hematoma or a neoplasm.

A portal to remove rolled gauze packed into the sinuses to prevent hemorrhage or to allow lavage of the sinuses after surgery can be created dorsolateral to the frontonasal flap, through a 2-cm long, longitudinal, cutaneous incision that extends through the periosteum. After reflecting the periosteum, a hole is created in the frontal bone into the conchofrontal sinus by using a 9.5-mm (3/8 inch) Galt trephine or drill bit. A portal can also be created in the maxillary bone into the caudal maxillary sinus in a similar manner, about 2 cm ventral and 2 cm rostral to the medial canthus of the eye. The end of a gauze roll packed into the sinuses can also be exited into the ipsilateral nasal cavity through a fenestration in the ventral or dorsal conchal sinus.

The flap is replaced at the end of surgery, and the subcutaneous tissue is apposed with 4–6, widely spaced, simple-interrupted, absorbable sutures, and the skin incision is closed with staples. The inelastic periosteum is difficult to impossible to suture. The bone in the flap need not be secured to the surrounding bone because the bevel on the bone prevents the flap from becoming depressed into the sinuses. The flap can be secured, if desired, by placing No. 2 polydioxanone at the corners of the flap. To place the suture, holes are drilled in the corners of the flap and at the adjacent bone by using a 3-mm-diameter Steinmann pin inserted into a Jacobs pin chuck. The sutured surgical site is compressed with a stent bandage or with gauze swabs anchored by elastic, adhesive tape placed in a figure-of-eight fashion rostral and caudal to the eyes. The arms of the bandage cross at the incision site and encompass the mandible.

Postoperative care

The bandage is removed in 5–7 days, and staples are removed in 12–14 days. Rolled gauze inserted into the sinuses can usually be removed within 12 hours. The cutaneous incision over the trephine hole is closed with staples after the gauze packing is removed or after lavage of the sinuses is no longer required. Decisions about postoperative or preoperative administration of antimicrobial and analgesic drugs are based on the nature of the disease treated through the osteoplastic flap.

References

Bardell D, Iff I, Mosing M. 2010. A cadaver study comparing two approaches to perform a maxillary nerve block in the horse. *Equine Veterinary Journal* 42(8):721–725.

Doherty T, Valverde A. 2006. Management of sedation and anesthesia. In: Doherty T, Valverde A, eds. *Manual of Equine Anesthesia and Analgesia* (pp. 206–208). Ames, IA: Blackwell Publishing.

Fletcher BW. 2004. How to perform effective dental nerve blocks. *Proceedings of the American Association of Equine Practitioners* 50:233–239.

Freeman DE, Orsini PG, Ross MW, Madison JB. 1990. A large frontonasal bone flap for sinus surgery in the horse. *Veterinary Surgery* 19(2):122–130.

Quinn GC, Kidd JA, Lane JG. 2005. Modified frontonasal sinus flap surgery in standing horses: Surgical findings and outcomes of 60 cases. *Equine Veterinary Journal* 37(2):138–142.

Schumacher J, Dutton DM, Murphy DJ, Hague BA, Taylor TS. 2000. Paranasal sinus surgery in sedated, standing horses. *Veterinary Surgery* 29(2):173–177.

Staszyk C, Bienert A, Baumer W, Feige K, Gasse H. 2008. Simulation of local anaesthetic nerve block of the infraorbital nerve within the pterygopalatine fossa: Anatomical landmarks defined by computed tomography. *Research in Veterinary Science* 85(3):399–406.

29 Frontonasal and Maxillary Sinusotomy Performed Under General Anesthesia

Warren Beard

Introduction

Flap sinusotomy of the frontonasal and maxillary sinuses is commonly performed for treatment of paranasal sinus cysts, neoplasia, ethmoid hematoma, repulsion of cheek teeth, sinusitis, and a variety of less common conditions (Freeman 2003; Hart and Sullins 2011; Tremaine and Dixon 2001). Although sinusotomy may be performed in the standing horse, (Schumacher and Crossland 1994; Schumacher et al. 2000; Quinn et al. 2005) the author prefers to perform these procedures under general anesthesia. Standing sinusotomy requires working in the sinus, nasal passages, and sometimes the oral cavity. Local anesthesia can be provided for the skin incision but it is difficult to get adequate desensitization of the nasal passages; therefore, standing restraint relies on repeat bolus injections or a continuous rate infusion of analgesics. This level of sedation necessitates the use of a head stand or cross tying, and often causes ataxia and movement. Head movement occurs despite sedation and requires constant shifting of the surgical lights. For

these reasons the author is able to complete a flap sinusotomy under general anesthesia faster, without distraction, and with less discomfort to the horse.

Advocates of standing sinusotomy usually cite the safety of general anesthesia as the principal reason and these concerns may be warranted, especially for conditions such as an ethmoid hematoma in which significant blood loss is expected. Careful planning, a solid understanding of the complicated anatomy of the equine sinuses, and expedited surgery can minimize the risk of general anesthesia. When significant blood loss is expected, the hemorrhage will not stop until the sinus is successfully packed with gauze. To this end, the procedure should not be started until all necessary materials for packing and closure are open and on the surgical table. Finally, any procedures that will result in hemorrhage should be performed last. A total surgical time of less than 25 minutes is expected for a flap sinusotomy and significant hemorrhage should occur for less than 5 minutes of this time with appropriate planning.

Advances in Equine Upper Respiratory Surgery, First Edition. Edited by Jan Hawkins.
© 2015 ACVS Foundation. Published 2015 by John Wiley & Sons, Inc.

Anesthesia and preoperative management

Anesthetic management for a flap sinusotomy is relatively straightforward. The anesthetist should be prepared to treat hypovolemia and hypotension associated with blood loss with crystalloid fluid administration and the use of vasopressors. Some authors recommend cross-matching to identify a compatible blood donor prior to surgery; however, this is usually unnecessary when the aforementioned steps to minimize blood loss and expedited surgery are followed.

Horses are positioned in lateral recumbency with the affected side up. The nose should be pointed downward at a slight angle to ensure that hemorrhage, exudates, and lavage solutions drain outward instead of accumulating in the nasopharynx and oral cavities. The dependent nasal passage may become edematous; therefore it is a good idea to place a nasotracheal tube prior to the development of nasal edema and to recover horses with a nasotracheal tube in place to maintain a patent airway. Remember that the operated nasal passage may be packed with gauze. Anecdotally, it seems that anesthetic recovery in horses with gauze packing of the sinus tends to be more rapid and rougher than desired. Presumably, the gauze packing of the nasal passages stimulates the horses to recover too quickly. Sedation with small doses of xylazine or acepromazine at the end of surgery will result in a longer and smoother anesthetic recovery.

Selection of surgical approach

A frontonasal flap sinusotomy is performed more commonly than a maxillary sinusotomy because it is a more versatile approach that provides better access to most of the sinus compartments (Freeman et al. 1990). A frontonasal approach is usually the best approach for conditions such as an ethmoid hematoma, paranasal sinus cyst, inspissated pus in the ventral conchal sinus, neoplasia, or in cases in which the preoperative diagnosis is uncertain (Schumacher et al. 1987). The flap may be made large enough for a surgeon to insert their entire hand which can be useful in removing large expansile masses. It allows exploration of both medial and lateral to the infraorbital canal

which is more difficult with a maxillary sinusotomy. A maxillary sinusotomy is superior for repulsion of cheek teeth contained within the sinus or for the repair of an orosinus fistula (Hawkes et al. 2008; Tremaine and Dixon 2001). The emphasis of this chapter is on performing a flap sinusotomy. Details on the specific lesions are addressed elsewhere.

Frontonasal flap sinusotomy

The following description is for a medial-based frontonasal flap sinusotomy. The horse is positioned in lateral recumbency with the affected side up. Landmarks for the frontal sinus are described in the preceding chapter. The caudal border of the incision is perpendicular to the midline and on a line from the supraorbital foramen to midline. The lateral border should not extend lateral to the medial canthus and is usually contoured to remain on the flat dorsal surface of the frontal and nasal bones. The rostral border is made so that the flap will be large enough to accommodate the surgeon's hand (Figure 29.1). The flap may be further enlarged rostrally; however, the bone becomes thicker and more difficult to fracture. The skin, subcutaneous tissue, and periosteum are incised such that the initial incision goes all the way to the bone. The periosteum is not elevated and the bone is cut to the same dimensions as the skin incision with either an oscillating bone saw or an osteotome and mallet. The author prefers an osteotome because the flap can be contoured in any shape desired. There is often a bony septa attaching to the ventral surface of the flap at the caudal border that must be transected with the osteotome before the flap can be fractured. One or more osteotomes can be used to elevate the lateral border of the flap so that the bone may be fractured.

Negligible hemorrhage should result from creation of the flap. A combination of saline irrigation and suction is used to remove any exudate that obscures visibility. Visual and digital exploration of the sinus should precede any disruption of the sinus architecture and starting hemorrhage. The thin floor of the conchofrontal sinus can be removed rostral to the ethmoid turbinates to expose the ventral conchal sinus and bulla, the caudal maxillary sinus, and the rostral surface of the ethmoid turbinates. The ventral conchal bulla may

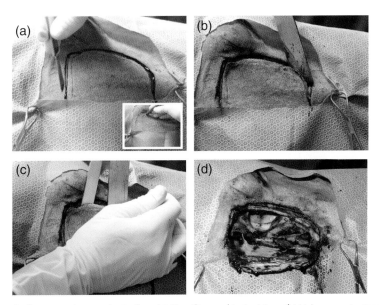

Figure 29.1   Creation of a frontonasal osteoplastic flap. (a) Curvilinear skin incision. (b) Using an osteotome to create a three-side bone flap. (c) Elevation of the flap with two osteotomes. (d) Completed and reflected osteoplastic flap.

be removed to expose inspissated pus contained within.

Any expansile mass within the sinus usually obliterates the normal architecture as it expands to occupy all of the sinus compartments. The infraorbital canal is often completely demineralized leaving the infraorbital nerve exposed in the maxillary sinus. The infraorbital nerve will palpate as a thick fibrous cord coursing from rostral to caudal in the maxillary sinus and the surgeon should recognize it as such and not damage it by pulling on it.

Following correction of the sinus lesion, two issues remain to be addressed, establishing effective drainage and packing of the sinus. Some cases require neither. Creation of an additional drainage portal into the nasal passages is beneficial for conditions in which the nasomaxillary aperture is expected to provide inadequate drainage. Examples would include expansile masses that have deformed the nasomaxillary opening, inspissated pus, granulation tissue formation within the sinus, and a thickened sinus lining from chronic sinusitis. A drainage portal may be made into the nasal passages through the medial wall of the sinus with rongeurs or sponge forceps providing effective long-term drainage. In many instances, this will prevent the need for a repeat sinusotomy. Cre-

ation of a drainage portal that is larger than necessary for exiting the packing is beneficial in cases of ethmoid hematoma so that transnasal sinoscopy may be performed through the portal postoperatively. This will allow intralesional formalin injections for small lesions within the sinus and eliminate the need for a second surgical procedure when there is a recurrence. Alternatively, drainage to the exterior may be made with a trephine into the maxillary or frontal sinus or by removing a corner of the bone flap. Drainage in this manner is preferred by some; however, these drainage portals are not permanent and sinus empyema may recur after the drainage portal heals.

Packing of the sinus postoperatively is necessary only if there is significant intraoperative hemorrhage. To pack the sinus, a uterine pipette is prepared with a curved tip and a 30-inch length of orthopedic wire inserted into the lumen (Figure 29.2). The surgeon advances the pipette up the ventral nasal meatus with one hand while the other hand palpates the medial wall of the sinus. The curved tip is directed toward the sinus wall as the pipette is advanced up the nasal passage so that the surgeon can feel the tip passing against the hand within the sinus. The sinus wall is perforated at this site and the hole enlarged as necessary. The

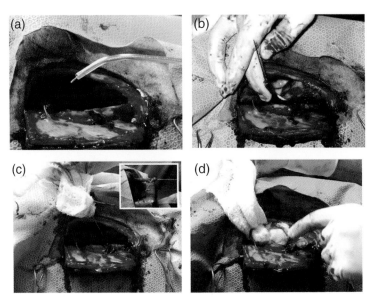

Figure 29.2   Placement of gauze packing into the sinus for control of hemorrhage. (a) Gigli wire inserted into a uterine pipette. (b) Insertion of the Gigli wire inside of the pipette via the ventral nasal meatus. (c) Tying of the wire onto the gauze packing and retrieval from the nares (inset photograph). (d) Packing of the sinus with gauze to control hemorrhage.

tip of the pipette is advanced into the sinus and the orthopedic wire is advanced through the pipette so that it may be tied to the gauze packing. The wire and pipette are withdrawn pulling the gauze packing into the nasal passage and exiting the nares. An alternative to the uterine pipette is to use a jointed Chambers catheter or in some horses, a sponge forceps can be used to retrieve the packing from the sinus and out the nares. The remaining gauze is accordion folded into the sinus from rostral to caudal making certain to fill the entire sinus thereby stopping hemorrhage by tamponade. The gauze exiting the nares is loosely secured to the floor of the nostril with a single suture. The gauze is typically removed in 48 hours resulting in transient hemorrhage that resolves without treatment.

The bone flap is replaced following completion of the procedure (Figure 29.3). A Jacobs chuck and Steinmann pin are used to drill small holes to secure each corner of the bone flap with a single stainless steel suture (Freeman et al. 1990). Many surgeons use an absorbable suture instead of wire and some elect not to wire the bone and rely solely on closure of the periosteum to hold the bone flap in place. All three methods appear to provide satisfactory results. The periosteum is closed with absorbable suture and the skin is closed with staples.

Horses are typically administered trimethoprim/sulfamethoxazole (15–30 mg/kg, PO, BID) for 10–14 days, and phenylbutazone (4.4 mg/kg, PO, q24h) for 5 days after surgery. Not surprisingly, since sepsis is a frequent indication for performing a flap sinusotomy, incisional infection occurs in about one-third of the cases. Infection usually occurs at the rostral corner of the flap and is managed by skin staple removal, local wound care, and systemic antimicrobials. The incidence of infections that necessitate removal of the wire is extremely low. Nasal discharge should decrease and become less purulent in the first week postoperatively. It is common to have the nasal discharge still present at the conclusion of antibiotic therapy. In this instance, antimicrobials are continued for another 10–14 days. Persistence of nasal discharge longer than 1 month after the initial surgery is an indication for further evaluation to include physical exam, endoscopy, and radiographic examination; however, interpretation of sinus radiographs following a flap sinusotomy can be difficult. Cosmetic results are usually excellent (Figure 29.4).

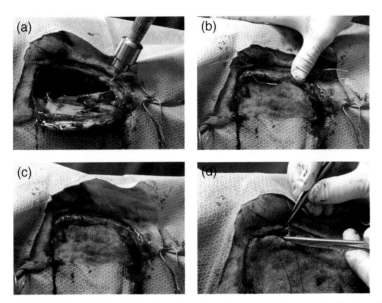

Figure 29.3   Replacement of the bone flap following completion of the procedure. (a) A Jacobs chuck and a 3-mm Steinmann pin is used to drill small holes at the corner of the bone flap. (b, c) Stainless steel wire (20–22 gauge) is used to secure the corners of the bone flap. (d) Finally, the periosteum and subcutaneous tissue is closed with absorbable suture material.

Some horses will develop a prominent bony callus, especially along the rostral transverse cut in the flap. The callus may initially be unsightly but remodeling occurs such that it is barely perceptible by 1 year after surgery.

Maxillary flap sinusotomy

A maxillary sinusotomy is most commonly performed for repulsion of cheek teeth, repair of orosinus fistulae, and neoplasia. Other conditions may be accessed through a maxillary sinus flap; however, surgical access is inferior to that provided with a frontonasal sinusotomy.

The borders of the maxillary sinus flap are roughly rectangular with the dorsal border being a line from the medial canthus of the eye to the infraorbital canal and the ventral border being the facial crest. The caudal limit of the maxillary flap is the medial canthus of the eye and the rostral limit is the rostral border of the facial crest. The angularis oculi artery and vein cross the rostral border of the maxillary flap at approximately the midpoint and require ligation. Otherwise, the maxillary flap is made in the same manner as a frontonasal sinusotomy. The flap may be rectangular or U-shaped depending on surgeon preference. The flap can be created with an osteotome and mallet or with an oscillating bone saw. The roots of the cheek teeth lie very close to the maxilla at the rostral border of the flap and can be inadvertently damaged with a bone saw or osteotome. The septum between the rostral and caudal maxillary sinus attaches to the underside of the flap and must be cut with an osteotome before the flap can be elevated. One final consideration in making the maxillary flap is the age of the horse and the reserve crowns of the cheek teeth. If tooth repulsion is the objective, the flap must be made large enough in a dorsoventral direction to allow access to the apices of the tooth roots. Otherwise, the tooth root will have to be cut with an osteotome to allow dorsal exposure for repulsing the tooth. The maxillary bone flap should be made so that the hinge of the flap is as far dorsal as possible without crossing a line connecting the medial canthus of the eye and the infraorbital canal. A lateral radiograph projection is useful to determine the position and dimensions of the maxillary bone flap with relation to the cheek teeth.

Long-standing sinusitis results in thickening of the sinus lining, which combined with granulation

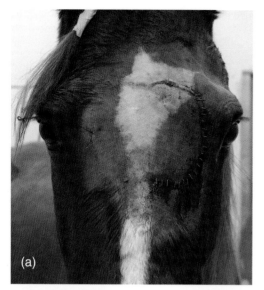

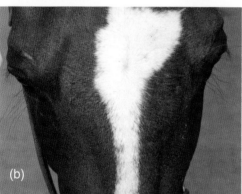

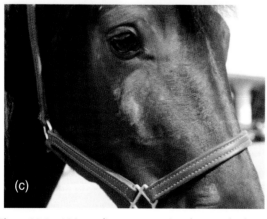

Figure 29.4 (a) Immediate postoperative photograph of a frontonasal osteoplastic flap and (b) after complete healing. (c) Postoperative photograph of a horse with a healed maxillary sinus osteoplastic flap.

tissue formation from the surgical procedure, can obliterate the small communication channels between sinus compartments and even the nasomaxillary opening itself. Surgical intervention to promote free communication between sinus compartments and provide adequate drainage may be required for resolution. The bony septum separating the rostral and caudal maxillary sinuses may be removed to enlarge the communication and improve drainage. A trephine can be used to create a hole in the bony shelf ventral to the infraorbital canal to establish a more ventral communication between the maxillary and ventral conchal sinuses. The ventral conchal bulla may be removed to prevent the accumulation of inspissated pus in that compartment. The ability to perform the preceding steps is somewhat dependent on the reserve crowns of the cheek teeth and many are not possible in a young horse. Creation of a drainage portal into the nasal passage should be performed if it is believed that the nasomaxillary opening will not provide adequate drainage. Criteria for deciding this and the method of creating the drainage portal are the same as for a frontonasal sinusotomy. A drainage portal into the nasal passages is cosmetic, permanent, and may likely prevent the need for a second sinus exploration. Alternatively, drainage to the exterior can be created by removing a corner of the bone flap or by a separate trephine hole into the maxillary sinus.

Packing of the sinus is not usually performed following a maxillary sinusotomy, if for no other reason than the conditions that result in extensive hemorrhage are usually corrected via a frontonasal sinusotomy. In instances in which packing is necessary; it is performed as described for the frontonasal sinusotomy. Closure of a maxillary sinusotomy is as described for a frontonasal sinusotomy and similar cosmetic results can be expected (Figure 29.4). Aftercare is identical to that described for a frontonasal sinusotomy.

Discussion

For many disorders of the sinus, a frontonasal or maxillary flap sinusotomy provides the best chance for resolution of clinical signs with a single surgical procedure. There has been an effort in recent years to develop less-invasive surgical procedures for treatment of sinus disorders and some techniques have been successfully developed to accomplish parts of the procedures described above. Laser vaporization of the dorsal conchal sinus has been described to access the conchofrontal sinus in standing horses (Morello and Parente 2010). A balloon sinuplasty technique has been developed to dilate the nasomaxillary opening and improve drainage although it has not yet been validated in clinical cases (Bell et al. 2009). Lastly, the ventral conchal bullae have been removed via a sinoscopic approach for treatment of inspissated pus in the ventral conchal sinus (Perkins et al. 2009). These techniques have a reasonable chance of success for primary sinusitis; however, the incidence of primary sinusitis is only 5–37% in retrospective studies of sinus disease (Hart and Sullins 2011; Lane et al. 1987; Perkins et al. 2009; Tremaine and Dixon 2001). In cases in which the diagnosis is uncertain, sinoscopic examination may provide useful information although the surgeon should be advised that sinoscopy performed beforehand usually initiates a cellulitis that complicates the subsequent sinusotomy procedure. If the clinical examination makes it clear that there is a surgical lesion, or that exploration of the sinus is indicated, then it is best to proceed with a flap sinusotomy.

References

Bell C, Tatarniuk D, Carmalt J. 2009. Endoscope-guided balloon sinoplasty of the equine nasomaxillary opening. *Veterinary Surgery* 38.791–797.

Freeman DE. 2003. Sinus disease. *The Veterinary Clinics of North America Equine Practice* 19:209–243.

Freeman DE, Orsini PG, Ross MW, Madison JB. 1990. A large frontonasal bone flap for sinus surgery in the horse. *Veterinary Surgery* 19:122–130.

Hart SK, Sullins KE. 2011. Evaluation of a novel post operative treatment for sinonasal disease in the horse (1996–2007). *Equine Veterinary Journal* 43:24–29.

Hawkes CS, Easley J, Barakzai SZ, Dixon PM. 2008. Treatment of oromaxillary fistulae in nine standing horses (2002–2006). *Equine Veterinary Journal* 40:546–551.

Lane JG, Gibbs C, Meynink SE, Steele FC. 1987. Radiographic examination of the facial, nasal and paranasal sinus regions of the horse: I. Indications and procedures in 235 cases. *Equine Veterinary Journal* 19:466–473.

Morello SL, Parente EJ. 2010. Laser vaporization of the dorsal turbinate as an alternative method of accessing and evaluating the paranasal sinuses. *Veterinary Surgery* 39:891–899.

Perkins JD, Windley Z, Dixon PM, Smith M, Barakzai SZ. 2009. Sinoscopic treatment of rostral maxillary and ventral conchal sinusitis in 60 horses. *Veterinary Surgery* 38:613–619.

Quinn GC, Kidd JA, Lane JG. 2005. Modified frontonasal sinus flap surgery in standing horses: Surgical findings and outcomes of 60 cases. *Equine Veterinary Journal* 37:138–142.

Schumacher J, Crossland LE. 1994. Removal of inspissated purulent exudate from the ventral conchal sinus of three standing horses. *Journal of the American Veterinary Medical Association* 205:1312–1314.

Schumacher J, Honnas C, Smith B. 1987. Paranasal sinusitis complicated by inspissated exudate in the ventral conchal sinus. *Veterinary Surgery* 16:373–377.

Schumacher J, Dutton DM, Murphy DJ, Hague BA, Taylor TS. 2000. Paranasal sinus surgery through a frontonasal flap in sedated, standing horses. *Veterinary Surgery* 29:173–177.

Tremaine WH, Dixon PM. 2001. A long-term study of 277 cases of equine sinonasal disease. Part 1: Details of horses, historical, clinical and ancillary diagnostic findings. *Equine Veterinary Journal* 33:274–282.

Surgery of the Paranasal Sinuses: Surgical Removal of the Cheek Teeth and Management of Orosinus Fistulae

Padraic M. Dixon

Introduction

Treatment of the different types of equine sinus disease, especially if chronic (>2 months duration) can be difficult, with many such cases not responding to conservative measures including rest, antimicrobial therapy, or sinus lavage (Tremaine and Freeman 2007). Such refractory cases of sinus disease require further clinical examination, endoscopy, sinoscopy, radiography, and advanced imaging (if available) to allow absolute confirmation of the cause of the sinusitis. Details of these clinical and ancillary diagnostic techniques have been recently described (O'Leary and Dixon 2011). The different causes of sinusitis include primary sinusitis that has been termed subacute (<2 months duration) and chronic (>2 months duration) (Dixon et al. 2012a, 2012b). Primary sinusitis was the main cause of sinus disease in two major UK studies (Dixon et al. 2012a, 2012b; Tremaine and Dixon 2001) followed by dental sinusitis (caused by apical "tooth root" infection) and sinus cysts. Less common causes of sinus disease include: sinus trauma, mycotic sinusitis, dental-related oromaxillary fistula, intrasinus progressive ethmoid hematoma, and sinus neoplasia (Dixon and Head 1999; Gerard et al. 2010;

McGorum et al. 1992; Schumacher et al. 1988, 1997; Walker et al. 1998; Woodford and Lane 2006).

Dental Sinusitis

Conservative treatment

Because of the major short- and long-term consequences of extracting an equine cheek tooth (CT), a conservative approach is warranted in cases where radiographic and clinical findings are not definitive for periapical infection and where scintigraphy or computed tomography are unavailable. It is advisable to initially treat a suspected case of dental sinusitis with antimicrobial therapy and lavage of the appropriate sinuses (often the two rostral sinuses are affected as CT Triadan 09 is commonly infected). The case should be radiographically reevaluated 6–8 weeks later, by which time radiographic dental changes may have become more convincing, if an apical infection is actually present. It is also worthwhile to clinically reassess for the presence of occlusal pulpar exposure, dental fractures, and other changes of the clinical crown of the suspected tooth or adjacent periodontal

Advances in Equine Upper Respiratory Surgery, First Edition. Edited by Jan Hawkins.
© 2015 ACVS Foundation. Published 2015 by John Wiley & Sons, Inc.

tracts by repeating a careful oral examination using a dental mirror and headlamp in the sedated horse. A small percentage of apical infections of caudal maxillary CT with secondary sinusitis may respond to antibiotic therapy (Dixon et al. 2012b). A combination of trimethoprim–sulfonamide and metronidazole has been recommended (Lowder and Mueller 1999). Recurrence of clinical signs in suspect cases of dental sinusitis following medical treatmentis usually an indication for dental extraction. Periapical curettage and retrograde endodontic treatment of cheek teeth apical infections have shown poor results to date (Simhofer et al. 2008), but a recent study using orthograde (from the occlusal surface) endodontic treatment shows promise (Lundström 2012).

Dental extraction

Oral extraction (Dixon 1997, 2005) is the technique of choice for dental extraction in horses and should always be attempted first, as the postoperative complication rates are very low with this procedure (Bienert et al. 2008; Dixon et al. 2000, 2012b). Oral extraction of cheek teeth is best performed in the standing sedated horse (Figure 30.1) which additionally removes the risks and costs of general anesthesia. In contrast, following cheek teeth repulsion, serious postoperative complications can occur, including sequestration (some-

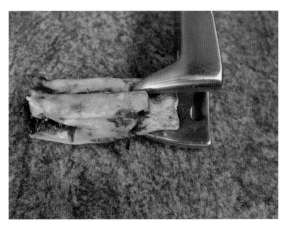

Figure 30.2   This infected maxillary cheek tooth has been completely removed, with all of its roots intact. There is damage to the clinical crown caused by the dental extractors, which is of no consequence. Most importantly in this case, the alveolus remained intact and so there is minimal risk of development of an oromaxillary fistula.

times delayed) of alveolar bone, persistent dental fragments, development of oromaxillary fistula, chronic sinusitis, chronic cutaneous draining tracts, and iatrogenic damage to adjacent CT.

Oral extraction (unlike repulsion) usually removes the complete dental apex (Figure 30.2) and postoperative digital and visual (using a dental mirror or endoscope) examination) will inevitably confirm the absence of any *gross* communication between the alveolus and overlying sinus. The alveolus should be gently lavaged of any remaining debris, a blood clot should be allowed to form and remain in its apical aspect (to promote alveolar healing), and the remaining alveolus is packed with 1 or 2 antimicrobial soaked gauze swabs. These should be removed after about 2 weeks, at which time the alveolus should be digitally checked for the presence of sequestered alveolus fragments, which should be removed if present.

Failure to orally extract an infected CT is usually due to iatrogenically fracturing the apically infected CT during the procedure, which is predisposed to by advanced caries or by the presence of preexisting "idiopathic" dental fractures. Less commonly, the horse's temperament, that is, suddenly moving its head and fracturing the clinical crown, or not tolerating this standing procedure precludes standing oral extraction. Regional anesthesia by

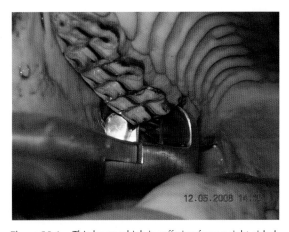

Figure 30.1   This horse which is suffering from a right-sided maxillary dental sinusitis is having dental separators placed on the rostral aspect of the affected tooth to loosen its periodontal ligaments during the start of an oral extraction procedure.

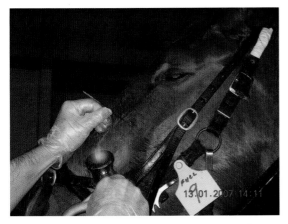

Figure 30.3   This horse has an apically infected maxillary cheek tooth that also has damage to its clinical crown that prevents oral extraction from being performed. A row of staples has been inserted at the estimated repulsion site to allow accurate radiographic determination of the Steinmann pin insertion site and also of its angulation in order to repulse the dental fragment.

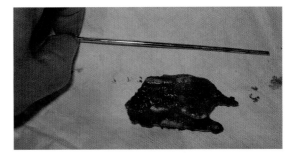

Figure 30.4   This image shows the repulsed dental fragment with an intact apex (roots) and the Steinmann pin.

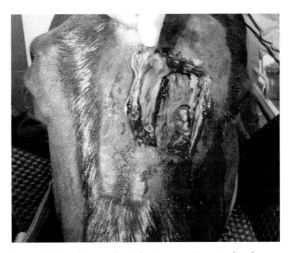

Figure 30.5   This nasofrontal osteotomy in a standing horse with empyema and mycotic growths in the frontal and caudal maxillary sinuses is a suitable portal for repulsion of the Triadan 10 and 11, especially in older horses. However, the alveolar damage caused by such repulsion can cause long-term continuing sinus infection and/or oromaxillary fistula formation.

maxillary nerve blocks improves the tolerance to surgery in some of these cases. Further loosening of CT with iatrogenic clinical crown fractures may be attempted using various long-bladed dental picks inserted between the alveolus and tooth (Zaluski and Davis 2006).

Depending on how loose the infected CT is by the time the clinical crown becomes damaged during oral extraction, the remaining dental fragment can be repulsed with a fine (e.g., 3-mm diameter) Steinmann pin for a loose fragment to a 10-mm diameter dental punch for a crown that is still firmly attached. This procedure can be performed under standing sedation in most horses. Pre- and intraoperative radiographs should be taken to ensure accurate rostrocaudal and lateromedial alignment of the punch with the affected tooth apex. Placing skin markers (e.g., a series of three parallel subcutaneous, 3.8-cm long, 18-gauge needles or skin staples) (Figure 30.3) is recommended before repulsing the tooth (Figure 30.4) to avoid iatrogenic damage to adjacent structures, especially the infraorbital canal and adjacent cheek teeth. If necessary, repulsion can be performed via a sinusotomy (Figure 30.5, which also allows the affected sinuses to be explored for the presence of inspissated exudate (Freeman et al. 1990; Hart and Sullins 2011; Quinn et al. 2005; Schumacher et al. 1987, 2000). However, the vast majority of dental sinusitis cases, even with inspissated pus in the two rostral compartments, can be dealt with by standing sinoscopy with fenestration of ventral conchal bulla and removal of all exudate (Figure 30.6). Poor sinus drainage is rarely a problem in dental sinusitis cases and so sinonasal fistulation is seldom warranted.

Following repulsion of an infected CT, the alveolus is palpated for the presence of residual dental or alveolar bone fragments, including the use of an intraoral mirror or endoscope (oroscope). Postoperative radiographs can identify the presence of

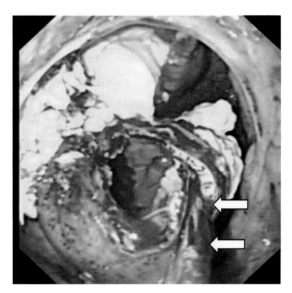

Figure 30.6   Sinoscopic view of the right frontomaxillary opening and the ventral conchal bulla (that has inspissated pus lying on top of it). The bulla is being opened with forceps (arrow) under sinoscopic guidance, revealing further inspissated pus within its lumen. Nearly all cases of sinus empyema (primary and secondary) can be treated by such sinoscopy techniques without performing an osteotomy.

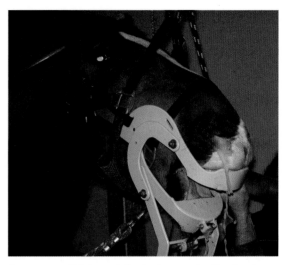

Figure 30.7   This horse is having lavage of a 107 alveolus that has incompletely healed with development of an oronasal fistula, resulting in the lavage fluid flowing down the right nostril.

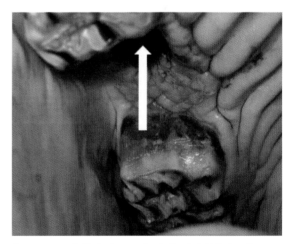

Figure 30.8   (left) An incompletely healed 108 alveolus which has an oromaxillary fistula on its rostral aspect (arrow). The adjacent teeth have a phosphoric acid gel (blue color) applied to etch them and so help retain a PMMA prosthesis.

intra-alveolar bone or dental fragments that are likely to act as persistent sequestra. If recognized, these are removed by alveolar curettage. When a tooth is repulsed with a fine punch (e.g., Steinmann pin), minimal alveolar damage will be present and the alveolus can be packed with antimicrobial soaked swabs, as if an oral extraction had been performed.

If extensive damage has been caused to the apex of the alveolus by use of a wide dental punch, a polymethyl methacrylate (PMMA) plug should be attached to the clinical crown of the two adjacent cheek teeth (that should protrude no more than 2–3 cm into the occlusal aspect of the alveolus) to prevent the development of an oromaxillary fistula. If an oronasal or oromaxillary fistula develops following repulsion (Figure 30.7), it can usually be treated under sedation by alveolar curettage; removal of any intrasinus food, sequestra, and exudate and sealing the oral aspect of the defect with PMMA (Figures 30.8 and 30.9). A sliding mucoperiosteal flap can be performed in refractory cases (Barakzai and Dixon 2005).

Lateral buccotomy technique

The lateral buccotomy technique can involve a very vascular site, always requires general anesthesia and carries the additional risk of causing temporary or permanent facial paralysis or parotid duct laceration. In addition, surgical access to the caudal maxillary CT is limited. Cases of chronic dental sinusitis

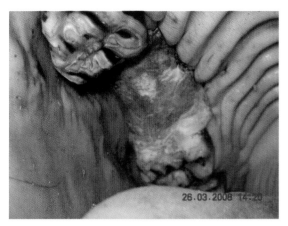

Figure 30.9   (right) Following curettage of the mucosal lining of the fistula, a PMMA prosthesis has been placed between the two adjacent teeth to prevent food contamination of the fistula, thus allowing it to heal. Note that the prosthesis does not have occlusal contact with the opposite teeth which would loosen it.

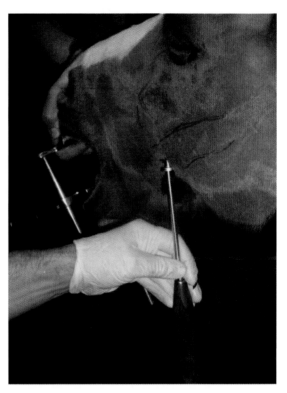

Figure 30.10   This sedated horse that has had its left maxillary nerve blocked, its facial nerves marked out on the side of its face, and its parotid duct cannulated, followed by transbuccal insertion of a small cannula. It is now having an elevator tapped into the periodontal space around an infected cheek tooth to loosen it.

where extensive cemental deposition has occurred on the affected apex, which prevents oral extraction or repulsion of the infected tooth, are suitable candidates for reduction of their enlarged apices by this technique.

A more recent technique to remove fractured cheek teeth is the minimally invasive transbuccal technique (Stoll 2011). Following identification and marking of the buccal nerves on the shaved face and *per os* catheterization of the parotid duct, a horizontal stab incision is made in the cheek at an appropriate site. A trocar with a short cannula is inserted through the cheek (Figure 30.10). Using this portal and under endoscopic (or oroscopic) guidance an elevator is pushed (or tapped) into the periodontal space around the fractured tooth until it is loosened (Figure 30.11). The tooth remnant is then drilled (Figure 30.12), the drill hole tapped, and a screw inserted into the tooth, allowing it to be withdrawn into the oral cavity where it is freed from the screw and removed. The intact alveolus can be treated as described above following an oral extraction. A single suture or staple is inserted into the cheek wound.

Dental-related oromaxillary fistulae

In addition to sinusitis caused by apical infection of the caudal maxillary cheek teeth (i.e., dental

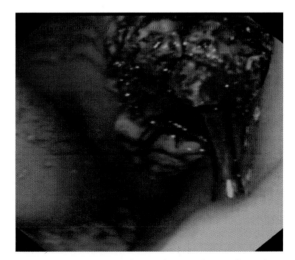

Figure 30.11   An intraoral view showing the transbuccal cannula. The elevator is inserted into the periodontal ligament of the infected tooth that has a fractured crown.

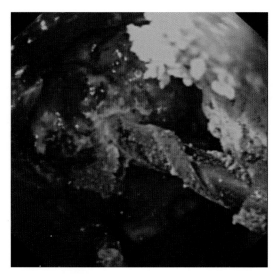

Figure 30.12   This intraoral image shows drilling into the apical aspect of a fractured, but now loosened tooth, to allow further manipulation and its eventual withdrawal into the oral cavity.

sinusitis), sinusitis can also be caused by dental-related oromaxillary fistulae (usually due to the presence of diastemata between the caudal maxillary cheek teeth) that allow food to enter the overlying maxillary sinus (Hawkes et al. 2008). In the absence of apical infection of the two teeth directly adjacent to the diastema, this type of sinusitis can be successfully treated by lavaging all food material from the sinuses (by sinoscopy) and fistula by high-pressure lavage *per os*, and sealing the oral aspect of the diastema with plastic dental impression material (3M ESPE, St Paul, Minnesota, USA) or PMMA.

Conclusions

Equine sinus surgery and dentistry have progressed greatly over the past couple of decades and current techniques, usually minimally traumatic and carried out in the standing horse, carry an excellent prognosis for dental sinusitis and oromaxillary fistula treatment.

References

Barakzai SZ, Dixon PM. 2005. Sliding muco-periosteal hard palate flap for treatment of a persistent oro-nasal fistula. *Equine Veterinary Education* 17:287–291.

Bienert A, Bartmann CP, Feige K. 2008. Comparison of therapeutic techniques for the treatment of cheek teeth in the horse: Extraction vs repulsion. *Pferdeheilkunde* 24:419–427.

Dixon PM. 1997. Dental extraction in horses: indications and preoperative evaluation. *Compendium Continuing Education Practicing Veterinarian* 19:366–375.

Dixon PM, Head KW. 1999. Equine nasal and paranasal tumours: Part 2: A contribution of 28 case reports. *The Veterinary Journal* 157:279–294.

Dixon PM, Tremaine WH, Pickles K, Kuhns L, Hawe C, McCann J, McGorum BC, Railton DI, Brammer S. 2000. Equine dental disease part 4: A long-term study of 400 cases: Apical infections of cheek teeth. *Equine Veterinary Journal* 32:182–194.

Dixon PM, Dacre I, Dacre K, Tremaine WH, McCann J, Barakzai S. 2005. Standing oral extraction of cheek teeth in 100 horses (1998–2003) *Equine Veterinary Journal* 37:105–112.

Dixon PM, Parkin TD, Collins N, Hawkes C, Townsend N, Tremaine WH, Fisher G, Ealey R, Barakzai SZ. 2012a. Equine paranasal sinus disease: A long term study of 200 cases (1997-2009): Ancillary diagnostic findings and involvement of the various sinus compartments. *Equine Veterinary Journal* 44(3):267–271.

Dixon PM, Parkin TD, Collins N, Hawkes C, Townsend N, Tremaine WH, Fisher G, Ealey R, Barakzai SZ. 2012b. Equine paranasal sinus disease: Long term study of 200 cases (1997- 2009): Treatments and long term result of treatments. *Equine Veterinary Journal* 44(3):272–276.

Freeman DE, Orsini PG, Ross MW, Madison JB. 1990. A large frontonasal bone flap for sinus surgery in the horse. *Veterinary Surgery* 19:122–130.

Gerard M, Pruitt A, Thrall DE. 2010. Radiation therapy communication: Nasal passage and paranasal sinus lymphoma in a pony. *Veterinary Radiology and Ultrasound* 51:97–101.

Hart SK, Sullins KE. 2011. Evaluation of a novel postoperative treatment for sinonasal disease in the horse (1996–2007). *Equine Veterinary Journal* 43:24–29.

Hawkes C, Easley J, Barakzai SZ, Dixon PM. 2008. Treatment of oromaxillary fistulae in nine standing horses (2002–2006). *Equine Veterinary Journal* 40:546–551.

Lowder MQ, Mueller POE. 1999. Periradicular dental disease in horses. *Compendium on Continuing Education for the Practicing Veterinarian* 21:874–877.

Lundström T. 2012. Orthograde endodontic treatment of equine teeth with periapical disease—a long-term follow-up. In: *Proceedings of the 51st British Equine Veterinary Association Congress.* (pp. 103–104). Birmingham, United Kingdom.

McGorum BC, Dixon PM, Lawson GHK. 1992. A review of ten cases of mycotic rhinitis. *Equine Veterinary Education* 4:8–12.

O'Leary JM, Dixon PM. 2011. A review of equine paranasal sinusitis. Aetiopathogenesis, clinical signs and ancillary diagnostic techniques. *Equine Veterinary Education* 23:148–159.

Quinn GC, Kidd JA, Lane JG. 2005. Modified frontonasal flap surgery in standing horses: Surgical findings and outcomes of 60 cases. *Equine Veterinary Journal* 37:138–142.

Schumacher J, Honnas C, Smith B. 1987. Paranasal sinusitis complicated by inspissated exudates in the ventral conchal sinus. *Veterinary Surgery* 16:373–377.

Schumacher J, Smith BL, Morgan SJ. 1988. Osteoma of paranasal sinuses of a horse. *Journal of the American Veterinary Medical Association* 192:1449–1450.

Schumacher J, Yarbrough T, Pascoe J, Woods P, Meagher D, Honnas C. 1997. Trans-endoscopic chemical ablation of progressive ethmoidal haematomas in standing horses. *Veterinary Surgery* 27:175–181.

Schumacher J, Dutton DM, Murphy DJ, Hague BA, Taylor TS. 2000. Paranasal sinus surgery through a frontonasal flap in sedated, standing horses. *Veterinary Surgery* 29:173–177.

Simhofer H, Stoian C, Zetner K. 2008. A long-term study of apicoectomy and endodontic treatment of apically infected cheek teeth in 12 horses. *The Veterinary Journal* 178:411–418.

Stoll M. 2011. Minimalinvasive Bukkotomie mit bukkaler Schraubextraktion nach Stoll. In: Vogt C, ed. *Lehrbuch der Zahnheilkunde beim Pferd.* (pp. 208–13). Stuttgart (Germany): Schattauer.

Tremaine WH, Dixon PM. 2001. A long-term study of 277 cases of equine sinonasal disease. Part 2: treatments and results of treatments. *Equine Veterinary Journal* 33:283–289.

Tremaine WH, Freeman DE. 2007. Disorders of the paranasal sinuses. In: McGorum BC, Robinson NE, Dixon PM, Schumacher J, eds. *Equine Respiratory Disorders. Equine Respiratory Medicine and Surgery.* (pp. 393–408). Oxford, England: Elsevier.

Walker MA, Schumacher J, Schmitz DG, McMullen WC, Ruoff WW, Crabill MR, et al. 1998. Cobalt 60 radiotherapy for treatment of squamous cell carcinoma of the nasal cavity and paranasal sinuses in three horses. *Journal of the American Veterinary Medical Association* 212:848–851.

Woodford NS, Lane JG. 2006. Long-term retrospective study of 52 horses with sinonasal cysts. *Equine Veterinary Journal* 38:198–202.

Zaluski P. Davis MH. 2006. The use of dental picks for difficult extractions. Proceedings of the AAEP Focus on Dentistry (pp. 322–324). Indianapolis, IN.

Section IV

Surgery of the Soft Palate, Epiglottis, Arytenoid, and Trachea

31 Surgical Repair of Cleft Palate

Lloyd P. Tate, Jr

Introduction

Cleft palate in the equine is a rare congenital defect usually limited to the soft palate (Figure 31.1). The etiology of cleft palate has not been determined but the author has observed mares bred to the same stallion have repeat foals with the defect. This suggests that there is a genetic component. Cleft palate is not restricted to a single breed but the Arabian horse has the highest incidence in the author's experience. Cleft palates can also be iatrogenic or secondary to trauma and penetrating wounds involving the soft and hard palate (Holcombe et al. 1994). Other respiratory diseases such as entrapment of the epiglottis and pharyngeal cyst can occur simultaneously with cleft palate (Figures 31.2a and 31.2b).

All cases have a guarded prognosis, which should be clearly stated to the owners (Bowman et al. 1982; Kirkham and Vasey 2002; Krause et al. 2008; Murray et al. 2013). Owners should be informed that if surgical repair fails, repeated attempts have a poor prognosis for success secondary to tissue fibrosis of the cleft edges and the additional tension required to oppose them. Foals

evaluated for surgical repair prior to 6 weeks of age appear to have fewer postoperative complications, heal rapidly, and provide the best surgical exposure. Older foals (>6 months of age), other than having increased risk for aspiration pneumonia, tend to have a higher incidence of dehiscence of the surgical repair. Older foals are capable of ingesting solid food and the formation of a food bolus plus swallowing places significant stress on the repair, resulting in failure.

Occasionally, a horse will be encountered that has survived to maturity (Figure 31.3) (Barakzai et al. 2013). These animals are frequently unthrifty and their growth is likely stunted. Dysphagia is always present but varies with severity. In the study by Barakzai et al. congenital defects of the soft palate were diagnosed in 15 horses older than 1 year (Barakzai et al. 2013). The most common clinical signs were nasal discharge, coughing, and abnormal exercising respiratory noise. Only one horse had evidence of aspiration pneumonia. They concluded that horses with cleft palate not affected by severe pneumonia or poor body condition may survive without surgical correction (Barakzai et al. 2013).

Advances in Equine Upper Respiratory Surgery, First Edition. Edited by Jan Hawkins.
© 2015 ACVS Foundation. Published 2015 by John Wiley & Sons, Inc.

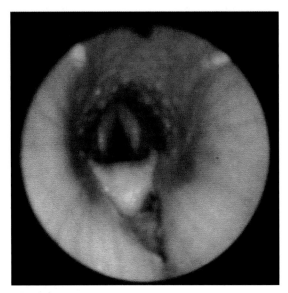

Figure 31.1   Endoscopic photograph of a cleft palate showing oral cavity ventrally and epiglottis and arytenoids in the background.

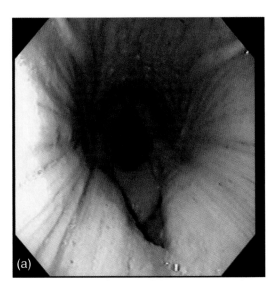

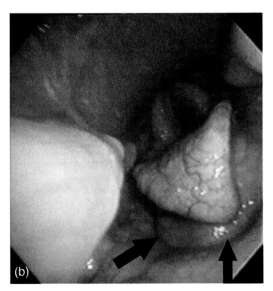

Figure 31.2   (a) Endoscopic photograph of a 6-month-old, Quarter Horse filly with a congenital cleft soft palate and epiglottic entrapment. (b) Endoscopic photograph of a Arabian foal with congenital cleft palate and a subepiglottic cyst (black arrows).

Clinical signs

The primary clinical sign of cleft palate immediately after birth is bilateral nasal discharge of mare's milk (Figure 31.4a). Other signs consistent with cleft palate that may appear as a foal ages include postprandial bilateral nasal discharge, dysphagia, and aspiration pneumonia (Figure 31.4b). Confirmation of cleft palate can be made by nasal endoscopy, which allows for evaluation of the extent and configuration of the cleft. Clefts are not always located on the midline but often deviate to one side (Figure 31.5). In foals, the nasal discharge contains milk, occurs immediately after birth and is persistent. Aspiration pneumonia develops quickly and is related to the foal's inability to suckle normally. This is the major reason not to prolong surgical repair because aspiration pneumonia can be life threatening and fatal. Thoracic radiography and auscultation can be used to assess the presence and severity of aspiration pneumonia.

Surgery: Soft palate

Historically, surgical correction of cleft palate has been attempted through an oral approach, buc-

cotomy, pharyngotomy, and laryngotomy. These approaches provided minimal surgical exposure and generally resulted in an unsatisfactory outcome. Repair made using an oral approach combined with a mandibular symphysiotomy has provided the best exposure and the highest incidence

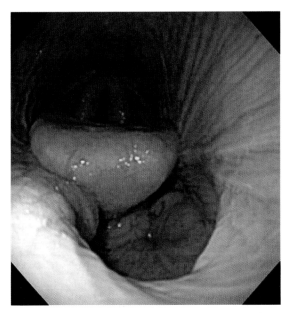

Figure 31.3   Three-year-old, Quarter Horse colt referred for surgical correction of epiglottic entrapment. Endoscopic examination revealed an incomplete cleft of the soft palate.

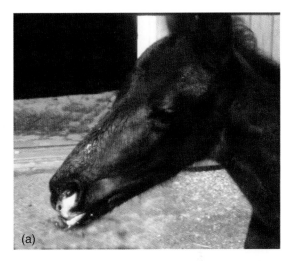

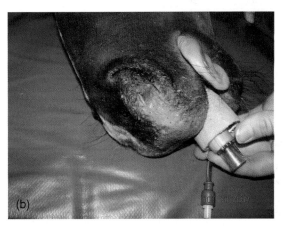

Figure 31.4   (a) Bilateral nasal discharge of milk from a 1-week-old foal with a congenital cleft palate. (b) Six-month-old, Quarter Horse foal with a cleft soft palate demonstrating clinical signs of dysphagia and nasal discharge of feed material.

of satisfactory results (Figure 31.6). Mandibular symphysiotomy can be combined with a laryngotomy and/or pharyngotomy and inhalant anesthesia is administered through a mid-cervical tracheotomy (Bowman et al. 1982; Holcombe et al. 1994; Kirkham and Vasey 2002; Murray et al. 2013; Nelson et al. 1971; Semevolos and Ducharme 1998). Additional methods which have been described to either surgically repair or manage cleft palate include repair via an intraoral approach or the use of the laryngeal tie-forward to manage small cleft palate defects in young horses (Krause et al. 2008; Roecken et al. 2013).

Mandibular symphysiotomy

It is not necessary to extensively fast the foal prior to surgery other than preventing nursing for 4–6 hours prior to anesthetic induction. Broad-spectrum antimicrobial therapy should be started several days prior to surgery and be continued up to 2 weeks post repair. When feasible, antimicrobials are selected based on the results of bacterial culture and sensitivity obtained from pharyngeal swabs or tracheal wash. In order to reduce lung and postsurgical inflammation, nonsteroidal anti-inflammatory drug (NSAID) therapy is combined with antimicrobial therapy.

Immediately prior to surgery the oral cavity should be thoroughly lavaged to remove food material. After anesthetic induction the foal is positioned in dorsal recumbency. The hair is clipped from the chin to thoracic inlet, and the area prepared for aseptic surgery. Tracheotomy is performed first so inhalant anesthesia can be administered through an endotracheal tube inserted

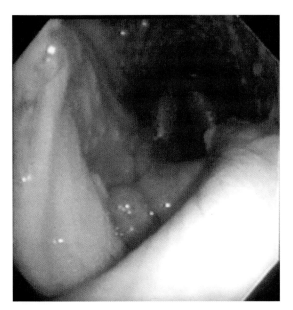

Figure 31.5   Six-week-old foal with an eccentric congenital cleft palate (toward right side).

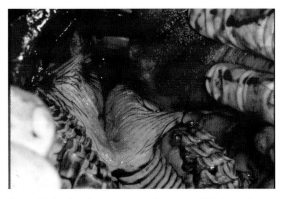

Figure 31.6   Surgical exposure of a congenital cleft palate in a 6-week-old foal through mandibular symphysiotomy.

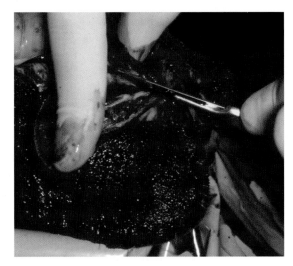

Figure 31.7   Incision of the entire lower lip in preparation for mandibular symphysiotomy.

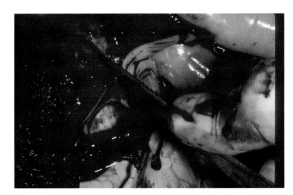

Figure 31.8   Division of the mandibular symphysis in a foal with an osteotome.

through the tracheotomy. Laryngotomy is then performed which will be used later in the surgical correction. Mandibular symphysiotomy is initiated by incising the lower lip, including the Mentalis muscle, on the midline using a full-thickness cut (Figure 31.7). The mandibles are then separated by splitting them between the two central incisors. In young foals, using a large scalpel blade, hardback scalpel, or osteotome is sufficient (Figure 31.8). In older foals, a hardback scalpel may need to be tapped with an orthopedic hammer or a 12–14 mm

osteotome is used to divide the mandibular symphysis. An osteotome or reciprocating bone saw will be required in foals older than 6 months or in adult horses. It has been reported that a horizontal incision made at the level of the gingiva can be used to spare cutting the lip and mentalis muscle. The author has found this to restrict separation of the mandibles and reduce access to the soft palate. Once the lip has been divided on the midline the skin is then incised along one side of the mandible staying approximately a centimeter medial to the lower portion of the ramus of the mandible (Figure 31.9). As the incision progresses caudally, it is directed more toward the lingual

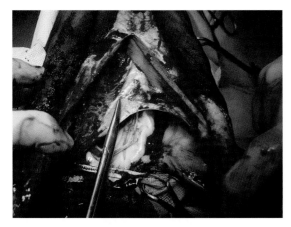

Figure 31.9   Photograph depicting the oral mucous membrane following mandibular symphysiotomy for surgical access of the soft palate.

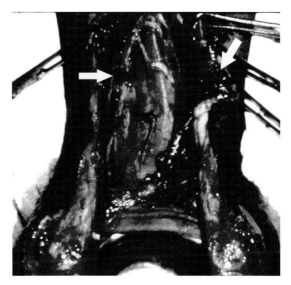

Figure 31.11   Incised geniohyoideus muscle with sufficient tissue present on both sides to fascinate reattachment (white arrows).

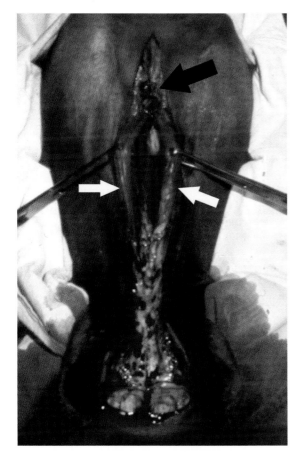

Figure 31.10   Full-length incision to the lingual process which is palpable through the soft tissue (black arrow) and bluntly divided mylohyoideus muscle (white arrows).

process of the hyoid bone, which is easily palpable (Figure 31.10). Termination of the skin incision at the lingual process is usually sufficient but later in the procedure it can be continued a short distance past this point, if required. Subcutaneous tissue can be incised by sharp dissection or with scissors. A finger is then used to bluntly divide the mylohyoideus muscle and mandibular lymph nodes. Traction is applied to each side of the mandible and the geniohyoideus and genioglossus muscle attachment is severed leaving sufficient tissue to reattach them to the mandible (Figure 31.11). Blunt finger dissection is conducted only until the oral mucous membrane or buccal mucosa remains. Any large vessels exposed, hypoglossal nerve, and the duct of the mandibular salivary gland should be preserved if encountered. With continued traction applied to each mandible, the buccal mucosa is incised using sharp dissection or scissors, between the tongue and molars, leaving a minimum of a 1-cm margin of oral mucosa adjacent to the cheek teeth for closure at the completion of the cleft repair. The tongue and both mandibles are wrapped in saline-soaked towels and periodically moistened throughout the surgery (Figure 31.12). Once the mandibles have been separated a Richardson or malleable retractor are used to lift the caudal oral cavity at the level of the hyoid apparatus. The cleft in the palate can be

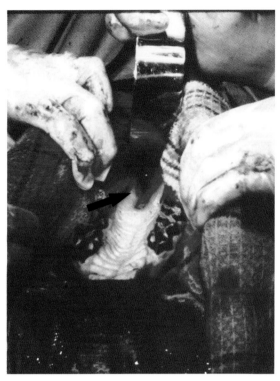

Figure 31.12   Progression of mandibular symphysiotomy through oral mucosa exposing cleft palate (black arrow) with blade retractor in place and mandibles protected by moist sterile towels.

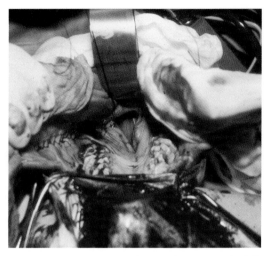

Figure 31.13   Intraoperative photograph depicting the full extent of the soft palate defect. Note stay sutures placed at the caudal extent of the cleft palate. A retractor is being used to elevate the tongue and an assistant is retracting the mandibles. Photograph courtesy of Dr. Dean Richardson.

visualized along with the epiglottis and arytenoids (Figure 31.13). The oral cavity should be swabbed to remove any remaining food material and blood clots that have settled there. The extent and direction of the cleft is easily evaluated at this point and repair can begin.

Long needle holders of 30-cm length, forceps, and suture scissors are required. Horses or foals older than 3 months will require even longer instruments to complete the repair. Sufficient surgical lighting, which is best provided by a surgical headlamp, expedites the surgery. To approximate the length of repair and provide correct alignment a stay suture of 3-0 nylon is placed in each side of the cleft 5 mm caudal to the point where the cleft will be surgically closed. Closure should be planned a centimeter past the desired level as some degree of failure is anticipated. If at all possible, every attempt should be made to oppose the margins of the cleft underneath or in contact with the epiglottis.

Unfortunately, the cleft is most likely at its thinnest at the most caudal extent of the cleft and the location most prone to failure (Murray et al. 2013).

The needle is placed from the nasal side to the oral with each suture. Each stay suture is then passed through the laryngotomy incision and the ends of each stay suture are placed in Kelly hemostats. The needle is left on the suture or a knot placed in the needle side to identify it. This will allow manipulation of the soft palate and consists of elevation, caudal traction, and alignment of the edges of the cleft by an assistant holding the hemostats. Both sides of the cleft are injected with 2% lidocaine and epinephrine to reduce hemorrhage. Following placement of stay sutures a No. 12 scalpel blade is used to split each side of the cleft to a depth of 1 cm (Figure 31.14). This is facilitated by keeping steady tension on the stay sutures and keeping the incision in the middle of each edge of the cleft. In most instances, the No. 12 blade, after being inserted, can be drawn rostrally in one even incision. The two incisions should be united at the edge of the hard palate.

When the cleft terminates at the hard palate, oral and nasal mucosa will need to be elevated off it for a centimeter or what is sufficient to allow approximating of the edges. The nasal mucosa can now be sutured in a simple interrupted pattern or

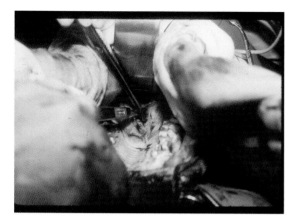

Figure 31.14 Intraoperative photograph depicting suture closure of the nasal mucosa (first layer) in a simple continuous pattern.

everting horizontal mattress pattern (Figure 31.15). The knots should be placed in the nasal pharyngeal passage with equal alignment of the sides provided by manipulating tension on the nylon stay sutures exiting the laryngotomy. Suture material is either 3-0 silk or polyglactin 910 (Vicryl) on a taper point needle. Knot security is sufficient using either type of suture material. When the nasal pharyngeal mucosa is closed, 5-cm relief incisions are made in the oral mucosa adjacent to and centered on the hamulus of the pterygoid bone parallel to the cleft and axial to the molars (Bowman et al. 1982). Again, injection of 2% lidocaine and epinephrine is performed before making the incision to control hemorrhage. A 5-mm osteotome is inserted into each incision and with manual pressure the hamulus is fractured at its base. This allows medial collapse of the levator palatine muscle. Fracturing the hamulus and formation of the relief incision produce hemorrhage; therefore, these are performed after completion of the nasal pharyngeal closure. Three to four horizontal or vertical mattress sutures are then placed from one relief incision across the cleft edges through the opposite relief incision and back to the origin and tied using 3-0 polyglactin 910 (Figure 31.16). The relief incisions are left to close by second intention healing. The oral mucosa is then closed using either suture material in an interrupted or everting pattern using 3-0 silk or polyglactin 910 (Figure 31.17). The nonneedle ends of the nylon stay sutures are tied together and the

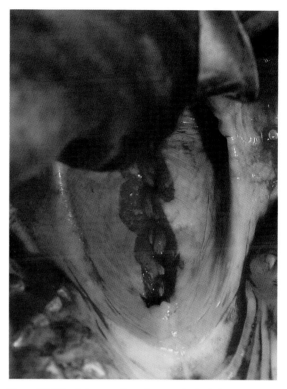

Figure 31.15 Intraoperative photograph depicting suture closure of the nasal mucosa (first layer) in a simple continuous pattern.

knot slid through the laryngotomy and centered on the nasal pharyngeal side of the repair. The remaining two ends (needle ends) are tied through the laryngotomy incision and are used as a tension suture for the most cranial portion of the repair. Some authors suggest the oral or nasal mucosa can be closed using a continuous suture pattern. The author has found that if any of the sutures fails, the entire suture line could be lost. This is a factor that could result in entire repair failure.

Closure mandibular symphysiotomy

The buccal mucosa along the molars is closed with 2-0 polyglactin 910 using a simple continuous suture pattern. This suture line is completed to the level of the first molar and will be finished after repair of the mandibular symphysis is complete. This is accomplished by placing two 4.5 mm ASIF

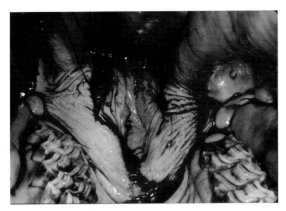

Figure 31.16   Relief incision with ends of one tension-relieving suture spanning cleft palate exiting the wound before being tied.

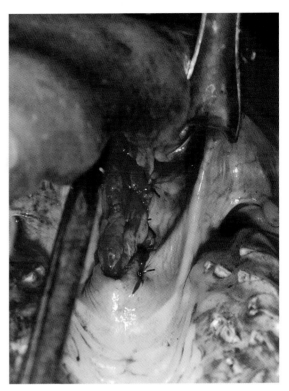

Figure 31.17   Intraoperative photograph of the second layer closure of the cleft soft palate using an interrupted vertical mattress pattern.

screws (cancellous or cortical) of appropriate length across the symphysis to stabilize it. Washers can be useful in distributing the tension of the screw heads on the soft mandibular bone. One screw is placed just caudal and ventral to the lateral incisor and the second 2 cm caudal to the first screw. The second may cross the intermandibular space, which is expected. The symphysis is further secured by placing an 18-gauge stainless steel suture around the two central incisors. Use 14-gauge needles driven through the gingiva to guide their placement. A second wire suture can be placed encompassing the two middle incisors if additional stability is needed.

The screws will become loose in 3–4 weeks and can be easily removed with the foal sedated. The wire surrounding the incisors should remain in place for 6 weeks before it is removed. An alternative to lag screw stabilization of the mandibular symphysis is to use a combination of Steinman pins inserted across the symphysis followed by a (Figure 31.8) tension band wire around the ends of the Steinman pins. However, the author feels that bone screws in combination with hemicerclage wire is the simplest and provides stability and compression to the repair. It is advantageous not to have the drill hole pierce the oral mucosa on the far side decreasing the potential for infection in the holding bone. When placing screws if the screw can be palpated through the mucosa it should be replaced with a shorter screw preventing ulceration and screw exposure (Figure 31.18). The screw heads generally cannot be covered by mucosa and most

screws loosen or demonstrate sufficient surrounding bone lysis to indicate they should be removed in 4–6 weeks. There is generally sufficient stability at that time and the wires can remain in place for 8 weeks. The oral buccal closure can now be finished. A Penrose drain should be placed between the buccal mucosa and the dorsal mylohyoideus, geniohyoideus, and genioglossus muscles. Its ends should exit at the level of the first molar and the last molar. The cut ends of the geniohyoideus and genioglossus muscles are sutured together, and a simple continuous suture of 2-0 polyglactin 910 is used to close the mylohyoideus muscle. A second Penrose drain is placed under the closure of the subcutaneous tissue and exited adjacent to the ends of the previously placed drain. A simple continuous suture of 2-0 or 3-0 polyglactin 910 is used to secure the subcutaneous layer. The skin is closed using suture and the pattern of choice. The author prefers skin staples for their ease and speed of placement.

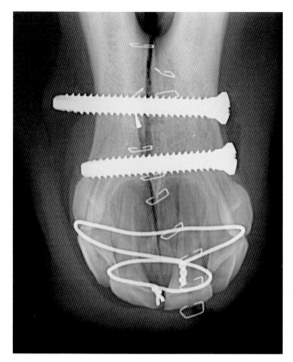

Figure 31.18 Photograph of a radiograph depicting closure of the mandibular symphysis with two bone screw and two bands of stainless steel 16-gauge wires around the corner and central incisors. The distal screw protrudes too far past the edge of the mandible and will be replaced with a shorter screw prior to recovery from general anesthesia.

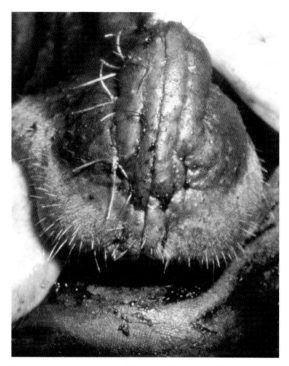

Figure 31.19 Completed closure of the lower lip following mandibular symphysiotomy incorporating tension-relieving sutures.

The mentalis is an area of movement and dehiscence is a frequent occurrence. It should be additionally sutured on the oral surface and reinforced with three to five tension sutures using a horizontal or vertical mattress pattern (Figure 31.19).

Surgery: Hard palate

Repair of clefts involving the hard palate are less likely to have a satisfactory outcome. Hard palate clefts that are over a centimeter wide generally fail after repair. Clefts discovered that are 2–3 cm in length and accompany a soft palate defect can be approximated using sliding mucoperiosteal flaps of the oral mucosa. To create the mucoperiosteal flap, a periosteal elevator or osteotome is used to elevate the tissue. Injection of 2% lidocaine with epinephrine will decrease bleeding and can be employed to provide better visualization. The tissue should be elevated a centimeter past the end of the cleft to provide mobility and sufficient coverage of the defect. If there is tension on approximating the edges of the sliding flaps then relief incisions should be made parallel to the maxilla. Care should be taken in forming the flap and creating relief incisions to not incise the palatine artery. Closure is facilitated using a simple continuous pattern on the nasal side of the repair followed by an interrupted pattern reinforced with mattress tension sutures on the oral side (Figure 31.20). All sutures are absorbable and relief incisions are left to heal by second intention.

Aftercare

Antimicrobial theory should be continued for 10–14 days and anti-inflammatory medication for a minimum of 4 days. The lungs should be monitored for resolution of aspiration pneumonia with

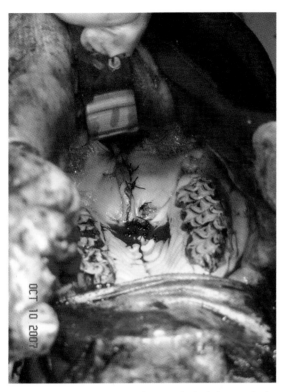

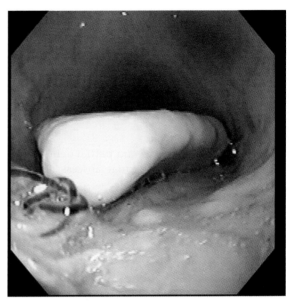

Figure 31.21   Endoscopic photograph of a foal 6 weeks post cleft soft palate repair. Note the presence of a suture material being extruded from the soft palate.

Figure 31.20   Intraoperative photograph depicting surgical repair of a cleft involving the soft and hard palates. The hard palate defect was bridged using sliding mucoperiosteal flaps. Note relief incisions made adjacent to the maxillary cheek teeth.

thoracic auscultation and radiography. The author has yet to have a foal demonstrate signs related to gastric ulcers, but these animals are highly stressed and prophylaxis against gastric ulceration should be considered. Most foals will attempt to nurse and are unable to take in all the milk that is offered by the mare. This is often dependent on the foal's ability to use their tongue. It is not unusual for the tongue to hang out of one side of the mouth or demonstrate partial paralysis for several days. This should improve by the end of the first week. There are reports of using pharyngostomy, esophagostomy, or nasogastric (NG) tube to provide hydration and nutrition. When extraoral alimentation is not used, hydration can be maintained intravenously. If total NPO is chosen, foals can meet their caloric needs via total parental nutrition (TPN). If extraoral alimentation is chosen, the NG tube should be placed into the esophagus prior

to closure of the nasal mucosa. Following completion of cleft palate repair the NG tube is advanced into the stomach. The tube should be of a small diameter, 1 cm or less, and be made of very pliable vinyl or rubber material. It should not be exited through the laryngotomy incision as this tends to cause continuous chewing which is detrimental to the repair. The NG tube should be removed as soon as the foal regains the ability to suckle normally. The Penrose drains should be left in place for 7 days. At 14 days, if the incisional discharge is purulent, gentle flushing of the wound with saline can be performed. Saline may be seen exiting the mouth in these situations. Buccal suture disruptions generally heal by second intention, and no additional treatment is required. The first endoscopic examination of the cleft palate repair can be performed a week after repair. It is not unusual to see several sutures displaced by 2 weeks (Figure 31.21). These areas of disruption will heal as long as the tension or nasal mucosa sutures remain. Skin staples or sutures are generally removed in 14 days, and the tension sutures in the mentalis at 21 days. The bone screws and cerclage wire encircling the incisors are removed in 4 and 6 weeks, respectively.

Complications

There are two classifications of complications—immediate and long term. Immediate complications occur within the first 6 weeks following surgical repair. These can be divided into those that will probably resolve on their own or require additional treatment and those which will remain present. Those, which resolve with treatment, are pneumonia, infection, osteomyelitis and partial dehiscence of the lower lip, submandibular abscess, tongue dysfunction, and gastric ulcers.

Complete or partial dehiscence of the palate repair is the primary failure that is long term. Caudal suture failure of the cleft can be approached through laryngotomy if performed before it heals. Foals may also demonstrate dorsal displacement of the soft palate and to a lesser degree expulsion of food material from the nostrils and presence of food material within the trachea on endoscopy. When this is noted they do appear to adapt and pneumonia persists as a subclinical infection. With complete dehiscence of the cleft repair, second attempts to correct it are not recommended. The palate appears to lose tissue following dehiscence or contracts to the point that reunion is not possible. The long-term problem with stunted growth does not have a specific etiology but is most likely related to multiple complications that persist following surgical correction. Sudden death can occur any time post repair and is most frequently attributed to bronchopneumonia. Any signs of colic is considered a surgical condition if abdominal distention is present. The author has observed foals which subsequently developed intestinal volvulus, jejunojejunal intussusception, and ileocecal intussusception following surgical repair. This has been attributed to the state of stress they are in. I do recommend that horses that have experienced variations of a successful repair not be used as breeding animals in hopes of limiting the future occurrence of the disorder. Owners should be counseled as to this before considering surgical repair of the cleft palate.

Prognosis

The prognosis for conservative management of cleft palate is poor in the foal with clinical signs of aspiration pneumonia and dysphagia. However, as previously noted some foals can grow to maturity with cleft palate defects and in one study the survival rate was 100% (Barakzai et al. 2013). Therefore surgical repair may not be required in all cases.

Foals with clinical signs of aspiration pneumonia and severe dysphagia are candidates for surgical management. The most recent information available regarding the survival rate of horses treated nonsurgically and surgically documented the following: dehiscence of the caudal edge of the soft palate following surgical correction was common, some horses can perform athletically without surgery, all horses that were discharged survived to 2 years of age or older, and that horses with cleft palate had a higher survival rate than previously reported (Murray et al. 2013).

Finally, in addition to surgical repair of cleft palate one additional surgical procedure which can be considered to manage either small clefts in the soft palate or small areas of dehiscence is a laryngeal tie-forward (Roecken et al. 2013). Roecken recently reported that a successful outcome can be achieved in young horses with a laryngeal tie-forward only.

References

Barakzai SZ, Fraser BS, Dixon PM. 2013. Congenital defects of the soft palate in 15 mature horses. *Equine Veterinary Journal* 46(2):185–188.

Bowman KF, Tate LP Jr, Evans LH, Donawick WJ. 1982. Complications of cleft palate repair in large animals. *Journal of the American Veterinary Medical Association* 180(6):652–657.

Holcombe SJ, Robertson JT, Richardson L. 1994. Surgical repair of iatrogenic soft palate defects in two horses. *Journal of the American Veterinary Medical Association* 205(9):1315–1317.

Kirkham L, Vasey JR. 2002. Surgical cleft soft palate repair in a foal. *Australian Veterinary Journal* 80(3):143–146.

Krause HR, Koene M, Rustemeyer J. 2008. Transoral endoscopically assisted closure of cleft palate in foals. *Plastic and Reconstructive Surgery* 122(5):166e–167e.

Murray SJ, Elce YA, Woodie JB, Embertson RM, Robertson JT, Beard WL. 2013. Evaluation of survival rate and athletic ability after nonsurgical or surgical treatment of cleft palate in horses: 55 cases (1986–2008). *Journal of the American Veterinary Medical Association* 243(3):406–410.

Nelson AW, Curley BM, Kainer RA. 1971. Mandibular symphysiotomy to provide adequate exposure for intraoral surgery in the horse. *Journal of the American Veterinary Medical Association* 159(8):1025–1031.

Roecken M, Barske K, Model G. 2013. Modified laryngeal tie-forward procedure for treatment of "small" cleft palates in the horse (abstract). *Proceedings American College of Veterinary Surgeons*, San Antonio, TX.

Semevolos SA, Ducharme NG. 1998. Surgical repair of congenital cleft palate in horses: eight cases (1979–1997). *Proceedings of the American Association of Equine Practitioners* 44:267–268.

32 Surgical Correction of Epiglottic Entrapment

Michael W. Ross and Jan Hawkins

Introduction

Epiglottic entrapment (EE) by subepiglottic tissue (SET), is a common abnormality of the upper respiratory tract and is widely considered a "surgical problem" necessitating management either by resection or by axial division of the entrapping tissue. Known by the misnomers, aryepiglottic or aryepiglottic fold entrapment and epiglottic fold entrapment (Boles et al. 1978), or entrapment of the epiglottis by the aryepiglottic folds, it is now known to be a mechanical entrapment of the epiglottis by SET, which is contiguous with the aryepiglottic folds. Most horses are diagnosed with EE during endoscopic examination for poor racing performance and in some, poor performance is accompanied by upper respiratory noise. However, a definitive causal effect of EE on performance is seldom made; EE may be an incidental endoscopic finding in some horses. Five of 678 normal Thoroughbred racehorses examined endoscopically had the incidental finding of EE (Sweeney et al. 1991). Four of 20 horses with EE managed surgically with transoral axial division under endoscopic guidance were diagnosed using post-race endoscopic examination for poor performance, rather than the presence of abnormal upper respiratory noise (Ross et al. 1993). The authors have examined numerous Standardbred racehorses with EE that was considered an incidental endoscopic finding. Horses were not managed or intermittently received medical management (Ross, unpublished data, 1981–2011). Many performed at elite, championship level without surgical correction (Ross, unpublished data, 1981–2011). While rebuffing the current ubiquitous concept that EE is considered an abnormality requiring surgery, others have advanced the impression that the condition may be incidental. Performance was unaffected by the presence of EE in 13 of 1005 TB racehorses (1.3%) examined after racing in South Africa (Saulez and Gummow 2009). In a prospective cross-sectional study in Australia, rhinolaryngoscopy was performed after racing in 744 TB racehorses, over a period of 35 months (Brown et al. 2005). EE was detected in seven (0.9%) horses and was significantly associated with superior performance and authors concluded that surgical management was likely not needed in horses performing as expected (Brown et al. 2005). In cadavers redundant SET can be easily rolled dorsally to manually induce EE in normal horses (Ross, unpublished data, 1981–2011). Lesions of the SET were prevalent, likely went undetected, and were unassociated with clinical disease in horses undergoing post-mortem examination for conditions unrelated to the upper respiratory tract (Diab et al. 2009). The authors suggest prudent investigation be performed in any horse detected with EE before undergoing surgical correction, particularly in those in which performance is not altered, there is no history of an upper respiratory noise, and those affected with other common causes of poor performance such as musculoskeletal abnormalities. Dynamic endoscopic examination should be used to confirm the presence of an actual mechanical obstruction of airflow.

Surgical techniques

For years, standard surgical management of horses with EE included laryngotomy and resection of redundant SET (Boles et al. 1978; Haynes 1978, 1983; Raker 1982). However, DDSP often developed in horses after undergoing subepiglottic resection without concurrent surgical management for DDSP. DDSP likely develops as a result of altered epiglottic function caused by scarring or excessive removal of SET, or altered function of the soft palate caused by contraction of healed pharyngeal tissue. The postoperative development of DDSP prompted the myriad of methods developed to preserve SET using axial division (see below). Laryngotomy and subepiglottic resection remains a viable technique to manage horses with EE, particularly those in which EE is chronic and entrapping tissue thick and ulcerated, in horses with subepiglottic abscesses, or those in which the tip of the epiglottis is adhered or necrotic. The technique can be used in any horse with EE but should always be combined with concurrent surgical management for DDSP, by using partial staphylectomy and sternothyroideus myotenectomy (if not already previously performed).

Laryngotomy

Horses are placed in dorsal recumbency under general anesthesia. An endotracheal tube is placed transorally and inserted completely with cuff inflated. Transoral intubation facilitates rather than impedes the surgical procedure. A transorally placed endotracheal tube often places tension on the SET or the tissue will be draped over the endotracheal tube, visible from the laryngotomy site. Sometimes the epiglottis will retrovert greatly assisting the surgeon in grasping the entrapping tissue. A minor disadvantage is that the tube decreases the effective size of the airway and may be slightly cumbersome around which to do the procedure. The surgery can be performed using nasotracheal intubation but I prefer oral intubation and later temporary tube removal to allow a partial staphylectomy to be performed. The surgery is best performed in an operating room with good surgical lighting; a head lamp can facilitate visibility within the incision, but good surgical lighting will suffice. In recent years, some have chosen to perform laryngotomy under less than ideal conditions such as in a barn or stall, or in a recovery stall under short-acting general anesthesia, but compromises such as these often result in rapid, incomplete surgical procedures done under less than ideal lighting conditions. The horse needs to be positioned precisely in dorsal recumbency with the head and neck extended; the head and neck should be straight and not tilted. For right-handed surgeons the surgery has to be performed from the right side of the horse and adequate room to maneuver the right hand and arm is necessary. Surgical lights need to be aimed from the surgeon's right obliquely toward the intermandibular space and focused to allow the pharynx to be illuminated. Indwelling endoscopic lighting can also be used. An area centered at the caudal aspect of the mandible is clipped and prepared for aseptic surgery. While this is considered a clean-contaminated surgical technique, general principles of asepsis should be observed. The contaminated airway will be entered but the inner layer of the incision will eventually be closed. Sterile surgical gloves and a surgeon's cap and mask are donned for the procedure. An assistant surgeon can be valuable but is not required. A single fenestrated drape is secured using towel clamps.

Laryngotomy is performed with commonly available instrumentation such as No. 3 scalpel handle (No. 10 surgical blade), thumb forceps (rat-toothed or Brown–Adson, Mayo (straight can be advantageous) and Metzenbaum scissors, Kelly forceps, and a Mayo-Hegar needle holder. A few key instruments are necessary to successfully perform subepiglottic resection and partial staphylectomy. The instruments required include: a blunt-tipped hinged self-retaining retractor (Adson Retractor, West Chester, PA), one straight and one curved (or two straight), Foerster Sponge Forceps (9 1/2", straight or curved, serrated, Sklar), long-handled Allis tissue forceps (9 1/2", 5 × 6 teeth, Sklar), and long-handled Satinsky scissors (Satinsky Scissors, 25.4 cm, S-curved, Integra™ Miltex®, Plainsboro, NJ; http://www.ssrsurgical.com/pages/pg27.html). An ample supply of gauze sponges (rarely suction is necessary), and 2-0 polyglactin 910 or polydioxanone suture material on a curved taper point needle should be available. With the horse in dorsal recumbency the most prominent palpable structure is the cricoid cartilage. The cranial aspect of the thyroid cartilage and occasionally the basihyoid bone can be palpated. Centered at a point where the vertical and horizontal rami of the mandible meet and approximately in the middle of the cricothyroid ligament, a 10–12 cm skin incision is made on the ventral midline of the cranial cervical region. It is important to judge the ventral midline correctly. While some surgeons plunge through the muscle layers without caution, the surgeon should carefully sharply dissect through the loose subcutaneous tissues without "scoring" the underlying muscles (combined sternohyoideus and omohyoideus muscles). At this stage the actual midline, the median raphe, can be seen. Rather than simply sharply incising the muscle layer, a straight Metzenbaum or Mayo scissors is used to carefully separate the median raphe (dissection parallel, in a cranial to caudal direction, to muscle bellies) deep to the level of the cricothyroid ligament. Once separated the rounded, smooth edge of the muscle bellies can be seen. Incision of the muscle layer is completed by placing one blade of the scissors to the depth of the cricothyroid ligament and pushing first cranially and then caudally, bluntly separating the muscles along the length of the incision. Care during this step avoids frayed, torn muscle fibers that can complicate incisional healing. The hinged retractor is then placed and opened (retractor handle is caudal) and the remaining medial fascia can be incised to the level of the cricothyroid ligament. Incision of the cricothyroid ligament must be made on the midline to avoid damage to the underling vocal folds. The midline is found by locating the origin of the paired cricothyroid muscles caudally and the cranial cornu of the thyroid cartilages (ventral prominence formed by the midline attachment of each thyroid cartilage). Before incising the cricothyroid ligament, it is important to ensure the endotracheal tube is well-positioned and the cuff is located caudal to the proposed incision in the mid-cervical region. A scalpel is positioned vertically on the ventral midline and with the back of the No. 10 blade at the cricoid cartilage, the scalpel blade is "plunged" into the laryngeal lumen, and in a "sawing-type" manner the entire cricothyroid ligament is incised to the level of the cranial cornu of the thyroid cartilage, from caudal to cranial. Beginning caudally obviates the potential to inadvertently incise the cricoid cartilage, which can be soft in young horses. The hinged retractor is then repositioned, with the blades placed into the laryngeal lumen, and opened.

Resection of subepiglottic tissue

Resection of SET using conventional surgical techniques remains a viable alternative to axial division of the entrapping SET, but surgeons are cautioned that signs of DDSP often develop if horses are not managed for this potential complication. Therefore, the author always combines resection of SET with partial staphylectomy and sternothyroideus tenectomy (STT). Once the laryngotomy has been completed and the hinged retractor is in place, the entrapping tissue is usually visible on the ventral aspect (surgeon side) of the orotracheal tube. If the tissue is not visible and the epiglottis is in normal anatomical position, a curved sponge forceps or digital manipulation can be used to retrovert the epiglottis. Alternatively, the aryepiglottic fold can be grasped on its midline using a sponge forceps under endoscopic guidance (Figure 32.1). The entrapping SET is grasped using a long-handled Allis tissue forceps and the epiglottis is retroverted using caudal retraction of the entrapping tissue. A straight sponge forceps is applied to the middle (axial aspect) of the entrapping tissue, which is often thick and ulcerated (Figure 32.2a). Occasionally in horses with chronic EE the rostral tip of the epiglottis is necrotic and protrudes through

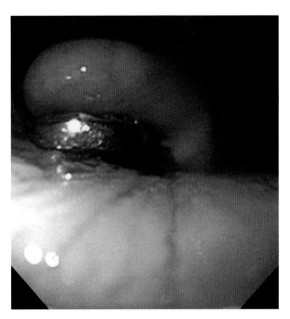

Figure 32.1   Intraoperative endoscopic photograph depicting the grasping of the aryepiglottic fold with a sponge forceps under endoscopic guidance.

the entrapping tissue; in these horses the author debrides (resects) the tip of the epiglottis. It is important to realize that ulceration seen endoscopically on the dorsal aspect of the entrapping tissue will be on the side of the tissue away from the surgeon; the ulcerated portion of the entrapping tissue will be in the portion incorporated by the axially placed sponge forceps. A long-handled Allis tissue forceps is placed on one edge of the entrapping tissue; the author usually places this on the horse's left side. The abaxial tissue is removed first from each side and the axial, midline tissue is removed last. With the straight sponge forceps axially and an Allis tissue forceps placed as far abaxial as possible on the horse's left, a three-step resection technique is then used. For the first step Satinsky scissors are used as much as possible to remove the entrapping tissue on the left side (from the corniculate process of the arytenoids to the left edge of the sponge forceps) (Figure 32.2b). Next, the same procedure is completed on the right side, to remove the entrapping tissue on the right lateral aspect, which is the second step (Figure 32.2c). The third step is completed by resection of the tissue incorporated in the sponge forceps, the axial or midline tissue (Figure 32.2d). Examination of this tissue will reveal an ulcer, if present, on the dorsal aspect. Resection is NOT a tissue preserving surgical procedure, and in fact as much SET as possible should be removed. Philosophically, if you are committed to managing these horses with a tissue-preserving approach, you should choose axial division rather than subepiglottic resection. Often an enormous amount of SET (often pieces of 1–2 × 1–2 cm) is removed. Once the middle of the entrapping tissue is resected, the epiglottis often returns to its normal anatomical position and may be difficult to re-retrovert (Figure 32.3). Thus, it is important to ensure adequate resection in each of the three steps. If as much tissue as possible is resected, the scalloped edges of the epiglottis are often visible. If the tip of the epiglottis is necrotic, it should be resected. Excessive removal of epiglottic cartilage should be avoided but the necrotic area should be debrided. Subepiglottic resection is always combined with partial staphylectomy. To retrieve the epiglottis use the procedures described above.

Partial staphylectomy

Partial staphylectomy is used to manage confirmed or potential DDSP. Unlike SET the soft palate cannot be seen through a laryngotomy until the oro-tracheal tube has been removed. With nasotracheal intubation the soft palate can be visualized on top of the endotracheal tube and does not require extubation. In horses with orotracheal intubation the tube is removed completely or at least far enough to completely clear the rostral end of the soft palate. The presence of an orotracheal tube places tension on the soft palate making it difficult to judge the length. Once the tube has been removed a straight sponge forceps is placed in the middle (axial aspect) of the soft palate (see Chapter 19). If an ulcer is present the ulcerated caudal free border of the soft palate will be incorporated in this bite. What is the correct amount of soft palate to resect? This is the art of the surgical procedure and is difficult to be precise. The authors do not perform the so-called "mini-trims" and do not resect only the middle of the soft palate. The authors prefer to trim the middle and both sides of the soft palate in a three-step procedure. The amount to be removed depends on the length and pliability of the palate.

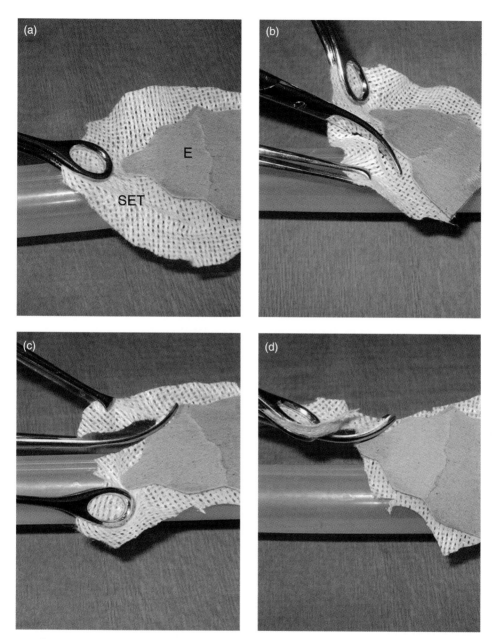

Figure 32.2   (a–d): Resection of subepiglottic tissue (SET) using laryngotomy and conventional surgical techniques is shown in (a–d) (horse is in dorsal recumbency, the horse's right is uppermost and caudal is to the left). (a) The epiglottis has been retroverted manually by grasping the SET using a straight sponge forceps. The dorsal surface of the epiglottis faces the surgeon. The endotracheal tube remains in place during SET resection. (b) A three-step resection is performed by first incising SET on the horse's left side. First, the SET is grasped with a long-handled Allis tissue forceps and resected using a Satinsky scissors. As much of the SET as possible is resected from the rostral margin to the base of the epiglottis. (c) Second, the SET on the horse's right is removed similarly. As much of the SET as possible is removed to the level of the scalloped edge of the epiglottis. (d) The third step involves resection of the apical portion of the SET. It is sometimes necessary to remove a necrotic tip of the epiglottis at this stage. Ulcers associated with the dorsal aspect of the SET will be removed at this stage. The resection should be completed as close as possible and follow the edge of the epiglottis.

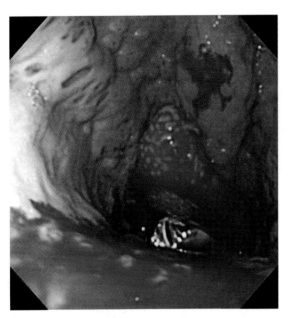

Figure 32.3 Intraoperative endoscopic photograph following surgical resection of the aryepiglottic folds (endoscope positioned in oral cavity).

Approximately one-half of the length of the tip of the sponge forceps is a reasonable amount (1-cm length). Grasp this amount, clamp the sponge forceps, and retract the palate. If the caudal free edge can easily reach the corniculate processes of the arytenoids then removing this amount is safe. If the palate seems short or under an unusual amount of tension the endotracheal tube may be withdrawn only to the rostral end of the palate, placing tension on the structure. There will be decreased tension on the soft palate if the horse's head is flexed and a tendency to remove more soft palate than is necessary; always ensure the horse's head is in a fully extended position. Occasionally the palate will be easily retracted to a position caudal to the corniculate processes of the arytenoids cartilages, and while elongation of the soft palate is unlikely to represent an authentic issue, in these horses as much as 1.25–1.5 cm is resected.

To perform a partial staphylectomy a three-step procedure is used. When SET is resected, the left and right sides of the tissue are resected before the middle, whereas when resecting the palate, the middle incision is made first. Once the correct amount of palate is grasped a Satinsky scissors is used to resect a semi-lunar piece of the midline of the palate, first incising from left-to-midline, and then reversing the scissors and incising from right-to-midline to complete the resection (Figures 32.4a,b). The incision is made right on the edge of the straight sponge forceps to ensure that more of the palate is not removed. Inspection of the dorsal side of this tissue will reveal an ulcer, if present. Next, the left lateral aspect of the caudal free border of the palate is resected by grasping the palate at the junction of the cut/uncut portion of the palate on the left side using a long-handled Allis tissue forceps (Figure 32.4c). A roughly triangular piece of the left lateral aspect of the palate is removed, taking care not to extend the incision all the way to the pharyngeal wall (leave 0.5–1.0 cm of palate intact on both lateral aspects). The third step is to resect a triangular piece of the palate from the right lateral aspect, once again leaving a small portion of the palate intact on the right lateral aspect (Figure 32.4d). Leaving intact palate on the lateral aspects may decrease scarring and potential contraction within the pharynx. Once the three-step incision is complete, the caudal aspect of the palate will be bleeding from the paired palatine arteries, and while hemorrhage may appear profuse, this rarely is a substantial problem. During intrapharyngeal surgery it is usually necessary to remove accumulated blood using a straight or curved sponge forceps or Allis tissue forceps with gauze sponges. The caudal border of the palate is inspected for any tags of tissue that develop if the three incisions have not conjoined. Once a final inspection is complete and the accumulated blood removed, a cuffed orotracheal or nasotracheal tube is reinserted and the cricothyroid ligament sutured.

Sternothyroideus tenectomy

There are various names for this surgery including sternothyroideus myectomy, myotenectomy, or as described, tenectomy depending on the level at which the muscle and tendon of the insert are either removed or cut. Given the many centimeters of extensive retraction that occurs, when the muscle or tendon of insertion is cut, I see no reason to remove an additional few centimeters. While scar tissue can repopulate, the vacated dead space at which the tendon or muscle once occupied the muscle and tendon do not reform either anatomically or functionally if not removed, so I simply cut the tendon of insertion.

STT is a modification of an older procedure known as a sternothyrohyoideus myectomy done most commonly with a horse in a standing position. In that procedure, a midcervical location is chosen and a 5–8 cm segment of the combined sternothyrohyoideus muscles is removed (Anderson et al. 1995; Tulleners et al. 1992). At the level of a laryngotomy, muscles through which the incision is made include the conjoined sternohyoideus and omohyoideus muscles; the paired ST muscles are no longer joined with the sternohyoideus muscles but have diverged craniodorsally to insert on the caudal edge of each thyroid cartilage. The procedure can be done as a standalone method to manage horses with DDSP or can be combined with partial staphylectomy. If combined with partial staphylectomy, once the laryngotomy is partially closed, the STT procedure is completed. The Adson retractor can be left in place but the procedure is more easily

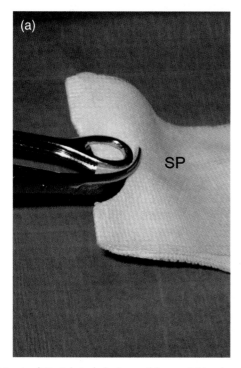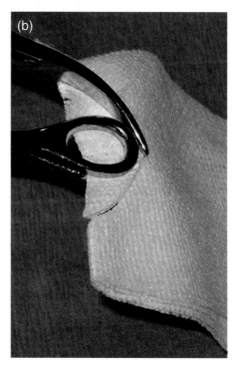

Figure 32.4   (a–d) Partial staphylectomy of the caudal border of the soft palate is shown in Figure 32.4 (a–d) (horse is in dorsal recumbency, the horse's right is uppermost and caudal is to the left). In order to perform partial staphylectomy the orotracheal tube must be removed (depicted). (a) Through a laryngotomy incision a straight sponge forceps is used to grasp the midline of the soft palate. Depth of incision depends on the judged length of the soft palate, which varies based on the head position. Head and neck should be completely extended. When grasped as shown, an approximate 1-cm portion of the middle of the soft palate is resected. A three-step resection is performed by first removing the middle of the caudal border of the soft palate. A curved Satinsky scissors is used to resect this portion of the soft palate by incising from the horse's left-to-right. (b) The first step of the resection is completed by incising from the horse's right-to-left. A half-moon shaped portion of soft palate is removed. If examined carefully, ulcers appearing endoscopically on the dorsal aspect of the caudal border of the soft palate will be incorporated in the resected tissue and are observed on the deep (dorsal) side. (c) The second step involves resection of the horse's left lateral border of the soft palate. A long-handled straight Allis tissue forceps is used to grasp the left edge of the soft palate at the caudal extent of the initial midline resection. A small, roughly triangular-in-shape piece is removed. Care should be taken to not extend the resection to the pharyngeal wall (a small portion of the soft palate on the lateral aspect is left intact). (d) The third step involves removing the horse's right lateral border of the soft palate. Once again, a triangular piece of the caudal free border of the soft palate is removed but the resection is not continued to the pharyngeal wall. The soft palate is inspected for any remaining tags of tissue, which are removed. The cricothyroid ligament is then closed primarily.

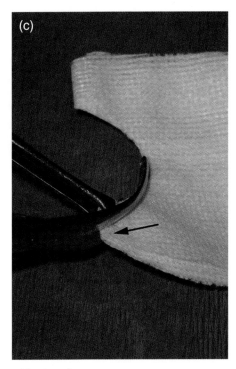 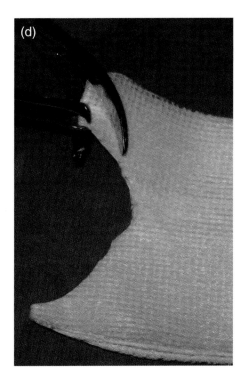

Figure 32.4   (Continued)

performed without it. Blunt digital dissection just caudal to each thyroid cartilage is used to isolate the tendon of insertion of the ST muscle. Dissection is performed at the depth of the cranial aspect of the trachea and parallel to the trachea. A finger can be inserted through the fascia dorsal to the ST tendon and the entire cranial aspect of the ST tendon/muscle is freed from the surrounding tissue and inspected. The ST tendon has a glistening appearance and should be clearly identified from surrounding tissues, such as the external jugular vein. A scissors is used to complete the tenectomy; once cut the muscle/tendon will retract for many centimeters. Occasionally there appears to be only muscle rather than tendon at the ST insertion and in these horses, occasionally, a mild amount of hemorrhage occurs.

Partial closure of the laryngotomy

Once the surgical procedures are completed an endotracheal tube is repositioned and the cuff inflated. The author (Ross) recommends partial closure of the laryngotomy. Historically, this incision is left open to heal by contraction and epithelialization, the so-called second intention healing. A strong recommendation to allow healing in this manner has been made for years (Turner and McIlwraith 1989). While healing can be achieved using the principle of contraction and epithelialization there are common complications, which develop, including, excessive swelling and drainage, foul odor (can smell your clinical cases before you see them), necrotic muscle necessitating debridement and excessive cleansing, anaerobic infections, abscessation, and necrosis of surrounding skin. Since 1987 the author has advocated partial closure laryngotomy, primary closure of the cricothyroid ligament, a procedure that was later modified and published (Beroza 1994); in this publication closure of both the cricothyroid ligament and muscle layers was advocated. Most if not all of the complications associated with second intention healing can be avoided. In addition, subjectively, there is less inflammation within the airway itself when compared to that seen when the laryngotomy is allowed to heal by second intention. Within

24 hours of surgery the mucosa appears sealed as judged from endoscopic examination and there is minimal inflammation within the larynx, both dramatically different observations than seen in horses in which the incision is left open to heal by second intention. The cricothyroid ligament is comprised of three layers, the mucosal layer, an adventitial/intermediate layer, and a dense, thick ventral fibrous layer. Simple interrupted sutures of 2-0 polyglactin 910 or polydioxanone suture on a taper-point needle are placed in the cricothyroid ligament by engaging the ventral fibrous layer and the submucosal tissues. Care should be taken to not penetrate the mucosa although untoward effects are minimal if penetration occurs. There is a fair amount of tension on this closure and cranially, the last suture bites are usually placed in the cranial, ventral aspect of each thyroid cartilage. The remainder of the incision including the muscle layer, subcutaneous tissues, and skin are allowed to heal by contraction and epithelialization, which usually occurs in 16–21 days. Minimal to no swelling, drainage, and lack of any malodor are the norms for laryngotomy healing using this technique.

Laryngotomy aftercare

Horses are maintained on procaine penicillin G (22 000 IU/kg, q12h), phenylbutazone (4.4 mg/kg, b.i.d for 3 days and then 2.2 mg/kg, q12h for 5–7 days), and dexamethasone (20 mg perioperatively, 10 mg, q24h on day 2, 3, 4, and 6 after surgery) and by cleansing of the surgical wound twice daily, ensuring fingers are not deliberately placed into the airway. Pharyngeal lavage (spray, flush) is optional, depending on the extent of intralaryngeal inflammation expected. Horses are given 1–2 weeks of stall rest with hand walking, followed by 1–2 weeks of walking either with a rider-up or in a jog cart, followed by 1–2 weeks of walking and light jogging, before returning to a normal training program. Postoperative endoscopic examination is recommended at 14 days after surgery.

Laryngotomy complications

Complications after laryngotomy using partial closure of the cricothyroid ligament are unusual.

Swelling is minimal, surrounding tissue is supple to the touch, and there is no odor, no necrosis of muscle edges, and little discharge. If care was taken to make the approach on the actual ventral midline and not through muscle the wound drains well without serum accumulation. If incisions through skin and muscle were staggered (in different planes) the wound may not drain well and seroma can develop. Seroma develops if muscle edges heal prematurely and can be alleviated by manually opening muscle edges and cleaning the site more frequently. Rarely the cricothyroid closure will dehisce. Dehiscence has occurred in two horses in which the author used a simple continuous suture pattern. Simple interrupted sutures are recommended. Sutures that penetrate the laryngeal mucosa may cause irritation and coughing but this complication is of minimal concern. However, care should be taken during cricothyroid closure to avoid luminal penetration.

Complications following resection of aryepiglottic folds

Complications can include recurrence, which is rare if adequate SET is removed as described. Occasionally horses affected with chronic EE in which a large amount of SET is removed, or in which the tissue was abscessed and chronically inflamed, will develop persistent DDSP; this usually occurs when partial staphylectomy was not done concurrently, but rarely occurs when the procedures are combined. Scarred SET likely prevents a normal position of the epiglottis relative to the soft palate, or interferes with normal epiglottal/palatal function. In these horses laryngohyoid reduction (tie-forward) can be contemplated but DDSP can remain a complication, given the restriction in the position. In three horses the author has performed hyoepiglotticus myotomy using a ventral midline approach cranial to the basihyoid (position for pharyngotomy). There is a distinct fibrous layer external to the actual hyoepiglotticus muscle that is incised as well. In two horses persistent DDSP resolved and horses raced after revision surgery. In one TB racehorse, the horse improved and raced but intermittent DDSP continued to occur.

Transoral axial division of EE

DDSP can be a complication after subepiglottic resection using the previously described surgical techniques, especially when not combined with concurrent surgical management for DDSP. This complication has prompted some surgeons to develop tissue sparing procedures. Axial division of the aryepiglottic fold preserves SET and obviates the potential for scarring and wound contraction that could potentiate mechanical problems or dysfunction with the soft palate. Techniques using transnasal approaches eliminated the need to use general anesthesia to perform laryngotomy, another criticism of performing conventional surgical management for EE. Transnasal axial division using a bistoury (Greet 1995; Honnas and Wheat 1988), transoral axial division using short-acting general anesthesia (Lumsden et al. 1994; Ross et al. 1993; Russell and Wainscott 2007), transoral axial division in standing horses (Perkin et al. 2007), and transnasal axial division using a shielded hook bistoury (Lacourt and Marcoux 2011) have been used. With the possible exception of the shielded hook bistoury technique, any of the approaches in conscious, standing horses, or any transnasal technique done in standing or recumbent horses, poses risks for inadvertent laceration of the soft palate, the most important and devastating of the possible complications. Iatrogenic damage to the soft palate cannot occur using a transoral technique. When compared to axial divisions performed using laser energy in standing horses, transoral axial division allows for a deeper (longer) incision in SET, obviates the potential for laser thermal damage to occur, and may cause less overall inflammation after surgery.

The technique was previously described in 20 horses (Ross et al. 1993). Horses were sedated with xylazine HCl (0.55–1.1 mg/kg of body weight, IV). Short-acting general anesthesia can be induced using ketamine HCl (2.2 mg/kg, IV) or glycerol guaiacolate (15–30 g/horse, IV) in combination with ketamine. If needed, anesthesia can be maintained with a continuous IV infusion of xylazine, ketamine, and glycerol guaiacolate (triple drip). Horses are placed in right lateral recumbency, with the head positioned on a pad, to allow the rostral 20 cm of the head to be elevated above floor or table level and free of the pad. A mouth

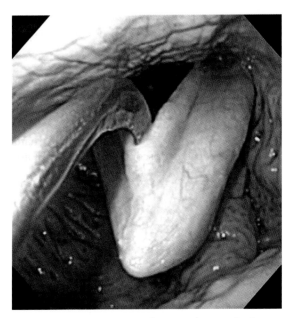

Figure 32.5   Intraoperative endoscopic photograph of a bistoury being used for oral axial division of the aryepiglottic fold under general anesthesia.

speculum is inserted, and the tongue is pulled from the right side of the mouth by an assistant. Tension is maintained on the tongue, a procedure which eases manipulation in the oral cavity. The soft palate is manually displaced, and a 1-meter flexible endoscope is inserted through the mouth to visualize the entrapped epiglottis. A custom-made stainless steel curved bistoury is used to incise the entrapping tissue (Figure 32.5). The bistoury can be constructed in the following manner. The handle, 90-cm long, is attached to a half-circle stainless steel cutting blade, 3 cm in diameter, with a sharp edge and tip. Beginning 30 cm from the cutting edge, the handle is curved downward 15° to allow the instrument to pass easily over the base of the tongue. The bistoury is positioned on the midline of the entrapping tissue under endoscopic guidance. If the bistoury is judged to be seated lateral to the axis, it can be repositioned. Care is taken to prevent the bistoury from entering the rima glottidis. Once the bistoury is properly seated, tension is placed on the handle (the surgeon uses the right hand to pull the handle) to maintain the position of the instrument. Tension on the handle is maintained while the endoscope is removed and the surgeon's left hand is inserted to the level of the caudal aspect of the tongue. Some horses can swallow during this stage of the procedure. Outward tension is maintained to prevent laceration of laryngeal and pharyngeal structures. The incision is completed while the surgeon maintained ventral pressure on the bistoury and ensured that the sharp tip does not penetrate the base of the tongue. The blade is carefully guarded in the surgeon's hand and removed. The endoscope is then inserted and used to ensure that the incision is complete. The procedure can be completed in 3–5 minutes.

Postoperative care

Immediately after recovery from general anesthesia, all horses are administered anti-inflammatories (phenylbutazone 4.4 mg/kg, IV and dexamethasone 20 mg/horse, IV). Pharyngeal spray (15 mL of a solution comprised of 750 mL nitrofurazone, 250 mL of DMSO, 100 mL glycerin, and 2 g of prednisolone), is administered to all horses after recovery, through a nasal catheter, 3 times daily for 7 days after surgery. Horses are housed in a box stall and hand walked, and are given phenylbutazone (3.3 mg/kg, PO, q12h) for 7 days after surgery. Endoscopic examination is performed immediately after surgery. Examining veterinarians are requested to perform endoscopic examinations on day 7 after surgery, and additional examinations are performed as needed. Horses are generally returned to race training on day 7 after surgery, if the epiglottis is free of entrapment and inflammation had subsided.

Complications are similar to any surgical procedure for EE including recurrence, development of DDSP after surgery, and continued poor racing performance despite surgical management for EE. Inadvertent laceration of the soft palate is not a complication of this procedure, although inadvertent laceration of aryepiglottic folds or other pharyngeal structures can occur if horses swallow. Once the bistoury is engaged in the SET, the surgeon must keep tension in a rostral direction at all times to prevent dislodgement of the bistoury. In the original manuscript, written by the first author, EE recurred in 2 of 20 horses (10%) but in practice, it appears that recurrence rate for any technique using axial division and tissue preservation may

be considerably higher. In addition, horses should have 2–3 weeks rest to allow resolution of inflammation before being placed back into race training. The 7-day period we originally recommended may place the horse at risk for early recurrence. Stall rest with hand walking for 7 days, walking in a jog cart or under tack for 7 days, and then light exercise for 7 days is my current recommendation.

Laser axial division of the aryepiglottic fold (Jan Hawkins)

Introduction

As previously mentioned, the three most common methods to surgically correct EE include: axial division with the laser, axial division with a transnasal or oral bistoury knife, and correction via laryngotomy. The method chosen varies with surgeon preference and experience with the three techniques. In the author's experience approximately 75–80% of horses with EE can be treated with axial division using the laser or bistoury knife. The remaining 20–25% of horses with EE are best treated with correction via laryngotomy. Laser axial division is chosen for horses with thin, non- to mildly ulcerated entrapments. It has been the author's experience that these horses respond well to axial division with a minimum of complications. Horses with thick, wide, and moderately to severely ulcerated entrapments are best treated with resection of the aryepiglottic fold via laryngotomy.

Standing laser correction of epiglottic entrapment

The equipment required for laser axial division of the aryepiglottic fold include: diode laser capable of generating 15–25 watts of laser energy, contact laser fiber, topical anesthetic, and bronchoesophageal grasping forceps. It is the author's preference to use a contact laser fiber rather than a noncontact laser fiber (Tulleners 1990, 1991). The main reason for this is that lower wattages and lower power density is required to incise the aryepiglottic fold. It has been the author's experience that noncontact laser incision is associated with increased edema, inflammation, and fibrosis

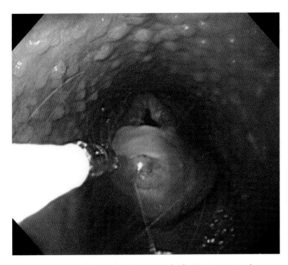

Figure 32.6 Endoscopic photograph depicting topical application of local anesthetic to the epiglottis via an endoscopic spraying device.

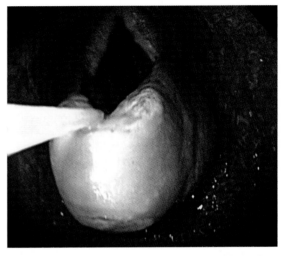

Figure 32.7 Endoscopic photograph depicting the initial positioning of the diode laser fiber at the caudal aspect of the aryepiglottic fold.

of the incision site following surgical correction. However, successful noncontact laser correction of EE has been described (Tate et al. 1990). The procedure begins with the horse restrained in stocks with the head secured in cross ties. The horse is sedated with detomidine hydrochloride (5–10 mg, IV) and butorphanol tartrate (5 mg, IV). The aryepiglottic fold is topically anesthetized with Cetacaine® (Cetylite Inc., Pennsauken, NJ) (Figure 32.6). A 600 μ laser fiber is passed down the biopsy channel of the endoscope and the sculpted fiber is placed in contact with the caudal aspect of the aryepiglottic fold (Figure 32.7). The laser is set to 15 watts and is delivered in a pattern of 3 seconds on and 1 second off. The fold is incised from caudal to rostral. The laser fiber is "dragged" across the fold to incise the uppermost layer of the fold (Figure 32.8). This is accomplished by both manual movement of the fiber and by an assistant who is manipulating the endoscope. The assistant must be aware that endoscopic movement needs to be subtle and deliberate to avoid excessive movement of the fiber. The surgeon has to communicate clearly when the endoscope is to be moved in or out by the assistant. The laser fiber is then used to incise the complete thickness of the fold starting at the caudal aspect (Figure 32.9). After each pass of the fiber the horse is triggered to swallow to cause retraction and stretch-

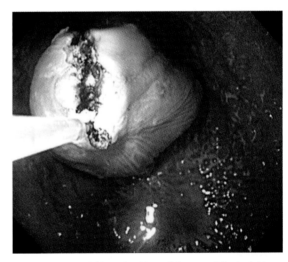

Figure 32.8 Initial laser incision of the aryepiglottic fold starting from the caudal to rostral. The incision should be centered as closely as possible down the center of the fold. It is important to incise the fold so that the incision terminates under the tip of the epiglottis.

ing of the fold (Figure 32.10). It is of paramount importance to identify the location of the epiglottic tip at all times (Figure 32.11). This is necessary to prevent iatrogenic damage to the epiglottic tip cartilage. In some cases of chronic EE the epiglottic tip can be folded up under the fold, resulting in

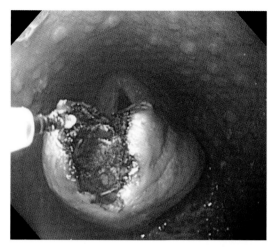

Figure 32.9   Once the fold has been incised through the superficial layer of the entrapping membrane the incision is progressively deepened. Starting caudally the edge of the fold is contacted with the laser fiber. At all points during the incision the epiglottic tip should be located and protected.

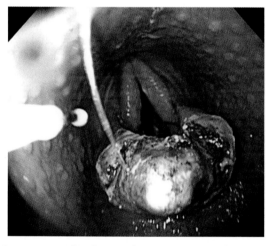

Figure 32.10   This photograph represents a critical point in the procedure because as the superficial layer of the fold has been completely incised, the epiglottic tip can be visualized through the deeper layer of the remaining portion of the aryepiglottic fold. Multiple swallowing attempts help stretch and tension the fold just prior to the final step in the correction.

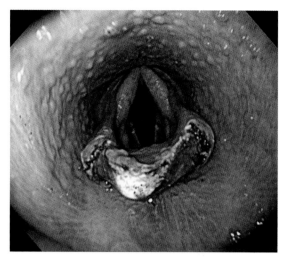

Figure 32.11   Final stages of the laser correction. A narrow "band" of aryepiglottic fold remains covering the epiglottic tip. Short bursts with the laser foot pedal and the induction of multiple swallowing attempts stretch the remaining portions of the fold and allow for complete correction. Extreme care should be taken by the surgeon to avoid iatrogenic damage to the epiglottic tip.

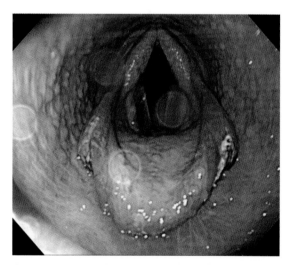

Figure 32.12   Completed diode laser correction of EE. Note: edema present along the sides of the incised aryepiglottic fold.

pressure necrosis. This can result in exposure of the epiglottic tip cartilage in the end. It is not difficult to iatrogenically damage the epiglottic tip cartilage. The risk for this can be minimized with careful incision and multiple swallowing attempts to gradually stretch the fold. Once the fold has been completely incised to correct the entrapment, the horse is triggered to swallow multiple times to make sure the epiglottis does not re-entrap (Figure 32.12).

In some cases complete retraction of the fold does not occur. Fortunately it is a rare case that does not resolve this problem with removal from exercise and administration of anti-inflammatory therapy. However, the author has had one horse which required surgical removal of the fold via laryngotomy. Bronchoesophageal forceps can also be used transnasally to facilitate grasping and excision of the section of the fold if needed. This is rarely needed.

Postoperative care

Horses are administered phenylbutazone (2.2–4.4 mg/kg, PO, q12h) for 7–10 days, pharyngeal spray (10 cc per transnasal catheter, q12h), and dexamethasone (20 mg, IV, q24h for 2 days; then 10 mg, IV, q24h for 2 days; then 10 mg q48h for two treatments). Antimicrobials are not routinely administered for routine laser correction of aryepiglottic fold entrapment. Removal from exercise is the most critical component for successful postoperative management. Horses must be stall confined with hand walking only following the surgical procedure. Horses should have an endoscopic examination performed within the first 7 days postoperatively to ensure that there is no excessive inflammation of the SETs. If after 7 days signs of subepiglottic inflammation are present, the horse should stay away from exercise for another 7 days. Returning to exercise before complete healing of the axially divided aryepiglottic fold only leads to continued edema and prolongs subepiglottic inflammation.

Complications of laser axial division EE

Approximately 5% of horses will develop recurrence of EE following the surgical procedure and 10% will develop DDSP. Horse which develops repeat EE can be treated with a second laser division of the aryepiglottic fold but the author would recommend surgical correction via laryngotomy if the EE recurs. DDSP can be treated with any of the previously described surgical methods (see Chapters 19–22).

The most common postoperative complication following laser correction of EE is excessive subepiglottic inflammation (Figure 32.13). The author has yet to predict which horses will

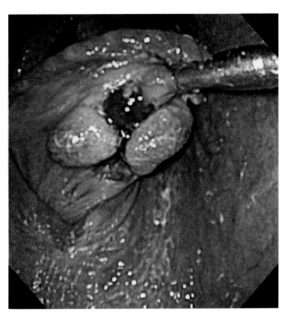

Figure 32.13   Endoscopic photograph of a Standardbred racehorse with excessive subepiglottic granulation tissue and granuloma formation following a diode laser correction of epiglottic entrapment.

develop excessive subepiglottic inflammation and which ones will not. Factors contributing to excessive subepiglottic inflammation include iatrogenic damage to the epiglottic tip, excessive number of joules (>5000) delivered to the fold, postoperative infection, and early return to exercise. This emphasizes the necessity for the administration of anti-inflammatory medication and frequent endoscopic monitoring of the epiglottis following surgery. Horses experiencing epiglottitis following laser axial division should be administered anti-inflammatories as detailed previously, antimicrobial therapy, and complete rest. Some horses require debridement of necrotic epiglottic tip cartilage and surgical resection of inflamed, granulating aryepiglottic fold via laryngotomy (Figure 32.14). In general, the author prefers to treat these horses conservatively rather than surgically because the prognosis may be subjectively worse following surgical debridement of the inflamed aryepiglottic fold. The prognosis following the development subepiglottic inflammation is guarded as most horses will almost certainly develop problems with soft palate function. Owners should be apprised of

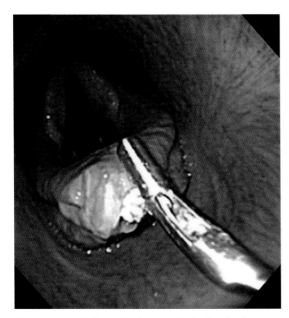

Figure 32.14   Endoscopic photograph of a Standardbred racehorse with excessive subepiglottic granulation tissue and exposed epiglottic tip cartilage following standing diode laser correction of epiglottic entrapment. The exposed epiglottic cartilage is being debrided with bronchoesophageal grasping forceps.

this as a possibility once epiglottitis postoperative has developed.

Conclusion

The method of surgical correction for EE depends on a variety of factors including: surgeon preference, standing versus correction under general anesthesia, thickness and degree of ulceration of the aryepiglottic fold, and potential for complications. In general, Hawkins prefers standing diode laser axial division for uncomplicated cases of EE and reserves correction via laryngotomy for those horses with a large amount of edema and ulceration involving the aryepiglottic fold. Each technique has its own advantages and disadvantages as previously discussed. However, the technique associated with potentially the most devastating side effects is improperly performed axial division with the diode laser.

References

Anderson JD, Tulleners EP, Johnston JK, Reeves MJ. 1995. Sternothyrohyoideus myectomy or staphylectomy for treatment of intermittent dorsal displacement of the soft palate in racehorses: 209 cases (1986–1991). *Journal of the American Veterinary Medical Association* 206:1909–1912.

Beroza GA. 1994. Partial closure of laryngotomies in horses. *Journal of the American Veterinary Medical Association* 204:1227–1229.

Boles CL, Raker CW, Wheat JD. 1978. Epiglottic entrapment by arytenoepiglottic folds in the horse. *Journal of the American Veterinary Medical Association* 172:338–342.

Brown JA, Hinchcliff DW, Jackson MA, Dredge AF, O'Callaghan RA, McCaffrey JR, Slocombe RF, Clarke AF. 2005. Prevalence of pharyngeal and laryngeal abnormalities in Thoroughbreds racing in Australia, and their association with performance. *Equine Veterinary Journal* 37:397–401.

Diab S, Pascoe JR, Shahriar M, Read D, Kinde H, Moore J, Odani J, Uzal F. 2009. Study of laryngopharyngeal pathology in Thoroughbred horses in southern California. *Equine Veterinary Journal* 41:903–907.

Greet TRC. 1995. Experiences in treatment of epiglottal entrapment using a hook knife per nasum. *Equine Veterinary Journal* 27:122–126.

Haynes PF. 1978. Surgical failures in upper respiratory surgery. *Proceedings of the American Association of Equine Practitioners* 24:233–249.

Haynes PF. 1983. Dorsal displacement of the soft palate and epiglottic entrapment: Diagnosis, management, and interrelationship. *Compendium on Continuing Education for the Practicing Veterinarian* 5:S379–S389.

Honnas CM, Wheat JD. 1988. Epiglottic entrapment: A transnasal surgical approach to divide the aryepiglottic fold axially in the standing horse. *Veterinary Surgery* 17:246–251.

Lacourt M, Marcoux M. 2011. Treatment of epiglottic entrapment by transnasal axial division in standing sedated horses using a shielded hook bistoury. *Veterinary Surgery* 40:299–304.

Lumsden JM, Stick JA, Caron JP, Nickels FA. 1994. Surgical treatment for epiglottic entrapment in horses: 51 cases (1981–1992). *Journal of the American Veterinary Medical Association* 205:729–735.

Perkins JD, Hughes TK, Brain B. 2007. Endoscope-guided, transoral axial division of an entrapping epiglottic fold in fifteen standing horses. *Veterinary Surgery* 36:800–803.

Raker CW. 1982. "Obstructive upper respiratory disease, the epiglottis." In: Mansmann RA, McAllister ES, eds. *Equine Medicine and Surgery.* (pp. 764–766). Santa Barbara, CA: American Veterinary Publishers.

Ross MW, Gentile DG, Evans LE. 1993. Transoral axial division, under endoscopic guidance, for correction of epiglottic entrapment in horses. *Journal of the American Veterinary Medical Association* 203:416–420.

Russell T, Wainscott M. 2007. Treatment in the field of 27 horses with epiglottic entrapment. *Veterinary Record* 161:187–189.

Saulez MN, Gummow B. 2009. Prevalence of pharyngeal, laryngeal and tracheal disorders in Thoroughbred racehorses, and effect on performance. *Veterinary Record* 165:431–435.

Sweeney CR, Maxson AD, Soma LR. 1991. Endoscopic findings in the upper respiratory tract of 678 Thoroughbred racehorses. *Journal of the American Veterinary Medical Association* 198:1037–1038.

Tate LP, Sweeney CL, Bowman KF, Newman HC, Duckett WM. 1990. Transendoscopic Nd:YAG laser surgery for treatment of epiglottal entrapment and dorsal displacement of the soft palate in the horse. *Veterinary Surgery* 19(5):356–363.

Tulleners E P. 1990. Transendoscopic contact neodymium: Yttrium aluminum garnet laser correction of epiglottic entrapment in standing horses. *Journal of the American Veterinary Medical Association* 196(12):1971–1980.

Tulleners EP. 1991. Correlation of performance with endoscopic and radiographic assessment of epiglottic hypoplasia in racehorses with epiglottic entrapment corrected by use of contact neodymium: Yttrium aluminum garnet laser. *Journal of the American Veterinary Medical Association* 198(4):621–626.

Tulleners EP, Schumacher J, Johnston J, Richardson DW. 1992. Pharynx. In: Auer JA, ed. *Equine Surgery*. (pp. 450–453). Philadelphia, PA: W.B. Saunders Company.

Turner SA, McIlwraith CW. 1989. *Techniques in Large Animal Surgery*, 2nd ed (pp. 222–229). Philadelphia, PA: Lea & Febiger.

33 Subepiglottic Cysts

Eric J. Parente

Introduction

Horses with subepiglottic cysts occasionally present as young animals with a history of dysphagia or respiratory noise or as mature performance horses with a history of exercise intolerance and/or respiratory noise. Subepiglottic cysts are uncommon and sometimes not easily diagnosed because of their variable position either above or below the soft palate (Figure 33.1). As a part of any resting endoscopic examination multiple swallowing attempts should be induced. This will sometimes cause a cyst in the oropharynx (under the soft palate) to reposition into the nasopharynx (over the soft palate) so it can be seen during endoscopic examination. Depending on the degree of attachment and size of the cyst, the cyst may remain within the oropharynx despite induced swallowing. In those situations, a small bulging from under the palate may be noted pushing upward toward the epiglottis. An adjunctive technique to allow endoscopic evaluation of the subepiglottic tissue is to use the bronchoesophageal grasping forceps to reflect/lift the epiglottis dorsally (Figure 33.2). In addition, if a subepiglottic cyst is suspected but not confirmed with standing endoscopy the horse can

be placed under general anesthesia. The base of the epiglottis can be palpated by inserting a hand in the mouth with the aid of a mouth speculum or the endoscope can be inserted into the oral cavity for direct visualization of the cyst (Figure 33.2). Infrequently a cyst may be associated with epiglottic entrapment or rarely the cyst can become large and loose enough that it can be swallowed by the horse resulting in obstruction of the glottis from the epiglottis pulled over it (Hay et al. 1997).

Although surgical resection is generally recommended, there is one case report of successful intralesional formalin treatment (Dougherty and Palmer 2008). This author has no personal experience with medical treatment of subepiglottic cysts and typically approaches them surgically. The surgical approach for removal is dependent upon the size, position, and the comfort level of the surgeon with the differents surgical options.

Subepiglottic cyst removal via laryngotomy

This technique is accomplished via laryngotomy and retroversion of the epiglottis toward the

Advances in Equine Upper Respiratory Surgery, First Edition. Edited by Jan Hawkins.
© 2015 ACVS Foundation. Published 2015 by John Wiley & Sons, Inc.

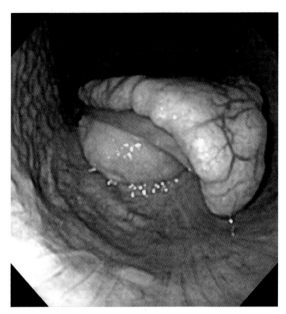

Figure 33.1   Standard endoscopic view of a subepiglottic cyst above the palate on the right side of the epiglottis.

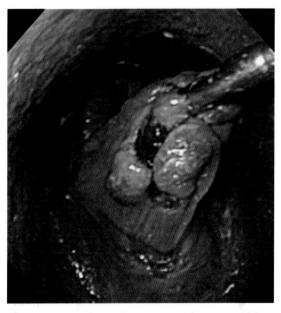

Figure 33.2   Standing endoscopic view of retraction of the epiglottis with bronchoesophageal grasping forceps inserted into the contralateral nasal passage caudally to allow for evaluation of the subepiglottic tissues connected to the epiglottis.

laryngotomy followed by surgical resection of the cyst (Stick and Boles 1980). This method would certainly be preferred if the surgeon does not have access to a surgical laser. With this technique the horse is anesthetized and positioned in dorsal recumbency and prepared for a ventral laryngotomy. To perform surgical resection of the cyst via laryngotomy the horse must not be intubated. The cyst can be retroverted along with the epiglottis by the surgeon or an assistant with a small hand can push the cyst toward the surgeon so that it can be grasped by the surgeon. Once the cyst has been retroverted toward the laryngotomy incision, an incision is made over the cyst with a scalpel blade and using a combination of sharp and blunt dissection the cyst is dissected free and removed. It is not unusual to rupture the cyst during the dissection but the surgeon should make sure the entire cystic lining has been removed to ensure against recurrence. The incision in the mucous membrane is left open to heal via second intention.

Transendoscopic laser resection using a transnasal approach

Most clinicians now advocate avoiding a laryngotomy by using a transnasal or an oral approach under endoscopic guidance. The standing transnasal approach has the advantage of being performed without general anesthesia and having a large area in the nasopharynx to manipulate tissue relative to the oropharynx. It requires experience with transendoscopic laser surgery and quality grasping instruments. Similarly the procedure can be performed with the horse nasotracheally intubated under general anesthesia and the cyst manipulated within the oropharynx. Although there is less concern about "losing" the cyst while trying to resect it, there is limited room within the oropharynx to work and smoke evacuation is required. Transnasal transendoscopic laser resection is the preferred technique of the author because of the advantages described above as well as having a better appreciation of tissues affected since the approach is made without distortion of tissues and the ability to assess the resection with normal anatomic perspective. When performing the resection with standing sedation and local anesthesia

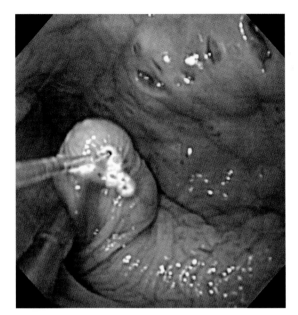

Figure 33.3   Transoral endoscopic laser ablation of a small subepiglottic cyst using a contact diode laser fiber. The fiber contacts the outer lining of the cyst at multiple sites to heat the interior of the cyst prior to puncture with the laser fiber.

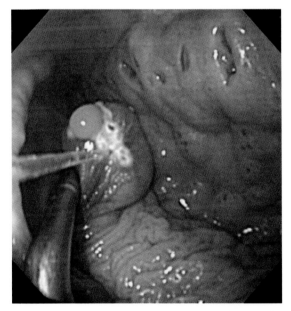

Figure 33.4   Endoscopic transoral approach to ablation of a subepiglottic cyst with a diode laser. The fiber has been used to penetrate the cyst and allow the escape of cystic fluid. The fiber is then discharged to cauterize the lining of the cyst. This will prevent cyst recurrence.

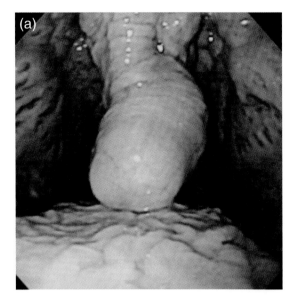

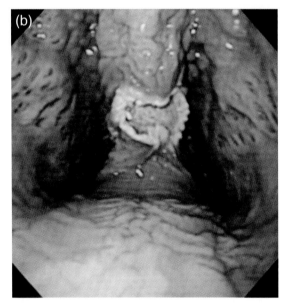

Figure 33.5   (a) Oropharyngeal view of the cyst at the base of the subepiglottic membrane. The horse is in dorsal recumbency with the palate at the bottom of the image and the epiglottis in the nasopharynx. (b) The image after resection by a transendoscopic diathermic loop.

it is critical to have a long bronchoesophageal grasping forceps, preferably with a locking mechanism to minimize the risk of losing a grasp on the cyst. Under videoendoscopic guidance the bronchoesophageal forceps are passed up the contralateral nostril to the endoscope and the cyst is held by the graspers. The diode laser is used in contact fashion set to 18 watts. Once grasped, the mass is retracted in multiple directions to best expose the base attachment and maintain tension on the target tissue to cut. The directions held cannot be predetermined, it is an intraoperative decision based upon the attachment of the cyst and exposure that can be achieved. Care must be taken to not get too close to epiglottic cartilage and to resect the least amount of tissue possible while removing the entire cyst. If the cyst is accidentally punctured the surgeon should continue to resect the tissue and estimate the remaining portions of cyst without resecting excessive subepiglottic tissue. The cyst is unlikely to recur with appropriate tissue resection. Perioperative treatment consists of antimicrobials and topical/systemic anti-inflammatories. A minimum of 4 weeks without exercise is recommended.

An alternative to standing laser removal is removal under general anesthesia. A mouth speculum is placed and the cyst is accessed through the oral cavity. The diode laser is set to 15–20 watts and a contact fiber is used to touch the outer surface of the cyst in multiple places to heat up the interior of the cyst (Figure 33.3). The cyst is then punctured with the laser fiber and the fiber is inserted into the interior of the cyst. Once deflated the laser is discharged to ablate the inner lining of the cyst (Figure 33.4).

Transoral snare removal of subepiglottic cysts

An alternative resection technique that can be performed through the oropharynx is snaring the cyst with obstetrical wire or using a transendoscopic diathermic (monopolar cautery) loop snare (Tulleners 1991) (Figure 33.5). Most snares are made by passing obstetrical wire through long tubing and manually manipulating or using bronchoesophageal grasping forceps to position the cyst into the snare for resection.

References

Dougherty SS, Palmer JL. 2008. Use of intralesional formalin administration for treatment of a subepiglottic cyst in a horse. *Journal of the American Veterinary Medical Association* 233:463–465.

Hay WP, Basket A, Abdy MJ. 1997. Complete upper airway obstruction and syncope caused by a subepiglottic cyst in a horse. *Equine Veterinary Journal* 29: 75–76.

Stick JA, Boles CW. 1980. Subepiglottic cysts in three foals. *Journal of the American Veterinary Medical Association* 177:62–64.

Tulleners EP. 1991. Evaluation of peroral transendoscopic contact neodymium: Yttrium aluminum garnet laser and snare excision of subepiglottic cysts in horses. *Journal of the American Veterinary Medical Association* 198(9):1631–1635.

34 Laser Resection of the Aryepiglottic Folds

Eric J. Parente

Introduction

Resection of the aryepiglottic folds is indicated when there is evidence of aryepiglottic fold collapse during exercise with overground or treadmill endoscopy. It can occur independently or in association with other abnormalities (Strand et al. 2012). The deviation of the aryepiglottic fold can be unilateral or bilateral (Figure 34.1) and the degree of obstruction is variable. Affected horses are usually younger (<3 years) and will typically make an inspiratory noise. While the diagnosis cannot be made based on resting endoscopy, some surgeons still may advocate resecting the aryepiglottic folds based on the presumption of dynamic collapse of the right aryepiglottic fold after laryngoplasty (Davidson et al. 2010; Rakesh et al. 2008). Deviation of the aryepiglottic folds has not been shown to occur in all horses after laryngoplasty, but it has been documented in some (Figure 34.2). Although younger horses can be treated with anti-inflammatories and rest with moderate success, surgical resection yields greater success and requires a shorter period of convalescence time (King et al. 2001).

Surgical technique

Transendoscopic laser resection of the aryepiglottic fold can be performed with a horse under general anesthesia (Figure 34.3) or standing. Standing surgical resection is preferred by the author. With the horse under general anesthesia the endotracheal tube within the glottis is a physical obstruction to manipulation of tissue during the procedure and smoke evacuation is required. It is a fairly simple procedure to perform transendoscopically in the standing, sedated horse since there is more space to mobilize the tissue without an endotracheal tube in the way, and smoke evacuation is accomplished by the horse's respiration.

Standing resection of the aryepiglottic folds

In preparation, the horse is sedated in stocks with detomidine (5–10 mg, IV) in combination with butorphanol (5 mg, IV). Having a way to support the head in a steady position with an overhead rope or a place to rest the horse's head (e.g., dental stand) is beneficial. After sedation, the

Advances in Equine Upper Respiratory Surgery, First Edition. Edited by Jan Hawkins.
© 2015 ACVS Foundation. Published 2015 by John Wiley & Sons, Inc.

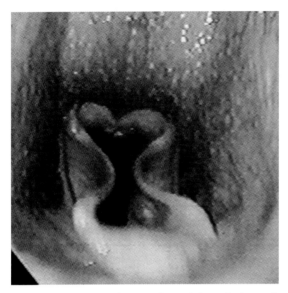

Figure 34.1   Endoscopic image obtained during high-speed exercise depicting bilateral axial deviation of the aryepiglottic folds.

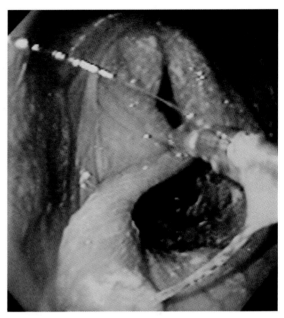

Figure 34.3   Intraoperative image of the right aryepiglottic fold being held by bronchoesophageal graspers and deviated axially to mimic the dynamic collapse and plan for surgical resection.

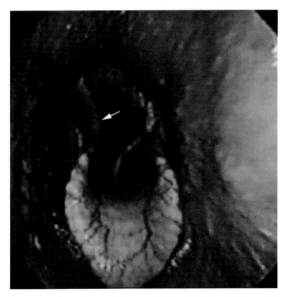

Figure 34.2   Endoscopic image obtained during high-speed exercise depicting right aryepiglottic fold deviation (and left vocal cord deviation) after laryngoplasty in a horse that continued to make abnormal noise during exercise.

nasal passage and the laryngeal region are locally anesthetized by using polyethylene tubing passed down the biopsy channel of the endoscope to apply anesthetic topically. Once anesthetized 600 mm bronchoesophageal forceps are passed up the contralateral nostril to the target fold. The videoendoscope with the laser fiber within the biopsy channel is passed up the ipsilateral nostril. The target aryepiglottic fold is grasped as close to the middle of the fold as possible and with rotation of the graspers the position of the fold mimics the dynamic axial deviation of the tissue (Figure 34.3). A triangular wedge of tissue is resected by contact fiber action with a setting of 18 watts. The triangular wedge of tissue that will be resected should be of similar size to the wedge of tissue obstructing the larynx dynamically. One incision line will be starting below the graspers (Figure 34.4) and one above. Generally the ventral incision is made first, but the area under greater tension should be cut first. There is little risk of damage to the adjacent tissue on the ventral cut, but care must be taken to not touch the corniculate with the laser fiber when

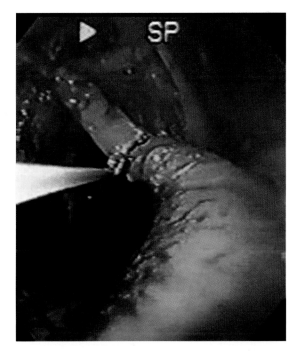

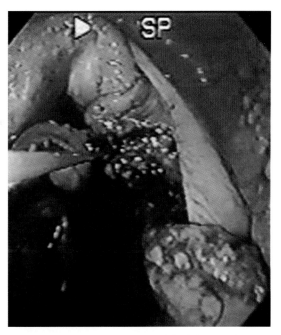

Figure 34.4 Intraoperative image of the left aryepiglottic fold being deviated axially and the laser fiber making the initial ventral cut into the fold.

Figure 34.5 Intraoperative image of the left aryepiglottic fold resection. The majority of the tissue has been transected and care must be exercised to remove the remaining portion of tissue without the fiber contacting the adjacent corniculate mucosa.

performing the dorsal cut (Figure 34.5). There is typically very little or no bleeding with this procedure and once one aryepiglottic fold is removed, the procedure is repeated on the opposite side for horses with bilateral obstructions. Several thousand joules are all that should be needed to perform a resection in this fashion.

Postoperatively the horse may be treated with systemic and topical anti-inflammatories and systemic antimicrobials for several days. Stall rest and hand walking for just 2–3 weeks is all that is recommended for mucosal cover and return to exercise. Once healed, the fold looks only slightly different than preoperatively to the untrained observer. It will be more recessed and scarred but not obviously different than a normal fold.

Resection of the aryepiglottic folds via laryngotomy

Resection of the aryepiglottic folds can be performed via laryngotomy. This is the only way to

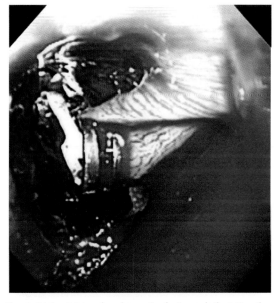

Figure 34.6 Intraoral endoscopic photograph depicting the "hooking" of the right aryepiglottic fold via laryngotomy. Once retracted toward the midline the fold is grasped with an Allis tissue forceps inserted through the laryngotomy incision.

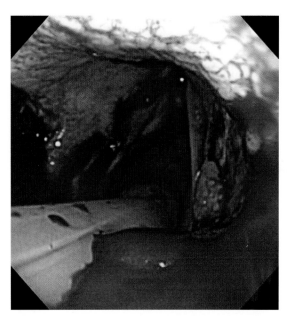

Figure 34.7   Endoscopic intraoperative view of the larynx via the oral cavity. Note the epiglottis is located toward the top of the photograph and the corniculate processes of the arytenoids are located toward the bottom. Both aryepiglottic folds have been resected via the laryngotomy incision as described.

perform the procedure if the surgeon does not have a diode or Nd:YAG laser available. The technique as described here was developed by Dr. Stephen B. Adams at Purdue University. A laryngotomy has been previously described in Chapter 32. To access the aryepiglottic fold a sharp Senn retractor is used to "hook" the fold (Figure 34.6). The fold is then retracted toward the midline of the larynx and then grasped with a long Allis tissue forceps. Once grasped the fold is then resected with curved Satinsky scissors (Figure 34.7). The procedure is then repeated for the contralateral fold if desired.

References

Davidson EJ, Martin BB, Rieger RH, Parente EJ. 2010. Exercising videoendoscopic evaluation of 45 horses with respiratory noise and/or poor performance after laryngoplasty. *Veterinary Surgery* 39(8):942–948.

King DS, Tulleners EP, Martin BB Jr, Parente EJ, Boston R. 2001. Clinical experiences with axial deviation of the aryepiglottic folds in 52 racehorses. *Veterinary Surgery* 30(2):151–160.

Rakesh V, Ducharme NG, Cheetham J, Datta AK, Pease AP. 2008. Implications of different degrees of arytenoid cartilage abduction on equine upper airway characteristics. *Equine Veterinary Journal* 40:629–635.

Strand E, Skjerve E. 2012. Complex dynamic upper airway collapse: Associations between abnormalities in 99 harness racehorses with one or more dynamic disorders. *Equine Veterinary Journal* 44:524–528.

35 Partial Arytenoidectomy with Mucosal Closure

Eric J. Parente

Introduction

Partial arytenoidectomy can be successful regardless of whether a primary mucosal closure is performed or not (Barnes et al. 2004; Parente et al. 2008). The main disadvantages of performing a primary mucosal closure are the increased intraoperative time and the risk of submucosal hematoma postoperatively (Dean and Cohen 1990). The main advantages observed by this author are the greater degree of control in maintaining a mucosal shelf to protect the airway from aspiration, the decreased appearance of postoperative granulation tissue, and the long-term success in the racehorse.

These advantages will not be recognized without a fairly meticulous surgical approach or if the appropriate surgical candidate is not chosen. Horses with any evidence of bilateral disease are unlikely to achieve an adequate airway for performance after unilateral partial arytenoidectomy (Tulleners et al. 1988a, 1988b) and may be more likely to suffer from aspiration if the remaining arytenoid adduction is affected. Thus partial arytenoidectomy should be reserved for horses with

bilateral disease only if the client is willing to accept a pasture sound animal or if permanent tracheotomy is not acceptable.

Clinical signs of arytenoid chondropathy

Horses with arytenoid chondropathy will initially present for increased respiratory noise or possibly respiratory distress. If the arytenoid is still in an active stage of inflammation then medical treatment should be initiated prior to surgical intervention. Surgery on edematous, inflamed tissue will create greater difficulty in achieving a mucosal closure. If the inflammation is so severe that it cannot be discerned whether the disease is unilateral or bilateral, the client should be advised that medical treatment will be required before surgery is recommended and a prognosis determined (Figure 35.1). Most horses should respond favorably within days (Figure 35.2). If there is no significant improvement after 2–5 days of medical management consideration should be given to the presence of a perilaryngeal abscess. Surgical intervention is recommended in these cases to

Advances in Equine Upper Respiratory Surgery, First Edition. Edited by Jan Hawkins.
© 2015 ACVS Foundation. Published 2015 by John Wiley & Sons, Inc.

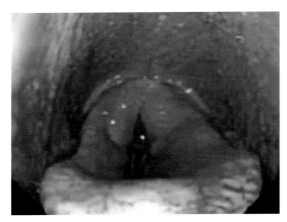

Figure 35.1 Endoscopic view of larynx at admission with induced maximal abduction. There is difficulty in determining whether bilateral or unilateral disease is present because of severe inflammation.

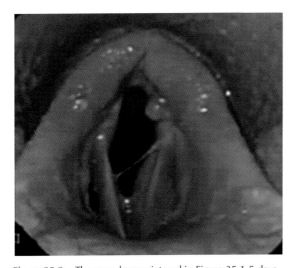

Figure 35.2 The same horse pictured in Figure 35.1 5 days after medical treatment. The photograph demonstrates the improved appearance of the airway, the ability of the right arytenoid to abduct, and the likely determination that the left arytenoid is solely affected.

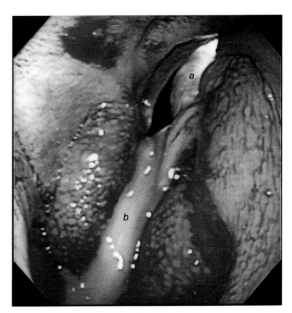

Figure 35.3 Intraoperative endoscopic view of the larynx. The horse is in dorsal recumbency and a finger (a) is pushing on the lateral aspect of the arytenoid through a laryngotomy causing purulent material to be expressed (b).

abnormalities of the shape of the corniculate process can usually be seen endoscopically. Cartilaginous protrusions are often endoscopically observed on the axial aspect of the arytenoid, just dorsal to the vocal process. There are often coexisting superficial ulcerated ("kissing") lesions, or granulation tissue, on the axial aspect of the opposing arytenoid, that may appear more significant than the lesion on the affected arytenoid. Rarely, lesions are absent at the opening of the glottis, but more caudally positioned ulcerative lesions are present within the laryngeal lumen that are difficult to observe without moving the endoscope into the laryngeal lumen. External laryngeal palpation of a chondritic arytenoid will demonstrate a less prominent or defined muscular process than the normal side.

Partial arytenoidectomy with mucosal closure

While different forms of arytenoidectomy have been described (Belknap et al. 1990; Hay et al. 1993; Tulleners et al. 1988a, 1988b), the partial arytenoidectomy has been shown to provide the

establish drainage (Figure 35.3), but an attempt to save a mucosal flap is not recommended. Laryngeal ultrasound can be very useful in the evaluation of the horse with arytenoid chondritis and should be considered for all cases (Garrett et al. 2013).

Although it is simple to make a diagnosis of arytenoid chondritis in the acute phase, it is sometimes more difficult to do so in chronic cases. In the chronic stage, there is no laryngeal edema, but least postoperative obstruction (Belknap et al. 1990; Lumsden et al. 1994). A temporary tracheotomy is required to administer the inhalant anesthesia for a partial arytenoidectomy, as the surgery is performed through a laryngotomy. There is usually a large enough glottic lumen to pass an endotracheal tube through the larynx after inducing anesthesia, and the tracheotomy can be performed under general anesthesia. The orotracheal tube is removed and a smaller endotracheal tube is placed through the tracheotomy site. A cleaner, smaller tracheotomy can be performed in this manner, but if there is any risk that endotracheal intubation may be difficult, then the tracheostomy should be performed in the standing horse before inducing general anesthesia. Caution should be exercised that the tracheostomy is not placed too far cranial when performed under general anesthesia. The relative position is deceiving with the horse in dorsal recumbency and the head extended. If the tracheotomy is placed too cranially it may become obstructed during recovery. The tracheotomy incision should be in the midcervical region of the neck.

To perform the arytenoidectomy, a standard laryngotomy approach is first made. A headlamp is useful for illumination while working within the larynx, and placing an endoscope transnasally with its tip placed in front of the larynx can also provide supplemental light.

Initially a dorsally based mucosal flap is created by making dorsoventral mucosal incisions at the caudal border of the arytenoid body, and at the rostral border of the body, just caudal to the corniculate. These incisions are connected with a horizontal incision along the ventral border of the arytenoid (Figure 35.4). The mucosa is dissected free from the arytenoid and left attached dorsally. If the contour of the medial surface of the arytenoid body is convex, more cartilage is left attached to the mucosa to minimize the risk of tearing the mucosa and those pieces are later removed. Once the flap is completely free of the cartilage, the abaxial border of the arytenoid is then freed of its soft-tissue attachments using primarily blunt dissection with a periosteal elevator to minimize hemorrhage. The muscular process is isolated and transected. The arytenoid is elevated with Allis forceps, and freed completely by first cutting the cricoarytenoid joint capsule caudally, then the remaining dorsal attachments and finally the remaining corniculate mucosa at the most rostral edge. Mucosa is positioned

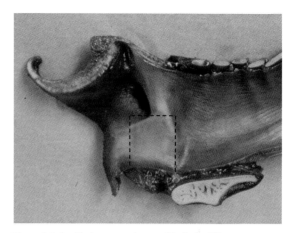

Figure 35.4   Cadaver specimen with dashed lines demonstrating the mucosal incisions to create a dorsally based mucosal flap.

together to plan its closure, and any excess mucosa is excised. The caudal edge of the mucosal flap is first reapposed to the laryngeal mucosa in a simple continuous pattern with 3-0 absorbable suture, in a dorsal-to-ventral direction. The rostral edge of the mucosal flap is apposed similarly to the remaining mucosa lying abaxial to the corniculate in a line parallel to the caudal edge. The most difficult part to suture is the very dorsal aspect of the vertical incisions, and closure of this area is most important for preventing the formation of postoperative granulation tissue. The ventral aspect of the mucosal wound is left open to drain. Bleeding should be minimal once the mucosal edges are sutured. After closure of the mucosal flap the vocal cord and ventricle are removed. This will leave an opening at the ventral aspect of the arytenoidectomy site for drainage of submucosal hemorrhage or blood clot lying abaxial to the final mucosal flap (Figure 35.5). Any granulating "kissing" lesions on the opposite arytenoid should be debrided at this time. At the conclusion of surgery, the endotracheal tube can be replaced with an equivalent-sized tracheotomy tube for recovery from general anesthesia.

Endoscopic examination should be performed the morning following surgery (Figure 35.6). A moderate opening to the glottis should be seen, and obstructing the tracheotomy tube should not create any difficulty for the horse to breathe. The tracheotomy tube can usually be removed the morning following surgery. The horse should be maintained on perioperative antimicrobials and

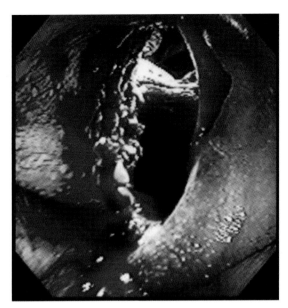

Figure 35.5   Intraoperative endoscopic view of the final mucosal closure after left partial arytenoidectomy with the horse in dorsal recumbency.

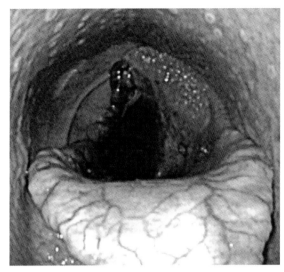

Figure 35.7   The same horse as imaged in Figure 35.6, 1 month postoperatively. Note the mucosal membrane just below the palatopharyngeal arch preventing aspiration and still providing a likely adequate laryngeal lumen for performance.

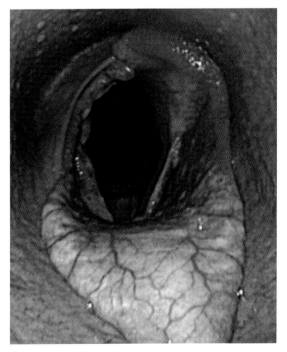

Figure 35.6   Endoscopic view of the larynx the morning after a right partial arytenoidectomy with primary closure. Moderate mucosal swelling, but glottic opening is adequate.

anti-inflammatories for 1 week and maintained in a stall for 1 month with only hand grazing. The tracheotomy and laryngotomy sites are left open to heal in by second intention. All feeding should be from the ground to minimize the risk of aspiration.

Endoscopy should be performed 1 month following surgery to examine for the presence of intralaryngeal granulation tissue. A thin rim of mucosa should be seen just under the palatopharyngeal arch that should minimize any risk of aspiration and still provide an adequate glottis for performance (Figure 35.7). If granulation tissue is present, it can be transendoscopically removed with a laser on an outpatient basis. Once there is complete mucosal healing, the horse should receive a second month with turnout before resuming exercise.

References

Barnes AJ, Slone DE, Lynch TM. 2004. Performance after partial arytenoidectomy without mucosal closure in 27 Thoroughbred racehorses. *Veterinary Surgery* 33:398–403.

Belknap JK, Derksen FJ, Nickels FA, Stick JA, Robinson NE. 1990. Failure of subtotal arytenoidectomy to improve upper airway flow mechanics in exercising

Standardbreds with induced laryngeal hemiplegia. *American Journal of Veterinary Research* 51:1481–1486.

Dean PW, Cohen ND. 1990. Arytenoidectomy for advanced unilateral chondropathy with accompanying lesions. *Veterinary Surgery* 19:364–370.

Garrett KS, Embertson RM, Woodie JB, Cheetham J. 2013. Ultrasound features of arytenoid chondritis in Thoroughbred horses. *Equine Veterinary Journal* 45(5):598–603.

Hay WP, Tulleners EP, Ducharme NG. 1993. Partial arytenoidectomy in the horse using an extra-laryngeal approach. *Veterinary Surgery* 22:50–56.

Lumsden JM, Derksen FJ, Stick JA, Robinson NE, Nickels FA. 1994. Evaluation of partial arytenoidectomy as a treatment for equine laryngeal hemiplegia. *Equine Veterinary Journal* 26:125–129.

Parente EJ, Tulleners EP, Southwood LL. 2008. Long-term study of partial arytenoidectomy with primary mucosal closure in 76 Thoroughbred racehorses (1992–2006). *Equine Veterinary Journal* 40:214–218.

Tulleners EP, Harrison IW, Raker CW. 1988a. Management of arytenoid chondropathy and failed laryngoplasty in horses: 75 cases (1979–1985). *Journal of the American Veterinary Medical Association* 192:670–675.

Tulleners EP, Harrison IW, Mann P, Raker CW. 1988b. Partial arytenoidectomy in the horse with and without mucosal closure. *Veterinary Surgery* 17:252–257.

36 Partial Arytenoidectomy without Mucosal Closure

Jan Hawkins

Introduction

The indications for partial arytenoidectomy (PA) have been previously described (Lumsden et al. 1994; Parente et al. 2008; Tulleners 1988a; Witte et al. 2009). PA with mucosal closure was detailed in Chapter 35. This chapter will concentrate on the technique of PA without mucosal closure (Barnes et al. 2004; Tulleners 1988b). PA without mucosal closure was initially described by Eric Tulleners (Tulleners 1988b). He reported that PA could be performed without mucosal closure with a similar outcome to PA with mucosal closure. Barnes et al has also reported on the surgical outcome of Thoroughbred racehorses treated with PA without mucosal closure (Barnes et al. 2004). The author prefers PA without mucosal closure because personal experience with mucosal closure has been associated with mucosal dehiscence, intralaryngeal granulation tissue formation, and in some cases excessive soft-tissue remnants which lead to postoperative noise and exercise intolerance. I have found PA without mucosal closure to be consistent and repeatable with a minimum of complications.

Surgical technique: Partial arytenoidectomy without mucosal closure

The horse is anesthetized and positioned in dorsal recumbency. Following induction of anesthesia a midcervical tracheotomy is performed and a suitably sized endotracheal tube is inserted into the trachea. Following aseptic preparation of the ventral aspect of the larynx a laryngotomy is performed. If necessary to improve exposure of the affected arytenoid the thyroid can be split on the midline. A three-sided incision is made to expose the body of the arytenoid. The incision begins along the corniculate process (rostrally), over the vocal process (ventrally), and the body of the arytenoid caudally (see Chapter 35). Following dissection of the mucosa away from the axial aspect of the arytenoid this mucosal flap is excised dorsally with scissors. Following the three-sided incision the author prefers to remove the laryngeal ventricle and vocal cord. This can be accomplished with a roaring burr. Once the ventriculocordectomy has been performed, a Freer elevator is used to dissect the mucosa from the arytenoid on the axial aspect, and the abaxial aspect is separated from the connective tissue with scissors. The body of the arytenoid is held with an Allis tissue forceps during the dissection. Once the body and corniculate process has been dissected from its attachments the muscular process of the arytenoid is incised with cartilage-cutting scissors and the arytenoid is removed. Additional portions of the muscular process can be removed with Ferris Smith rongeurs to ensure the remaining cut edge of the cartilage is below the level of the laryngeal mucosa. Any loose pieces of mucosa or connective tissue are excised and any remaining mucosa should be trimmed level with the dorsal aspect of the larynx. The final step of the procedure is to determine how much of the corniculate mucosa to remove. The goal is to leave a 3-mm portion of corniculate mucosa to "protect" the laryngeal lumen and decrease the risk of postoperative aspiration of feed material. Through trial and error the author has found the best way to consistently ensure the ideal amount of corniculate mucosa remains is to perform intraoperative endoscopy (Figures 36.1 and 36.2). The endoscope is inserted into the oral cavity with the aid of a mouth speculum and the mucosa is directly visualized. This can be complicated by hemorrhage but this can generally be controlled with suction and digital pressure with gauze sponges. The corniculate mucosa is grabbed with two Allis tissue forceps and under endoscopic guidance the desired amount of mucosa is resected with scissors. This completes the procedure and the horse is recovered from general anesthesia with an indwelling tracheotomy tube.

Aftercare and postoperative monitoring

Horses are treated with perioperative antimicrobials and anti-inflammatories. The author prefers to use potassium or procaine penicillin G and gentamicin sulfate for antimicrobials. A combination of phenylbutazone and dexamethasone are used as anti-inflammatories. The laryngotomy is cleaned twice daily until healed. An endoscopic examination is performed the day following surgery to evaluate whether or not the tracheotomy tube can be removed. In almost all cases the tube can be removed the day following surgery. In some cases it may be obvious that "too much" corniculate

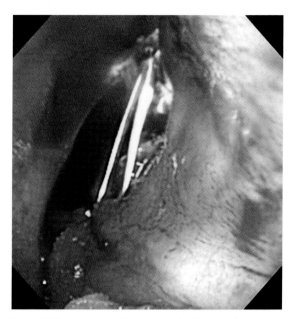

Figure 36.1   Intraoperative endoscopic photograph depicting removal of remaining corniculate mucosa following partial arytenoidectomy. This photograph is obtained by inserting the endoscope into the oral cavity. Ventral is located toward the top of the photograph and dorsal is located toward the bottom of the photograph. An Allis tissue forceps is being used to retract the remaining corniculate mucosa toward the surgeon. Then the corniculate mucosa is trimmed by the surgeon under endoscopic guidance.

mucosa was left and the surgeon may elect to resect additional tissue either by a pair of scissors inserted through the laryngotomy incision or with the aid of diode laser used endoscopically (Figure 36.3).

Additional endoscopic examinations are performed at 3–5 day intervals to evaluate for the development of intralaryngeal granulation tissue. Generally a "wait and see" approach is elected as granulation tissue formation to some degree is not unusual. If the granulation tissue protrudes into the laryngeal lumen I generally favor removal to keep it level with the laryngeal lumen. If granulation tissue removal is elected and if the laryngotomy is still open a Ferris Smith rongeur can be inserted and the granulation tissue is removed under endoscopic guidance (Figure 36.4). If the laryngotomy is closed a contact diode laser fiber is used to remove the granulation tissue mass. Once excised, granulation tissue does not generally regrow and mucosal healing occurs uneventfully (Figure 36.5).

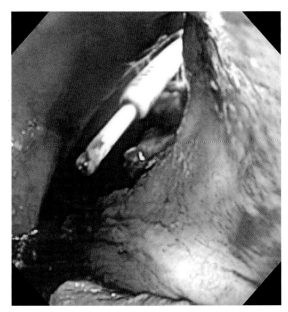

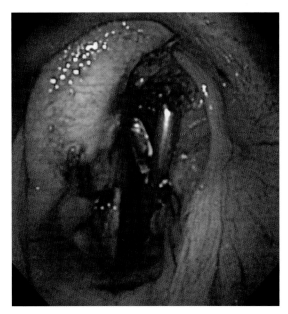

Figure 36.2   The same horse as pictured in Figure 36.1. This is the final appearance of the remaining section of corniculate mucosa left to heal via second intention. The white structure is a Poole suction tip.

Figure 36.4   Endoscopic photograph depicting removal of excessive granulation tissue with a Ferris Smith rongeur inserted through the laryngotomy incision. Removal is performed under endoscopic guidance.

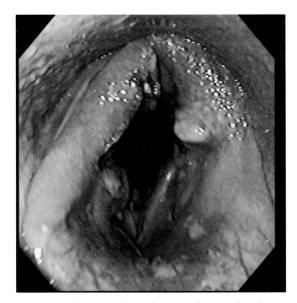

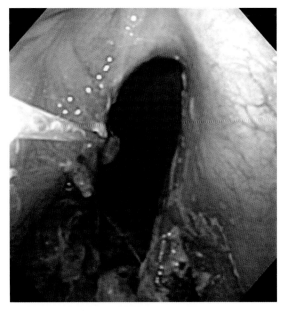

Figure 36.3   Postoperative endoscopic photograph 1 day following partial arytenoidectomy. The remaining portion of right corniculate mucosa is more than the author would like to see in a horse used for racing. If needed, this portion of corniculate mucosa can be trimmed with scissors inserted through the laryngotomy incision or can be excised with a contact diode laser fiber.

Figure 36.5   Endoscopic photograph depicting diode laser excision of intralaryngeal granulation tissue located on the axial aspect of the right hemilarynx following right partial arytenoidectomy.

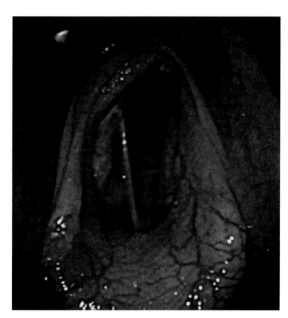

Figure 36.6   Endoscopic photograph depicting complete epithelialization of the left hemilarynx following left partial arytenoidectomy without mucosal closure.

Horses are returned to exercise once complete mucosal healing has taken place. This generally occurs within 45–60 days of the surgical procedure (Figure 36.6). Horses that experience excessive respiratory noise or exercise intolerance post arytenoidectomy should be examined on the high-speed treadmill as some horse develop collapse of remaining corniculate mucosa or the ipsilateral aryepiglottic fold. Horses that develop this complication may be successfully treated with laser resection of collapsing soft-tissue structures.

References

Barnes AJ, Slone DE, Lynch TM. 2004. Performance after partial arytenoidectomy without mucosal closure in 27 Thoroughbred racehorses. *Veterinary Surgery* 33:398–403.

Lumsden JM, Derksen FJ, Stick JA, Robinson NE, Nickels FA. 1994. Evaluation of partial arytenoidectomy as a treatment for equine laryngeal hemiplegia. *Equine Veterinary Journal* 26:125–129.

Parente EJ, Tulleners EP, Southwood LL. 2008. Long-term study of partial arytenoidectomy with primary mucosal closure in 76 Thoroughbred racehorses (1992–2006). *Equine Veterinary Journal* 40:214–218.

Tulleners EP, Harrison IW, Raker CW. 1988a. Management of arytenoid chondropathy and failed laryngoplasty in horses: 75 cases (1979–1985). *Journal of the American Veterinary Medical Association* 192:670–675.

Tulleners EP, Harrison IW, Mann P, Raker CW. 1988b. Partial arytenoidectomy in the horse with and without mucosal closure. *Veterinary Surgery* 17:252–257.

Witte TH, Mohammed HO, Radcliffe CH, Hackett RP, Ducharme NG. 2009. Racing performance after combined prosthetic laryngoplasty and ipsilateral ventriculocordectomy or partial arytenoidectomy: 135 Thoroughbred racehorses competing at less than 2400 m (1997–2007). *Equine Veterinary Journal* 41(1):70–75.

37 Management of Guttural Pouch Tympanites

Lloyd. P. Tate, Jr

Introduction

Tympany or tympanites of the guttural pouches is defined as entrapped air within the guttural pouch resulting in parotid region dilatation (Figure 37.1). It is most common in foals 1–4 months of age but can occur in older animals. The highest incidence is in the Arabian and Quarter Horse, but it has been reported in almost all breeds and is believed to be hereditary in Arabians and German Warmblood (Blazyczek et al. 2004a, 2004b; Metzger et al. 2012; Zeitz et al. 2009). It is more common for a single guttural pouch to be affected, but cases of bilateral tympany have been reported. More frequently, in unilateral cases, both guttural pouches can demonstrate distention which may be interpreted incorrectly as a bilateral condition. The distention can be seen by endoscopy as pharyngeal collapse and the foal will frequently experience respiratory stridor (Figure 37.2). Lateral radiographs of the throatlatch region show excessive distention of one or both guttural pouches with some fluid (milk) contained in the lower portions, and ventral deviation of the trachea. Dorsoventral radiographs are also useful in determining whether or not one or both pouches are involved. In unilateral tympany one pouch will be obviously distended with air (Figure 37.3). Tracheal deviation, pharyngeal collapse, and dysphagia often produce secondary aspiration pneumonia which can be appreciated on auscultation of the lung fields and thoracic radiography.

The etiology of guttural pouch tympany is unknown, but an inability of the pharyngeal opening to properly dilate or improper function of the plica salpingopharyngea results in a one-way valve that traps air within the pouch but does not allow it to exit. The dysfunction is considered to be a congenital lesion which probably has a genetic origin (Blazyczek et al. 2004a and 2004b; Metzger et al. 2012; Zeitz et al. 2009). I have seen mares bred to the same stallion produce more than one affected foal, which will not occur when the mare is then bred to a different stallion.

Diagnosis

Determining whether the foal has a unilateral or bilateral condition is a simple task. Originally, decompression of the guttural pouch involved choosing the side with the largest distention and

Advances in Equine Upper Respiratory Surgery, First Edition. Edited by Jan Hawkins.
© 2015 ACVS Foundation. Published 2015 by John Wiley & Sons, Inc.

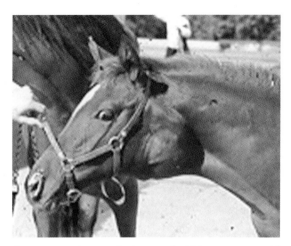

Figure 37.1   Photograph of a 6-week-old Quarter Horse with left-sided guttural pouch tympanites.

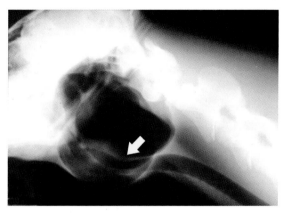

Figure 37.3   Lateral radiograph of a foal with guttural pouch tympanites demonstrating excessive distention of both guttural pouches and ventral displacement of the trachea (white arrow).

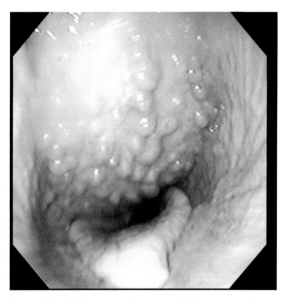

Figure 37.2   Endoscopic photograph of pharyngeal collapse associated with right-sided guttural pouch tympanites.

then percutaneously inserting a large gauge needle (16 or 14 gauge) into the guttural pouch to relive the distention. When needle decompression resulted in deflation of both guttural pouches, unilateral tympanites of that side was diagnosed. When only one side was deflated, it was assumed the tympanites were bilateral, which would require a slightly different surgical correction. Because of the risk for

iatrogenic damage of the numerous neurovascular structures within the guttural pouch, percutaneous needle decompression is no longer recommended. This technique has been largely replaced with endoscopic techniques.

Endoscopic decompression of the guttural pouches

In all cases, endoscopic examination of the pharynx should be performed to determine if any additional abnormalities are present. Endoscopy frequently requires sedation and manual restraint. The nasal passage on the more dilated side can then be anesthetized by using a lubricant containing a local anesthetic, or a local anesthetic can be sprayed out the biopsy channel of the endoscope. In either case, a section of polyethylene tubing can be passed from the biopsy port of the endoscope into the guttural pouch through the pharyngeal opening to evacuate the trapped air. Alternatively the pouch perceived to have the greatest amount of distension can be catheterized with a Chamber's catheter inserted under endoscopic guidance, or the endoscope may be inserted into the pouch directly (Figure 37.4a). Suction may be required and will speed the process of air removal. In either case, diagnosis can be made by deflation as was with percutaneous needle placement. Generally, tympanites will reoccur after deflation, usually within 24 hours.

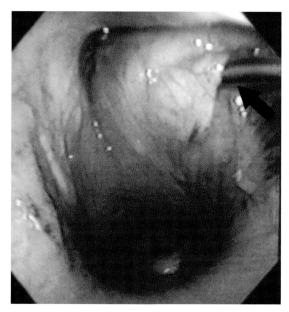

Figure 37.4   Insertion of a Chambers catheter (black arrow) into the left guttural pouch to decompress the pouch of air in a horse with left-sided guttural pouch tympanites.

Treatment

Conservative treatment for unilateral tympanites consists of placing a No. 24 or larger Foley catheter in the affected guttural pouch for 7–10 days. In a few cases, reoccurrence of the condition has not been seen but most will reoccur within 30 days. The other complication is that the Foley catheter may irritate the lining of the pharyngeal canal which will be sealed close permanently as it heals.

Surgical correction can be performed with the foal anesthetized and positioned in lateral recumbency for surgical excision of the median septum or plica salpingopharyngea or can be performed with the horse standing. Standing surgical correction involves the use of a diode or Nd:YAG laser delivered endoscopically.

Fenestration of the median septum and removal of the plica salpingopharyngea

In the absence of a laser, surgical correction for unilateral and bilateral tympanites requires the foal to be under general anesthesia in lateral and/or dor-

sal recumbency (Adams and Fessler 2000; McCue et al. 1989; Sparks et al. 2009). The side which is largest is prepped for aseptic surgery. In that there is a large amount of distention, major vessels are displaced ventrally. The lining of the guttural pouch is just beneath the subcutaneous tissue facilitating easy incisional entrance to the lateral compartment. Either a modified Whitehouse or Viborg's triangle approach can be used to access the interior of the guttural pouch. Prior to the surgical approach, a Chamber's catheter should be introduced in the opposite guttural pouch either blindly or under endoscopic guidance. Once the guttural pouch is surgically entered, the Chamber's catheter is then rotated. This speeds identification of the median septum by palpation of it through the opened guttural pouch (Figures 37.5a and 37.5b). The median septum is then fenestrated with scissors, creating a hole of a minimum of 4 cm in diameter. Fenestrations that are not of sufficient size may heal over resulting in reoccurrence of the tympanites. The fenestration will allow the pharyngeal opening of the normal guttural pouch to provide a means of escape for gases contained in either guttural pouch.

Foals that suffer from bilateral tympanites will require partial resection of the mucous membrane flap (plica salpingopharyngea) forming the pharyngeal opening in addition to median septum fenestration. Resection of the plica salpingopharyngea is easily performed with the foal in dorsal recumbency and accessed via a modified Whitehouse approach. The medial aspect of the plica is grasped with a thumb forceps and a 3 cm × 2 cm wide section of the plica is excised with scissors. After resection of the plica the medial laminae and cartilaginous flap are digitally palpated. The cartilaginous flap is inverted into the guttural pouch with the aid of a sharp-pronged Senn retractor. The flap is then grasped with an Allis tissue forceps and a 1 cm × 2 cm segment is resected with scissors. This widens the pharyngeal opening of the guttural pouch.

Standing laser median septum fenestration

Standing median septum fenestration can be successfully performed for unilateral tympanites (Blazyczek et al. 2004; Tate et al. 1995). The foal is sedated with xylazine hydrochloride (50–100 mg, IV) and butorphanol tartrate (2.5–5 mg, IV), and

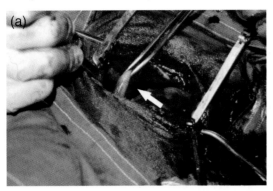 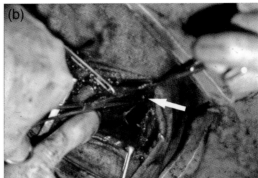

Figure 37.5 (a) Guttural pouch exposed through a Viborg's triangle approach with the median septum (white arrow) of the guttural pouch elevated by sponge forceps for resection. (b) The Chambers catheter (white arrow) held by Allis tissue forceps exposed in the opposite guttural pouch after a 4–6 cm diameter section of the median septum was resected.

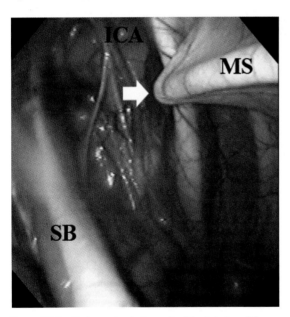

Figure 37.6 Endoscopic photograph of the interior of the right guttural pouch. A Chambers catheter placed into the left guttural pouch is being used to tent (white arrow) the median septum (MS) of the guttural pouch. ICA, internal carotid artery; SB, stylohyoid bone.

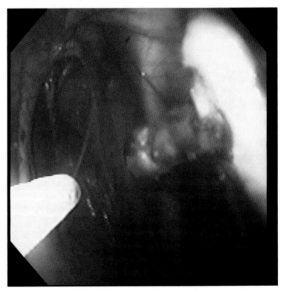

Figure 37.7 Endoscopic photograph of the right guttural pouch. A noncontact Nd:YAG laser fiber is being used to create a medial septum fenestration over a Chambers catheter inserted into the left guttural pouch.

a Chambers catheter is introduced into either guttural pouch. For convenience, the author generally places the Chambers catheter in the affected side to deflate it and reduce the parotid enlargement. It will be necessary to increase the arc or bend at the tip of the Chamber's catheter by an additional 20–30%. The arc must be enough to tent the median septum mucosa well into the opposite guttural pouch when the catheter is rotated and the tip pointed away from the affected guttural pouch

(Figure 37.6). The silhouette of the ball tip of the catheter should easily be seen when an endoscope is introduced into the other guttural pouch. A large fenestration of 4-cm diameter or greater can then be created using electrocautery, noncontact, or contact laser irradiation (Figure 37.7). To maximize the size of the fenestration, the Chamber's catheter is first pulled as far rostrally as possible. It is then moved in a caudal direction as the hole is enlarged, along with rotation, to gain a large vertical to dorsal component.

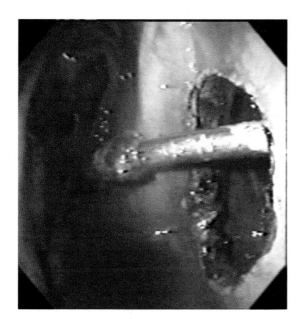

Figure 37.8   Completed fenestration of the guttural pouch median septum leaving a 4-cm opening with the Chambers catheter still in place.

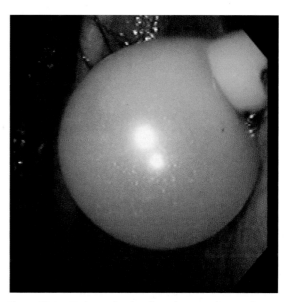

Figure 37.9   Endoscopic view from the normal guttural pouch demonstrating the placement of a Foley catheter through the laser fenestration to maintain the opening.

When a noncontact laser fiber is employed, usually an Nd:YAG, the ball tip acts as a backstop to prevent the beam from reaching other structures within the guttural pouches. Noncontact laser techniques use a high wattage output (60–100 watts) and generate large amounts of heat and smoke. It is therefore necessary, approximately every 10 seconds, to stop and let the cooling gasses of the coaxial fiber flow for 20 seconds to clear the smoke and decrease the temperature within the guttural pouches. The author has not seen any complications from the heat generated within the guttural pouch due to laser irradiation, but I have always employed the on/off cycle as previously described above. Sufficient smoke can be produced by contact laser fenestration to impede visibility, which will require suction. Noncontact laser fenestration is faster than electrocautery or contact laser application (Figure 37.8). If a contact diode laser fiber is used, the laser is set to 15 watts and delivered in a continuous wave (3 seconds on and 1 second off). The foal's sedation and attitude must be constantly monitored to be assured that the procedure is well tolerated (Figure 37.9). Following creation of the fistula, a Foley catheter is used to stent the opening for a minimum of 2–3 weeks after the surgical procedure (Figure 37.10). Transendo-

scopic laser fenestration can also be performed with the foal under general anesthesia held in a sternal position. In this situation, there is some collapse of the walls of the guttural pouches, which impairs visibility but not as much as when the procedure is attempted with the foal in lateral recumbency. Therefore, if a prolonged standing procedure appears not to be tolerated, the author recommends switching to general anesthesia with the foal in a sternal position. For such a short procedure, general anesthesia using only intravenous drugs such as a combination of xylazine and ketamine is sufficient without an endotracheal tube. Inhalant anesthesia enriched with oxygen should be avoided as it is more conducive to an airway fire, which would be fatal. General anesthesia may exacerbate any pneumonia that is present but is safer than risking damage to nerves or vessels within the guttural pouch.

Laser creation of a salpingopharyngeal fistula

An alternative to median septum fenestration is transendoscopic formation of a salpingopharyngeal fistula. The author has only performed this for unilateral tympanites. The procedure could be performed for bilateral tympanites or used in conjunction with median septum fenestration to provide relief from bilateral disease. The creation of a salpingopharyngeal fistula is faster than what has already been described and is not as technically challenging. The foal is sedated and maintained in the standing position, and a Chambers catheter is introduced into the guttural pouch that is most distended. The endoscope is introduced into the rostral pharynx through the opposite nostril. Placement of the catheter can be viewed endoscopically. It is necessary to increase the arc of the ball tip of the Chamber's catheter greater than that required for median septum fenestration. The catheter is pulled rostrally until the ball tip can be seen adjacent to the dorsal pharyngeal recess tenting the mucosa. One should be able, by feel, to appreciate the ball tip sliding off the cartilaginous portion of the inner opening medially as traction is applied. It is critical that the fistula into the guttural pouch be performed behind the plica salpingopharyngea. If the cartilaginous flap only is fenestrated, tympany will not resolve.

The laser fiber, introduced through the biopsy channel of the endoscope, is advanced forward and the mucosa is irradiated until the ball tip can be visualized (Figure 37.11). This is easily accomplished using noncontact delivery of irradiation from the Nd:YAG laser set at 100 watts output or a diode 810 or 980 um laser set at 50 watts output. Contact delivery at 15–18 watts can be used but it takes longer and a hole must be created of sufficient size that the ball tip is visualized endoscopically. The Chambers catheter is then removed.

A 24–26 French Foley catheter threaded onto a slightly bent stylet to stiffen is introduced through the freshly created salpingopharyngeal fistula (Figure 37.12). The balloon of the Foley is inflated with 5 cm^3 of water. The endoscope is then passed up the same side and into the guttural pouch and retroflexed to assure that the position of the Foley is just medial to the cartilage flap forming the inner os of the pharyngeal opening (Figure 37.13). If the Foley is placed through the cartilage, or lateral to it, within the pharyngeal passage, formation of a healed fistula will take longer to achieve and intermittent reoccurrence of the tympanites may occur. A fistula should allow visualization of the inner structures of the guttural pouch when an endoscope is later placed at the outer aspect of

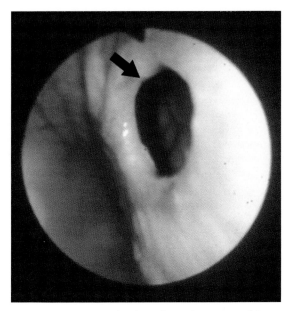

Figure 37.10   Two weeks after Foley catheter removal from a foal which had a noncontact laser fenestration demonstrating healed edge of the median septum (white arrow).

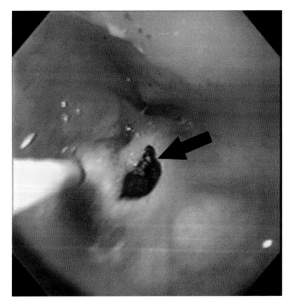

Figure 37.11   Noncontact laser fiber directed at the ball of the Chambers catheter (black arrow) positioned behind the plica salpingopharyngea and directed caudal and dorsal to the pharyngeal opening of the guttural pouch.

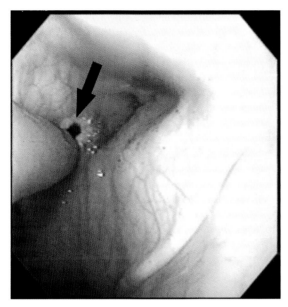

Figure 37.12   Foley catheter in the pharynx directed to the laser-created salpingopharyngeal fistula (black arrow).

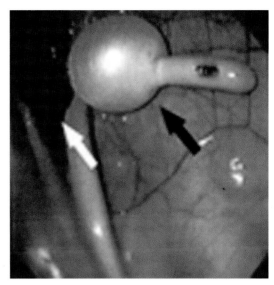

Figure 37.13   Endoscope (white arrow) inside the guttural pouch retroflexed showing placement of the inflated Foley catheter (black arrow) dorsal and medial to the plica salpingopharyngeal situated between the two.

the hole. Any tissue preventing this will require additional laser application and Foley replacement.

The proximal end of the Foley may be secured to the foals halter, but it must be constantly observed to be assured that the foal does not displace it by rubbing or nursing. A well-tolerated method of decreasing the chance of dislodging it is to make a small incision in the false nostril and bring the distal end of the Foley catheter out through it, and then secure it to a halter. The Foley catheter should remain in place a minimum of 2 weeks and preferably 3 weeks before removal. When removed, the salpingopharyngeal fistula should be observed weekly by endoscopy for an additional 4 weeks for signs of closure. If closure appears to be occurring, the Foley catheter should be replaced for an additional 2 weeks. The incision into the false nostril heals well and leaves only a small scar. The author is aware of one horse in which it is believed the salpingopharyngeal fistula was responsible for respiratory stridor, but the size of the fistula is not known. The majority of horses end up with a fistula of approximately a centimeter in size which has not been associated with respiratory stridor or other diseases that may affect the guttural pouches (Figure 37.14).

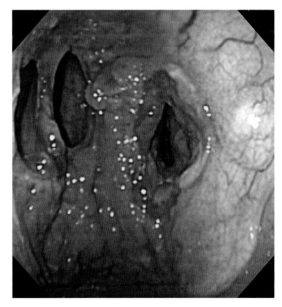

Figure 37.14   Endoscopic photograph of healed bilateral salpingopharyngea fistulas created with a contact diode laser.

Complications

The most common complication following surgical correction of guttural pouch tympanites is recurrence. Stricture post laser fenestration of either the median septum or plica salpingopharyngeal has been observed. It may also take 1–2 months for the foal's external conformation or appearance to return to normal. Foals may appear to retain partial distension which may appear pronounced at times. This emphasizes the importance of frequent follow-up endoscopic examinations. Finally, the editor has observed one case of permanent dysphagia post laser fenestration of the median septum of the guttural pouch. This same occurrence following surgical correction has also been reported by Bell (2007). For this case the endoscope was inserted via Viborg's triangle (previously the pouch has been catheterized with a Foley catheter for management of severe guttural pouch empyema) and the median septum was fenestrated with a contact Nd:YAG laser fiber. Dysphagia was immediately evident following laser fenestration and the foal was later euthanized. Aspiration pneumonia does occasionally develop prior to surgical correction but does lengthen postoperative treatment and adds expense for the owner.

References

Adams SB, Fessler JF. 2000. Median septum fenestration and pharyngeal orifice enlargement for guttural pouch tympany. In: *Atlas of Equine Surgery* (pp. 175–179). Philadelphia, PA: W.B. Saunders Company.

Bell C. 2007. Pharyngeal neuromuscular dysfunction associated with bilateral guttural pouch tympany in a foal. *The Canadian Veterinary Journal* 48:192–194.

Blazyczek I, Hamann H, Deegen E, Distl O, Ohnesorge B. 2004a. Retrospective analysis of 50 cases of guttural pouch tympany in foals. *The Veterinary Record* 154:261–264.

Blazyczek I, Hamann H, Ohnesorge B, Deegen E, Distl O. 2004b. Inheritance of guttural pouch tympany in the Arabian horse. *Journal of Heredity* 95(3):195–199.

McCue PM, Freeman DE, Donawick WJ. 1989. Guttural pouch tympany: 15 cases (1977–1986). *Journal of the American Veterinary Medical Association* 194(12):1761–1763.

Metzger J, Ohnesorge B, Distl O. 2012. Genome-wide linkage and association analysis identifies major gene loci for guttural pouch tympany in Arabian and German Warmblood horses. *PLoS One* 7(7):e41640.

Sparks HD, Stick JA, Brakenhoff JE, Cramp PA, Spirito MA. 2009. Partial resection of the plica salpinogopharyngeus for the treatment of three foals with bilateral tympany of the auditory tube diverticulum (guttural pouch). *Journal of the American Veterinary Medical Association* 235(6):731–733.

Tate LP Jr, Blikslager AT, Little ED. 1995. Transendoscopic laser treatment of guttural pouch tympanites in eight foals. *Veterinary Surgery* 24(5):367–372.

Zeitz A, Spotter A, Blazyczek I, Diesterbeck U, Ohnesorge B, Deegen E, Distl O. 2009. Whole-genome scan for guttural pouch tympany in Arabian and German Warmblood horses. *Animal Genetics* 40(6):917–924.

38 Treatment of Hemorrhage Associated with Guttural Pouch Mycosis

Daniel F. Hogan

Introduction

Hemorrhage from guttural pouch mycosis (GPM) is a severe and life-threatening clinical condition caused by fungal invasion through the mucosal lining of the guttural pouch with plaque formation directly on one of the major arteries as they course within the guttural pouch (Figure 38.1). *Aspergillus* spp. are the most common organisms but others have been reported too (Cook et al. 1968; Freeman and Donawick 1980a and 1980b; Guillot et al. 1997). Clinical signs of GPM include epistaxis, nasal discharge, dysphagia, and otic discharge (Caron et al. 1987; Freeman et al. 1989; Greet 1987; Smith and Barber 1984).

While the fungal plaque is the underlying etiology in these cases, the immediate concern is the profuse hemorrhage caused by erosion into the adjacent artery which not uncommonly is severe and can result in exsanguination (Edwards and Greet 2007). While the hemorrhage may be the most immediate concern with GPM, complete vascular occlusion of the affected artery is required to result in successful resolution of the fungal plaque (Speirs et al. 1995). However, it is critical to remember that both normograde and retrograde flow must be addressed as elimination of normograde flow (cardiac side of lesion) only will not result in resolution of the hemorrhage due to the cerebral arterial circle (circle of Willis) (Freeman et al. 1989; Hardy et al. 1990). For this reason, arterial flow must be stopped both proximal (cardiac side) and distal (rostral) to the fungal plaque (Church et al. 1986; Greet 1987; McIlwraith 1978; Owen 1974).

There are multiple techniques to eliminate arterial flow in these cases including ligation of the common carotid artery, thrombectomy catheter placement, detachable balloon placement, coil embolization, and the Amplatzer® vascular plug (AVP) (Delfs et al. 2009; Kauffman 1992; Leveille et al. 2000; Partington et al. 1993; Snaps et al. 1995). This chapter will focus on the following techniques: thrombectomy catheters, embolization coils, and the AVP.

Thrombectomy catheters

The use of thrombectomy catheters has traditionally been considered the standard of care for

Advances in Equine Upper Respiratory Surgery, First Edition. Edited by Jan Hawkins.
© 2015 ACVS Foundation. Published 2015 by John Wiley & Sons, Inc.

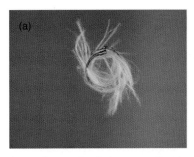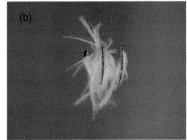

Figure 38.1   Picture of a stainless steel embolization coil with polyester fibers in cross-section (a) and longitudinal orientation (b).

arterial occlusion in horses with GPM (Caron et al. 1987; Freeman and Donawick 1980a,b). With this approach, the affected artery(ies) must be surgically accessed where one or two catheters are inserted to occlude flow both proximally and distally to the fungal plaque. Additional arterial access and catheters may be required in complex lesions (Freeman and Donawick 1980a,b; Freeman et al. 1989). Given the typical absence of intraoperative imaging, there is the possibility of inserting the catheters into the wrong artery or an aberrant branch (Bacon Miller et al. 1998; Freeman et al. 1993). When this happens, the arterial flow will not be adequately reduced and continued hemorrhage can occur. In addition, the catheters then need to be buried under the skin or left to exit the skin at the site of surgical access or from the mucous membranes of the mouth. This can lead to incisional infection at these sites. In some instances the catheters may require removal if surgical site infection occurs or the catheter erodes through the catheterized artery. Catheter removal can lengthen the hospital stay and increase cost to the owner. If catheter removal is required catheters should remain in place for a minimum of 7 days to allow sufficient thrombus formation within the catheterized artery.

Coil embolization

In an attempt to avoid some of these issues, an alternative method for vascular occlusion was developed (Kauffmann et al. 1992; Leveille et al. 2000; Partington et al. 1993; Snaps et al. 1995). This technique uses either platinum or stainless steel coils which are covered by polyester fibers (Figure 38.2). The goal is to fill up the internal lumen of the

artery with the coil where the polyester fibers help with acute thrombus occlusion and endothelialization. Embolization coils have been used for vascular occlusion in humans for a variety of conditions. Complications with coil embolization have included coil migration, coil embolization of the cerebral arterial circle, meningitis, and recannulation of the embolized artery(ies) (Ha and Calcagno 2005; Rossi et al. 2006). Reported complications associated with coil embolization in horses include death secondary to incomplete resolution of the fungal plaque, blindness, laryngeal hemiplegia, facial hemiparesis, and the potential for coil migration if the coil is not properly sized or deployed in the correct location (Caron et al. 1987; Freeman and Donawick 1980; Freeman et al. 1989; Hardy et al. 1990).

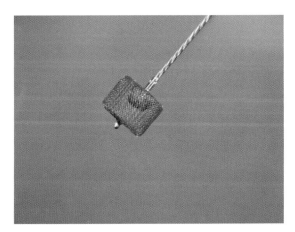

Figure 38.2   Picture of an Amplatzer® vascular plug attached to the threaded delivery cable. From Hogan et al. 2006.

As with the use of Fogarty catheters, one or more coils must be used to occlude the arterial supply both distal and proximal to the fungal lesion. A report of coil embolization in 31 horses reported that 2–12 coils were required for complete occlusion (Lepage and Piccot-Crezollet 2005). Expertise in vascular interventional procedures, fluoroscopic guidance, and a table that allows diagnostic imaging is required with this technique.

The external common carotid artery ipsilateral to the guttural pouch where the hemorrhage is originating is approached via surgical cut down. The vessel is approached at the middle to upper third of the cervical region. The vagosympathetic trunk is dissected off the external carotid artery and the external carotid artery is isolated and elevated by using an umbilical tape, a Penrose drain, or other suitable material. A vascular access sheath of appropriate size (typically 5–7 Fr) is inserted into the external carotid artery through a modified Seldinger technique so angiographic and coil delivery catheters can be inserted with minimal blood loss. An angiogram is performed proximal enough in the external carotid artery to adequately visualize the arterial supply and branching anatomy to the head to identify the vessel responsible for the hemorrhage (usually the internal carotid or maxillary artery). Once the vessel is identified, a delivery catheter of appropriate size and distal shape (multipurpose or Judkins right coronary work particularly well) is advanced using a guide wire to approximately 10 mm distal to the site of hemorrhage with fluoroscopic guidance. One or more embolization coils are deployed into the vessel with the use of the guide wire. After each coil is deployed, a small volume of radiographic contrast is injected by hand through the delivery catheter to determine if the vessel is completely occluded. Once complete occlusion is verified, the delivery catheter is withdrawn to a level approximately 10 mm proximal to the site of hemorrhage where one or more additional embolization coils are deployed in a similar manner to the distal arterial location to obtain complete occlusion of the vessel proximal to the lesion. Complete occlusion of arterial flow proximal (cardiac) and distal (rostral) to the fungal plaque has now been obtained. The small opening in the external carotid artery is closed using a purse string suture of 5–0 polyglactin 910. Additional simple

interrupted sutures are occasionally necessary to close the catheter insertion site. The remainder of the incision is closed in a routine fashion.

Amplatzer vascular plug

The AVP (St. Jude Medical Corp, St. Paul, MN, USA) has been used for the occlusion of various vascular abnormalities in humans and dogs as well as horses for GPM (Delfs et al. 2009; Fischer et al. 2007; Hogan et al. 2006; Smith and Martin 2007; Tabori and Love 2008). The AVP is a self-expanding, cylindrical device of nitinol wire mesh secured on both ends with platinum marker bands (Figure 38.2). The AVP is attached to a delivery cable and is flexible enough to be deployed through relatively small guiding catheters or vascular sheaths. Given the design and flexibility of the AVP, it can be accurately positioned, have controlled deployment, and can be recaptured after deployment. The AVP is designed to fully fill the targeted vessel, similar to a cork in a bottle, rather than relying on interlacing coils of wire and polyester fiber as with embolization coils.

After correct positioning is confirmed through fluoroscopy and angiography, the AVP is deployed from the delivery catheter and released by counterclockwise rotation of the delivery cable. The AVP is available in seven sizes ranging from 4 to 16 mm in 2-mm increments and should be 130–150% of the targeted vessel diameter. To date, all affected vessels associated with GPM have been completely occluded with either 10 mm or 12 mm AVP although this should be confirmed via angiography prior to AVP placement. The 10 mm and 12 mm AVP can be deployed through a 5 Fr vascular sheath or a 6 Fr guiding catheter. If the AVP is appropriately sized, the risk for migration or to become dislodged from the vessel after deployment appears to be extremely low.

At the author's institution, we prefer to have endoscopic visualization of the guttural pouch to visualize the affected vessel during the occlusion procedure. We feel this gives us good guidance and helps us to most accurately determine the location of the vascular hemorrhage. This is highlighted by the fact that many horses do not have active bleeding at the time of occlusion and vascular changes such as aneurysms are often absent. The procedure for deploying the AVP is essentially identical to that for embolization coils. The external common carotid artery ipsilateral to the guttural pouch where the hemorrhage is originating is utilized and vessel isolation is the same. A 7 Fr vascular access sheath is inserted into the external carotid artery through a modified Seldinger technique and an angiogram is performed to adequately visualize the arterial supply and branching anatomy to the head to identify the vessel responsible for the hemorrhage.

An appropriately sized guide wire is inserted into a 5 Fr Judkins right coronary catheter and the catheter is inserted into a 5 Fr vascular sheath of at least 70 cm in length such that approximately 50 mm of guide wire is exiting the 5 Fr catheter and 30 mm of the catheter is exiting the 5 Fr vascular sheath. The guide wire, catheter, and 5 Fr sheath are then inserted as a unit into the 7 Fr vascular access sheath and advanced to close proximity of the appropriate vessel using fluoroscopic guidance. The guide wire and 5 Fr catheter are then used to navigate the vasculature to a location approximately 10 mm distal to the site of the hemorrhage. The 5 Fr vascular sheath is advanced over the 5 Fr catheter and guide wire to the vascular location approximately 10 mm distal to the site of the hemorrhage. The guide wire and catheter are removed and the AVP is inserted into the 5 Fr vascular access sheath and advanced to the tip of the access sheath. The AVP is held in a stable manner while the 5 Fr vascular access sheath is withdrawn, deploying the AVP. At this point a small volume of radiographic contrast is injected by hand through the 5 Fr vascular access sheath to determine if the vessel is completely occluded. Once complete occlusion is verified, the AVP is released by rotating the deliv-ery cable counterclockwise. The 5 Fr vascular access sheath is then withdrawn to a level approximately 10 mm proximal to the site of hemorrhage where another AVP is deployed in a similar manner to the distal arterial location. Complete occlusion of arterial flow proximal (cardiac) and distal (rostral) to the fungal plaque has now been obtained. Closure of the vascular access site in the common carotid artery and skin incision is closed in a manner as described for placement of embolization coils.

Summary

In the author's opinion the AVP is the preferred technique for vascular occlusion in GPM. This opinion is based on the fact that the AVP can be delivered more precisely and quickly along with greater safety than embolization coils. This opinion on the AVP is shared within the human literature where some physicians favor the use of the AVP over embolization coils to reduce the risk of migration of the embolic device from the location of interest (Fischer et al. 2007; Ha and Calcagno 2005; Rossi et al. 2006).

The major advantages of the AVP over embolization coils in the author's opinion include the ability to occlude the affected vessel with one plug on each side of the fungal erosion compared to multiple embolization coils, the ability to retrieve a deployed AVP, complete luminal filling of the vessel, and the AVP is very unlikely to become dislodged due to the radial tension it exerts on the vascular wall (Figure 38.3).

The disadvantages of the AVP compared to surgical ligation or use of Fogarty catheters is the

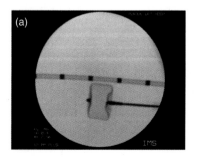 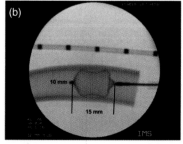 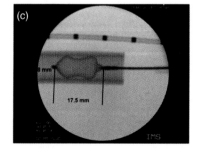

Figure 38.3   (a) *In vitro* pictures of a 12-mm Amplatzer® vascular plug in its native or unrestrained shape. (b) After deployment in a 10-mm tube approximating 130% oversizing of a vessel. (c) After deployment in an 8-mm tube approximating 150% oversizing of a vessel. Note how the AVP takes on a "dog bone" appearance when oversized compared to the native, unrestrained shape and that linear length of the AVP increases as it is progressively oversized.

need for specialized equipment and the expertise of an interventional cardiologist or individual knowledgeable with interventional peripheral vascular techniques; limiting this technique to specialty or university teaching hospitals. However, it could be argued that surgical expertise is required for surgical ligation or using thrombectomy catheters, which would also limit these techniques to specialty or university teaching hospitals. The need for specialized equipment and expertise is also required for embolization coils. A potential limitation for the AVP compared to embolization coils is that slightly larger delivery equipment (guiding catheters or vascular sheaths) is required. However, the vessels routinely involved with GPM are of sufficient size where this slight difference in delivery equipment is of no consequence.

Embolization coils and the AVP appear to be comparable in price. The AVP costs approximately $400 where embolization coils cost approximately $100 each. However, given that multiple embolization coils are typically required to completely occlude a leaking vessel compared to two AVP, there may be negligible difference in price for most cases.

References

Bacon Miller C, Wilson DA, Martin DD, Pace LW, Constantinescu GM. 1998. Complications of balloon catheterization associated with aberrant cerebral arterial anatomy in a horse with guttural pouch mycosis. *Veterinary Surgery* 27:450–453.

Caron JP, Fretz PD, Bailey JV, Barber SM, Hurtig MB. 1987. Balloon-tipped catheter catheter arterial occlusion for prevention of hemorrhages caused by guttural pouch mycosis: 13 cases (1982–1985). *Journal of the American Veterinary Medical Association* 191:345–349.

Church S, Wyn-Jones G, Park AH, Ritchie HE. 1986. Treatment of guttural pouch mycosis. *Equine Veterinary Journal* 18:362–365.

Cook WR, Campbell RSF, Dawson C. 1968. The pathology and aetiology of guttural pouch mycosis in the horse. *Veterinary Record* 83:422–428.

Delfs KC, Hawkins JF, Hogan DF. 2009. Treatment of acute epistaxis secondary to guttural pouch mycosis with transarterial nitinol vascular occlusion plugs in three equids. *Journal of the American Veterinary Medical Association* 235:189–193.

Edwards GB, Greet TR. 2007. Disorders of the guttural pouches. Guttural pouch mycosis. In: McGorum BC,

Dixon PM, Robison NE, Schumacher J, eds. *Equine Respiratory Medicine and Surgery*, 1st ed. (pp. 424–430). Philadelphia, PA: W.B. Saunders Company.

Fischer G, Apostolopoulou SC, Rammos S, Kiaffas M, Kramer HH. 2007. Transcatheter closure of coronary arterial fistulas using the new Amplatzer vascular plug. *Cardiology in the Young* 17:283–287.

Freeman DE, Donawick WJ. 1980a. Occlusion of the internal carotid artery in the horse by means of a balloon tipped catheter: Clinical use of the method to prevent Epistaxis caused by guttural pouch mycosis. *Journal of the American Veterinary Medical Association* 176:236–240.

Freeman DE, Donawick WJ. 1980b. Occlusion of the internal carotid artery in the horse by means of a balloon tipped catheter: Evaluation of a method designed to prevent Epistaxis caused by guttural pouch mycosis. *Journal of the American Veterinary Medical Association* 176:232–235.

Freeman DE, Ross MW, Donawick WJ, Hamir AN. 1989. Occlusion of the external carotid and maxillary arteries in the horse to prevent hemorrhage from guttural pouch mycosis. *Veterinary Surgery* 18:39–47.

Freeman DE, Staller GS, Maxson AD, Sweeney CR. 1993. Unusual internal carotid artery branching that prevented arterial occlusion with a balloon-tipped catheter in a horse. *Veterinary Surgery* 22:531–534.

Greet TRC. 1987. Outcome of treatment in 35 cases of guttural pouch mycosis. *Equine Veterinary Journal* 19:483–487.

Guillot J, Collobert C, Gueho E, Mialot M, Lagarde E. 1997. Emericella nidulans as an agent of guttural pouch mycosis in a horse. *Journal of Medical Veterinary Mycology* 35(6):433–435.

Ha CD, Calcagno D. 2005. Amplatzer vascular plug to occlude the internal iliac arteries in patients undergoing aortoiliac aneurysm repair. *Journal of Vascular Surgery* 42:1058–1062.

Hardy J, Robertson JT, Wilkie DA. 1990. Ischemic optic neuropathy and blindness after arterial occlusion for treatment of guttural pouch mycosis in two horses. *Journal of the American Veterinary Medical Association* 196:1631–1634.

Hogan DF, Green HW, Sanders RA. 2006. Transcatheter closure of patent ductus arteriosus in a dog with a peripheral vascular occlusion device. *Journal of Veterinary Cardiology* 8:139–142.

Kauffmann SI, Martin LG, Zuckermann AM, Koch SR, Silverstein MI, Barton JW. 1992. Peripheral transcatheter embolization with platinum microcoils. *Radiology* 184(2):369–372.

Lepage OM, Piccot-Crezollet C. 2005. Transarterial coil embolization in 31 horses (1999–2002) with guttural pouch mycosis: A 2 year follow-up. *Equine Veterinary Journal* 37:430–434.

Leveille R, Hardy J, Robertson JT, Willis AM, Beard WL. 2000. Transarterial coil embolization of the internal and external carotid and maxillary arteries for prevention of hemorrhages from guttural pouch mycosis in horses. *Veterinary Surgery* 29:389–397.

McIlwraith CW. 1978. Surgical treatment of acute Epistaxis associated with guttural pouch mycosis. *Veterinary Medicine Small Animal Clinician* 73:67–69.

Owen RR. 1974. Epistaxis prevented by ligation of the internal carotid artery in the guttural pouch. *Equine Veterinary Journal* 6:143–149.

Partington BP, Partington CR, Biller DS, Toshach K. 1993. Transvenous coil embolization for treatment of patent ductus venosus in a dog. *Journal of the American Veterinary Medical Association* 202:281–284.

Rossi M, Rebonato A, Greco L, Stefanini G, Citone M, Speranza A, David V. 2006. A new device for vascular embolization: Report on case of two pulmonary arteriovenous fistulas embolization using the Amplatzer vascular plug. *Cardiovascular Interventional Radiology* 29:902–906.

Smith DM, Barber SM. 1984. Guttural Pouch hemorrhages associated with lesions of the maxillary artery in two horses. *Canadian Veterinary Journal* 25:239–242.

Smith PJ, Martin MW. 2007. Transcatheter embolization of patent ductus arteriosus using an Amplatzer vascular plug in six dogs. *Journal of Small Animal Practitioner* 48:80–86.

Snaps FR, McEntee K, Saunders JH, Dondelinger RF. 1995. Treatment of patent ductus arteriosus by placement of intravascular coils in a pup. *Journal of the American Veterinary Medical Association* 207:724–725.

Speirs VC, Harrison IW, van Veenendaal JC, Baumgartner T, Josseck HH, Reutter H. 1995. Is specific antifungal therapy necessary for the treatment of guttural pouch mycosis in horses? *Equine Veterinary Journal* 27:151–152.

Tabori NE, Love BA. 2008. Transcatheter occlusion of pulmonary arteriovenous malformations using the Amplatzer vascular plug II. *Catheter Cardiovascular Intervention.* 71:940–943.

39 Surgical Management of Temporohyoid Osteoarthropathy

Norm G. Ducharme, Thomas J. Divers, and Nita Irby

Introduction

The temporohyoid articulation is a synchondrosis between the stylohyoid bone and the petrous temporal bone. There is a degenerative process that frequently occurs at this articulation with age (Naylor et al. 2010). A clinical disease occurs when degeneration of this synchondrosis leads to enlargement and fusion of this articulation and compression of the adjacent nerves. In addition, fracture of the petrous temporal bone may occur associated with swallowing or forced movement of the hyoid apparatus during veterinary manipulation (i.e., nasogastric intubation, dental procedures). The bony proliferation associated with osteoarthropathy of the temporomandibular joint eventually leads to compression of cranial nerves VII and VIII and of the parasympathetic fibers traveling with the facial nerve; the clinical signs are associated with deficits of the aforementioned nerves. In addition, this osteoarthropathy is painful leading to head shaking, resentment of the bit, ear rubbing, and pain during eating (Blythe 1997; Divers et al. 2006). The etiology of this disease appears mainly to be a degenerative process rather than an otitis media

and/or interna. Originally it was reported that temporohyoid osteoarthropathy (THO) was secondary to an infectious process (Blythe 1997). Otitis media and/or interna result from a hematogenous source or result from an ascending infection from the respiratory tract with the resulting bulla osteitis incorporating the temporohyoid joint but appears to be a less common cause of THO (Blythe 1997). Indeed, evidence is mounting that the cause of this disease is a degenerative condition. Indeed, the advent of CT evaluation in the last 15 years has revealed THO with only rare evidence of fluid accumulation in the middle ear of horses (Divers et al. 2006; Hilton et al. 2009; Pease et al. 2004). Furthermore, the report of an age-related (Naylor et al. 2010) or behavior-related (i.e., cribbing (Grenager et al. 2010)) degenerative process in horses argues against infectious origin as a common cause for this condition.

Clinical signs

The clinical signs are generally related to deficits of facial nerve paralysis with deviated lips and eyelid muscle paresis and decreased innervation

Advances in Equine Upper Respiratory Surgery, First Edition. Edited by Jan Hawkins.

of the lacrimal gland resulting in decreased tear production. Affected horses may thus experience corneal ulceration from exposure keratitis created by keratoconjunctivitis sicca combined with exposure keratitis. In addition, deficits of the vestibulo-cochlear nerve result in proprioceptive ataxia causing difficulty with balance and spatial orientation and a head tilt. If nearby meninges are sufficiently inflamed, depression and occasional seizures may be noted. Pain is exhibited through dysphagia and cessation of cribbing when present. Pain can be elicited by palpation at the base of the ear, digital pressure on the basihyoid bone, and manipulation of the tongue. Rarely a septic exudate may drain from the ear. On occasions the petrous temporal bone is fractured, potentially leading to death (Walker et al. 2002). The diagnosis of THO is made from the clinical signs and the detection of an enlargement of the proximal stylohyoid bone either by endoscopic examination of the guttural pouch or by imaging of the temporohyoid region.

CT is an important diagnostic test when considering surgery. It confirms the diagnosis, identifies bilateral versus unilateral disease (Figure 39.1) and provides details on hyoid bone involvement relevant to the surgery. Further value of CT in support of surgical management is discussed under management.

Management

Conservative management of this condition is best and consists of anti-inflammatory medication, frequent ocular medications as indicated, and antimicrobial therapy. Although primary septic otitis media/interna is a rare cause of the disease, hematomas that develop secondary to acute fracture at the THO site may be susceptible to infection. The symptoms to be alleviated by surgery include treatment of conjunctivitis, pain, and deficits associated with neural compression. Keratoconjunctivitis sicca and exposure keratitis are managed by performing a reversible tarsorrhaphy. The eyelid margins of the lateral two-thirds of eyelids are incised with a No. 15 blade, and buried simple interrupted sutures are used to suture the upper and lower eyelids together using 5-0 absorbable suture. This protects the cornea until 4–36 months after surgery when facial nerve function and tear

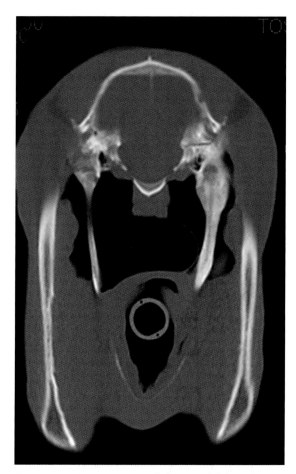

Figure 39.1   CT examination of a horse with bilateral temporohyoid osteoarthropathy.

production return at which time the tarsorrhaphy can be reversed. If tear production does not return as measured by Schirmer's test, then the tarsorrhaphy is maintained permanently. The tarsorrhaphy is usually done during the same anesthetic episode as the one required for ceratohyoidectomy and CT but can be performed with the patient standing.

THO results in an enhanced transfer of forces (i.e., lever arm effect) from the basihyoid bone to the petrous temporal bone during swallowing and other movements of the hyoid apparatus. This may lead to fracture of the petrous temporal bone and may cause death (Grenager et al. 2010). Articular enlargement and/or swelling and callus at the fracture site may cause damage to cranial nerves VII or VII. Surgical treatments were developed to

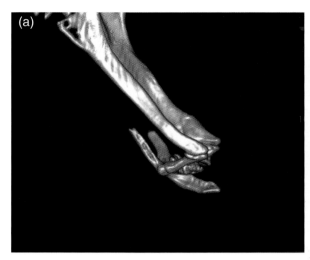 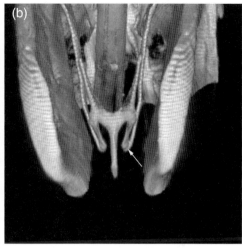

Figure 39.2   (a,b) CT examination showing orientation of stylohyoid articulation with ceratohyoid bone after 3D reconstruction. (a) From the lateral view the articulation is horizontal and (b) from the caudal view the articulation is oblique.

remove the lever arm forces on the temporohyoid articulation by either resecting a 2–5 cm section of stylohyoid bone or by removal of the ceratohyoid bone. Because of the technical difficulty of performing the partial stylohyoid bone resection, the increased likelihood of hypoglossal nerve or linguofacial artery injury with this approach, and the recurrence of the disease through bony union at the stylohyoidectomy site, unilateral or bilateral ceratohyoidectomy is now the preferred treatment (Pease et al. 2004).

Ceratohyoidectomy immediately removes the pressure on the temporohyoid articulation and thus reduces pain, especially while eating. It has been speculated that removing the pressure on the articulation favors a more rapid resorption of the enlargement of the temporohyoid area with a subsequent decrease in pressure (and its negative effect) on the adjacent nerves. There is no evidence-based data to support that hypothesis at this time. Most recently, it has been documented that bilateral involvement is present in 94% of horses evaluated by CT (Hilton et al. 2009). However, not all enlargements of the THO joint is associated with clinical signs. Therefore only moderate-to-severe bilateral THO lesions are treated surgically bilaterally. Bilateral treatment may be performed during the same anesthetic period or be staged. The morbidity of ceratohyoidectomy (i.e., possible damage to the hypoglossal nerve) should be considered before

electing to perform the procedure bilaterally. If ceratohyoidectomy is performed bilaterally the horse should be fed at shoulder height after surgery and attempts at an early return to feeding to decrease postoperative incisional swelling. Standing ceratohyoidectomy has also been reported. However, ceratohyoidectomy is preferentially performed by the authors under general anesthesia with the horse in dorsal recumbency to minimize the possibility of hypoglossal nerve damage. For this procedure it is important to know from the CT if there is petrous temporal bone fracture; if so traction on the ceratohyoid bone during surgery must be minimized as to not worsen the condition. It is also useful to know from the CT the plane of the stylohyoid bone articulation (Figures 39.2a and 39.2b) to guide the disarticulation between ceratohyoid and stylohyoid bones with cartilage scissors. Finally it is important to know if the ceratohyoid bone is also affected (i.e., enlarged; Figure 39.3); in those cases the resection is done at the fracture site and a hyoglossus muscle graft is placed between the basihyoid bone and the remnant of the ceratohyoid bone.

Ceratohyoidectomy

With the horse in dorsal recumbency the procedure is done as follows: a 10-cm incision is made immediately medial to the linguofacial vein on the

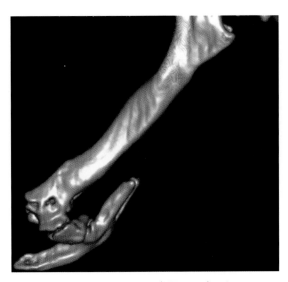

Figure 39.3   3D reconstruction of CT scan showing involvement of the ceratohyoid bone. Note the enlargement of the ceratohyoid bone with fracture in its mid portion (Compare to Figure 39.2a).

affected side. The incision extends rostrally from the caudal aspect of the basihyoid bone. The incision is extended dorsally immediately lateral to the geniohyoid muscle. The basihyoid articulation with the ceratohyoid bone is identified and opened with a curved hemostat or a curved scissor. The joint capsule is then transected so that the caudal aspect of the ceratohyoid bone can be grasped with an instrument. Using blunt dissection the hyoglossus muscle is freed from the lateral aspect of the ceratohyoid bone and the hypoglossal nerve is identified as it runs on the lateral aspect of the ceratohyoid bone near the stylohyoid—ceratohyoid articulation (Figure 39.4). After isolating the hypoglossal nerve, the ceratohyoid is mobilized to identify the articulation with the stylohyoid bone. Using a cartilage scissor in the acute angle formed by the stylohyoid and ceratohyoid joint the ceratohyoid bone is freed. The geniohyoid is reattached to the fascia near the linguofacial vein and the subcutaneous tissue and skin closed routinely. Recovery is assisted as many of

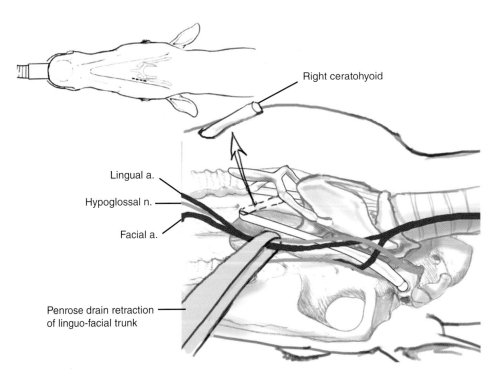

Right ceratohyoid

Lingual a.

Hypoglossal n.

Facial a.

Penrose drain retraction of linguo-facial trunk

Figure 39.4   Anatomical drawing showing the position of hypoglossal nerve, lingual nerve, and linguofacial artery in relation to ceratohyoid bone resection procedure (Redrawn from Divers TJ, Ducharme NG, de Lahunta A, Irby NL, Scrivani PV. 2006. Temporohyoid osteoarthropathy. *Clinical Techniques in Equine Practice* 5:17–23).

these horses are ataxic from the neurologic deficits associated with THO.

Supportive care is given until discharged 4–5 days after surgery. Eating is usually much improved within 48 hours of surgery. Patients are confined to a box stall with careful hand walking starting depending on the improvement of their level of ataxia usually within 2–4 weeks. They often can be turned out into a small paddock within 2 months of surgery. Re-evaluation is done at 4 months postoperatively to assess the return of lacrimal gland and eyelid motor function, as well as their neurological state. Return to exercise is usually around 6 months postoperatively. The prognosis for THO is fair to guarded but appears to be improved in most horses following ceratohyoidectomy.

References

Blythe LL. 1997. Otitis media and interna and temporohyoid osteoarthropathy. *The Veterinary Clinics of North America Equine Practice* 13:21–42.

Divers TJ, Ducharme NG, de Lahunta A, Irby NL, Scrivani PV. 2006. Temporohyoid osteoarthropathy. *Clinical Techniques in Equine Practice* 5:17–23.

Grenager NS, Divers TJ, Mohammed HO, Johnson AL, Albright J, Reuss SM. 2010. Epidemiological features and association with crib-biting in horses with neurological disease associated with temporohyoid osteoarthropathy (1991–2008). *Equine Veterinary Education* 22(9):467–472.

Hilton H, Puchhalski SM, Aleman M. 2009. The computed tomographic appearance of equine temporohyoid osteoarthropathy. *Veterinary Radiology Ultrasound* 50:151–156.

Naylor RJ, Perkins JD, Allen S, Aldred J, Draper E, Patterson-Kane J, Piercy RJ. 2010. Histopathology and computed tomography of age-associated degeneration of the equine temporohyoid joint. *Equine Veterinary Journal* 42(5):425–430.

Pease AP, Van Biervliet J, Dykes NL, Divers TJ, Ducharme NG. 2004. Complication of partial stylohyoidectomy for treatment of temporohyoid osteoarthropathy and preliminary results of an alternative surgical technique. *Equine Veterinary Journal* 36(6):546–550.

Walker AM, Sellon DC, Cornelisse CJ, Hines MT, Ragle CA, Cohen N, Schott HC. 2002. Temporohyoid osteoarthropathy in 33 horses (1993–2000). *Journal Veterinary Internal Medicine* 16(6):697–703.

40 Surgery of the Trachea

Lloyd P. Tate, Jr

Introduction

Surgical lesions of the trachea are rare (Freeman 2005; Mair and Lane 2005; Saulez and Gummow 2009). Causes may include intra-tracheal masses or extra-tracheal trauma. Both may result in obstruction of air flow, exercise intolerance, and on rare occasions death. The most common cause is iatrogenic and occurs when tracheal rings are cut during a tracheotomy. When transected tracheal rings tend to overlap or form cicatrix as healing progresses (Figure 40.1). Less common etiologies of tracheal narrowing are crushing injuries, over inflation of endotracheal tube cuff and infection followed by granuloma formation associated with large needle puncture of the trachea (Mair and Lane 2005) (Figure 40.2).

Tracheal obstruction presents as inspiratory and expiratory stridor. It is initially subtle, but over time may progress to being audible at rest or with minimal exercise. Early recognition and diagnosis is essential to a successful resolution. When early surgical intervention is not performed, lesions may expand and luminal space may become signifi-

cantly compromised to a point that surgical reconstruction is not possible (Figure 40.3).

Diagnosis of tracheal obstruction

Diagnosis will usually include a history of trauma or a previous surgical or diagnostic procedure. Physical examination will include a cough or resentment during tracheal palpation and irregularity of one or more rings. Lateral radiographs and an endoscopic examination should be performed to ascertain the size and shape of the lesion and determine the airway diameter (Carstens et al. 2009). Computed tomography can also be used to evaluate the trachea for extraluminal and intraluminal obstruction (Wong et al. 2008). The extent of tracheal obstruction is essential in determining which surgical technique should be used, assuming that a surgery will actually be able to enlarge the horse's airway.

Severe narrowing of the trachea necessitates a temporary tracheotomy prior to reconstruction. In such circumstances, the temporary tracheotomy

Advances in Equine Upper Respiratory Surgery, First Edition. Edited by Jan Hawkins.
© 2015 ACVS Foundation. Published 2015 by John Wiley & Sons, Inc.

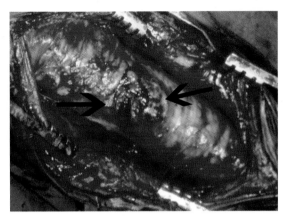

Figure 40.1   Tracheal cicatrix indicated by black arrows shown at the time of exploratory surgery resulting from disruption of two tracheal rings.

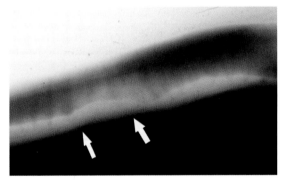

Figure 40.2   Lateral view radiograph demonstrating circumferential narrowing of the tracheal lumen involving three tracheal rings (between the two white arrows) secondary to over inflation of an endotracheal tube cuff.

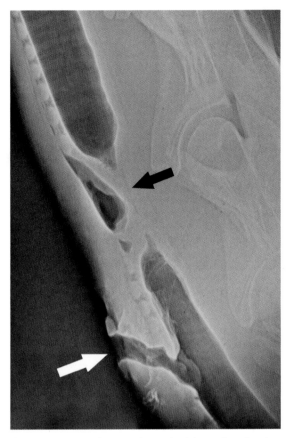

Figure 40.3   Lateral view radiograph of the trachea showing total loss of the tracheal lumen (black arrow) as a result of a chronic intraluminal abscess from a traumatic injury. A tracheal fistula (white arrow) has been maintained with a tracheotomy tube. The tube was removed so as not to obscure the extent of the lesion when the radiograph was taken.

should be performed as far distally as possible to the lesion. The same is true if the horse has a lesion that may require a permanent tracheostomy to maintain life. A granulomatous lesion in the dorsal trachea just caudal to the arytenoids can be associated with a previous prosthetic laryngoplasty and should not be treated as a primary tracheal lesion (Bienert-Zeit et al. 2013) (Figure 40.4). Similar masses occurring in the mediastinal area and bronchi frequently have an extra luminal origin and are not amenable to tracheal reconstructive procedures or endoscopic laser ablation (Figure 40.5). Primary tracheal tumors are extremely rare, and if suspected, an endoscopic biopsy should be performed

to determine the cell type. Circumferential tracheal cicatrices are rare in horses but can occur as a result of overinflated endotracheal tube cuffs. These usually involve large segments of the trachea, three to five rings (Figure 40.2), and may or may not be an indication for tracheal resection and anastomosis.

Laser ablation of tracheal masses or neoplasia

Granulomas found within the trachea can be solitary or multiple and are associated with an underlying fungal or bacterial etiology (Collins et al. 2005;

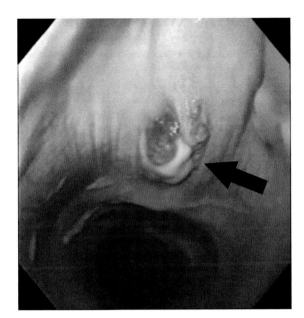

Figure 40.4   Endoscopic image of the dorsal trachea just distal to the pharynx demonstrating a suture granuloma (black arrow) associated penetration of the laryngeal lumen following prosthetic laryngoplasty.

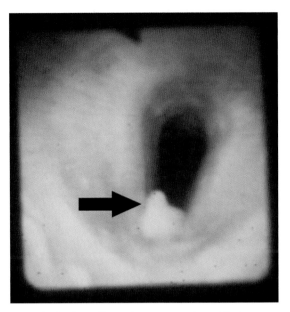

Figure 40.6   A small granuloma present (arrow) in the ventral trachea secondary to a transtracheal wash performed with a 10-gauge needle and introduction of tubing into the tracheal lumen.

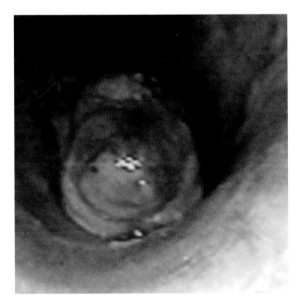

Figure 40.5   Endoscopic image of a distal tracheal mass responsible for partial airway obstruction. The mass proved to be an extra luminal squamous cell carcinoma that had eroded through the ventral floor of the trachea.

Lankveld 2001; Spanton et al. 2008). These have an irregular surface, are grey to green in color, and may bleed if the surface is disturbed. Small cicatrix lesions can be the result of needle puncture secondary to transtracheal lavage and aspiration (Figure 40.6). These are nodular in appearance and slightly lighter in color than the normal mucosa, if mature. A developing cicatrix may present as granulation tissue, being red in appearance and easily bleeding if manipulated.

Transendoscopic laser ablation can be performed using contact or noncontact techniques (Lankveld 2001). The procedure is routinely performed with the horse sedated, in standing stocks with additional topical aesthetic applied using endoscopic technique. If the procedure is to be performed under general anesthesia a low oxygen gas mixture or injectable anesthesia is required to prevent the possibility of an airway fire.

Application of contact diode or Nd:YAG laser fiber is directed at the base of the lesion. Typical contact laser settings range from 15–20 watts. The fiber is used to resect the lesion away from the tracheal mucosa creating a crater in the mucosa

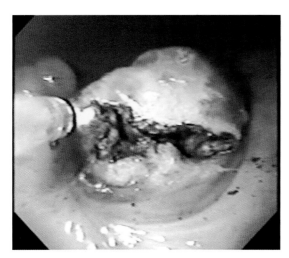

Figure 40.7   Fungal luminal tracheal granuloma being ablated with Nd:YAG laser using a noncontact fiber seen in the left side of the endoscopic picture.

just below its surface. Generally, a snare or endoscopic grasper is used to retrieve the freed tissue for histopathologic examination. Noncontact fiber ablation uses a different technique to apply laser energy. The laser is directed at the center of the lesion initially, and the center is vaporized creating a crater (Wattages ranges from 25–50 watts) (Figure 40.7). The crater is then enlarged until the lesion is reduced in size producing a mucosal deficit that is slightly below its surface. The author recommends cycling the laser on and off with 10–15 seconds between activation of the laser. This allows for smoke to be exhaled and cooling of the air and adjacent mucosa within the trachea. Some lasers, especially those used in the noncontact application, produce latent thermal necrosis. The base of lesions that do not immediately appear to vaporize should not have laser irradiation continuously directed at them. To prevent tracheal disruption to deeper layers due to the latent thermal effect, the lesion should be treated over an extended time period. There is no exact time schedule to recommend. I prefer to reapply the laser every 3–4 days and observe the damage that is produced. Similar healing should be monitored on a 7–10 day basis. Initially, the laser treated area will appear suppurative, but will then be replaced by granulation tissue. Mucosa will slowly migrate inward, and complete healing often appears as a slightly raised area in 2–4 weeks.

Surgical reconstruction of the trachea

When surgical reconstruction is necessary, aesthetic delivery is important to consider. An endotracheal tube of sufficient length is needed so that the cuff will inflate well past the location of the lesion. The tube's diameter must allow it to pass easily past the lesion. When a temporary tracheotomy has been performed, it may be necessary to direct the endotracheal tube through it in order to prevent anesthetic leakage.

Reconstruction of the trachea that involves removal of more than one ring requires that the horse become accustomed to having its head held in a flexed position (Figure 40.8) (Kirker-Head and Jakob 1990; Tate et al. 1981). The horse will have to recover from anesthesia with the head held flexed and remain so for 2 weeks post surgery. A martingale-type harness is used which is attached to the girth portion of a surcingle. This reduces the tension on the trachea and prevents the repair from being stretched. Allowing the horse to extend its head will place great tension on the repair and will result in surgical failure. The horse should wear the apparatus for 5–7 days before a planned surgery.

Prior to anesthetic induction the horse should be started on a broad spectrum antimicrobial which should continue for 5 days following surgery. To reduce tracheal secretions, Atropine Sulfate (0.01 mg/kg) can be administered 1 hour prior to surgery.

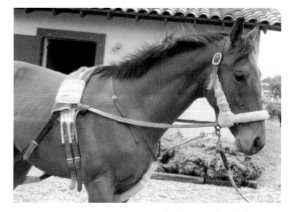

Figure 40.8   Horse wearing a surcingle combined with a martingale to maintain the head in a flexed position to acclimate to the restricted range of motion necessary for successful tracheal resection and anastomosis.

The horse is positioned in dorsal recumbency, the hair removed from the mandible to the thoracic inlet, and surgical scrub performed. Ventral midline skin incision is centered over the lesion and if reconstruction will not require the removal of any rings then a length of 25–30 cm is usually sufficient. Anastomosis after ring resection will require mobilization of as much trachea as can be reached, therefore the incision will be 40 cm or greater. The muscle bellies of the sternohyoideus and sternothyroideus are separated exposing the trachea and surrounding fascia. If an anastomosis is required, the trachea will need to be freed up from the cricoid cartilage to the thoracic inlet. This will require removing the fascia from the trachea and transecting and ligating vessels that enter the trachea, which are primarily found dorsally and on either side.

Non-anastomosis repair

Traumatic lesions to the trachea that produce abnormal tracheal conformation without intraluminal mass formation can be treated by tracheoplasty. This involves using a stent external to the trachea as a scaffolding to hold the rings in a circular formation. The scaffolds may consist of sterile polypropylene rings, stainless steel springs, or titanium mesh screens that closely match the outside diameter of the trachea (Figure 40.9) (Busschers et al. 2010; Epstein 2008; Graham et al. 2010; Mair and Lane 2005). The misshapen tracheal ring(s) are sectioned at multiple locations, taking care not to penetrate the mucosa (Figure 40.10). Segments of the ring are then sutured to the scaffold using a nonabsorbable suture. Suture should utilize a depth of half the ring cartilage, and attachment to the scaffold should be under little tension. At the conclusion of the procedure, endoscopic appearance of the trachea should closely represent a normal round lumen. Contamination from piercing the tracheal mucosa or from external sources can result in chronic drainage or luminal narrowing as a result of infection (Figure 40.11). Repairs should be monitored radiographically and by endoscopy for a year post surgery.

Tracheal collapse can also be managed with intraluminal stenting but is most commonly performed in miniature horses (Aleman et al. 2008; Couetil et al. 2004; Wong et al. 2008). Dynamic tracheal

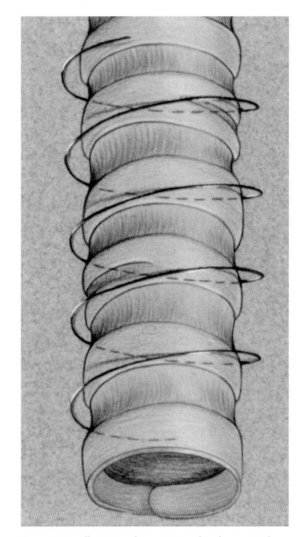

Figure 40.9   Illustration demonstrating the placement of a stainless steel spring in close contact to the tracheal rings to be used as a scaffold for a tracheoplasty.

collapse can also cause exercise intolerance during exercise (Tetens et al. 2000).

Tracheal resection and anastomosis

Tracheal ring resection and anastomosis case selection should include horses with dramatic tracheal narrowing from external trauma and those that present with intraluminal lesions causing airway obstruction (Robertson and Spurlock 1986; Tate

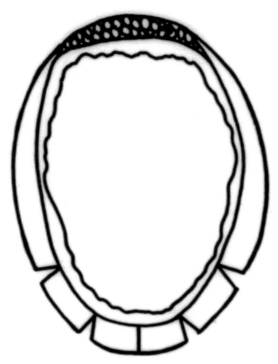

Figure 40.10   Diagram depicting multiple cuts sectioning a trachea ring in preparation to having tracheoplasty performed to reconstruct its normal conformation.

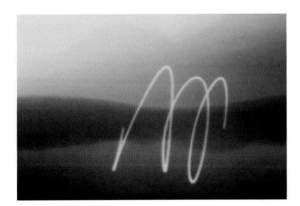

Figure 40.11   Lateral view radiograph of the trachea taken 4 months after tracheoplasty surgery showing extra luminal and intraluminal thickening attributed to infection caused by sutures being placed through the tracheal mucosa during the procedure in which a stainless steel spring was used as a scaffold. The spring also does not conform to the external diameter of the trachea which contributes to the thickening seen by causing physical irritation.

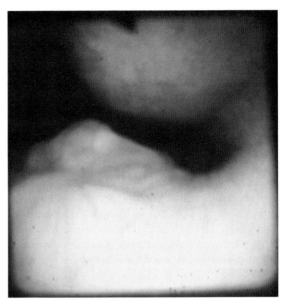

Figure 40.12   Endoscopic image indicating narrowing of the tracheal lumen of a horse with tracheal ring overlap from the cutting of tracheal rings and accompanying cicatrix formation.

et al. 1981). These include, but are not restricted to cicatrix formation, tumors, and cartilage ring overlap from ring cutting from a previous tracheotomy (Figure 40.12). In most instances, usually just one to two rings are involved. Suture tension following five-ring resection, is double of that following three-ring resection; thus the possibility of repair failure is greatly increased.

In order to mobilize the entire trachea, an incision is made over it from the cricoid cartilage to the thoracic inlet. A horse's trachea has a good collateral vascular supply arising from the proximal arteries and feed from the inferior thyroid artery and distally from the bronchial arteries. Vessels entering the tracheal segment on either side and dorsally can be ligated and transected as the trachea is separated from its surrounding fascia. After the entire trachea has been mobilized, ring(s) to be resected are identified. Traction sutures that will be used to manipulate the proximal and distal tracheal segments once rings have been removed and prevent the tracheal mucosa from tearing are then applied. Four traction sutures consisting of No. 2 absorbable suture material are placed around the ventral tracheal ring two rings proximal to the planned resection site and two in a similar location distally (Figure 40.13). The

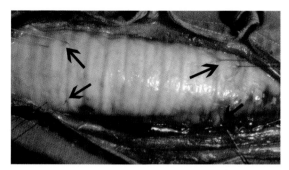

Figure 40.13   Four large stay sutures (arrows) are placed around tracheal rings to allow easy manipulation of the ends when cut and to prevent over separation.

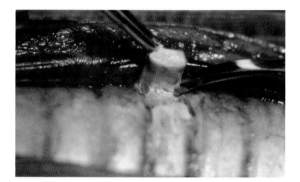

Figure 40.14   Bisected tracheal ring being elevated away from the tracheal mucosa.

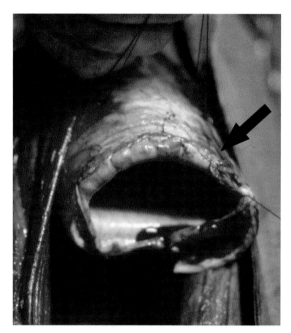

Figure 40.15   Photograph demonstrates the tracheal mucosa being folded back over the edge of the tracheal ring (arrow) as it is sutured in place.

resection is initiated by bisecting a tracheal ring on its ventral surface. This is performed on a normal tracheal ring on either side of the tracheal ring or rings to be removed. The ends of the bisected cartilage are elevated and separated from its mucosa using sharp scissors (Figure 40.14). In performing the bisection of the rings and elevating them, care is taken not to pierce or cut the mucosa. Similarly, the inflated cuff of the endotracheal tube should not be situated at this location. The head, if it has not been flexed to the 90° position, should be at this time, to reduce tension on the trachea. The lesion is resected by cutting the mucosa 360° immediately adjacent to the cartilages to be removed. A sterilized endotracheal tube is then inserted into the distal trachea to maintain anesthesia. The freed tracheal mucosa is folded back over the next tracheal ring and sutured to the adventitia using 2-0 or 3-0 absorbable suture in a continuous pattern (Fig-

ure 40.15). The traction sutures are used to approximate the two ends of the trachea, and the first endotracheal tube is passed distally after the second one has been removed. ASIF reduction forceps or four Bacchus towel clamps that were previously heated, and tips spread and resterilized, are used to hold the ends of the trachea in apposition (Figure 40.16). Anastomosis is completed using 25-gauge stainless steel wire suture swaged to a curved cutting needle using a simple interrupted pattern. Sutures are first placed on the dorsal portion where the cartilage is the thinnest. The suture pattern encompasses half the thickness of the tracheal cartilages. In performing placement care is taken not to pierce the mucosa except where it had been folded back over the tracheal ring. The anastomosis is completed by placing sutures 0.5–1 cm apart for 360°. The anastomosis is examined for air leaks by flooding the surgical area with saline and pulling the endotracheal tube proximal to the anastomosis while the horse is ventilated. Areas of leakage identified by air bubbles can be further tightened with additional interrupted or cruciate sutures. The sutures used for manipulating the tracheal ends can be removed or

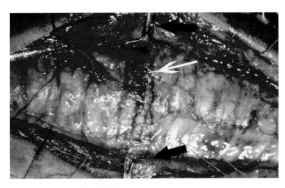

Figure 40.16   Tracheal rings with the mucosa folded over their edges to provide an air seal are held in place by Bacchus towel clamps (black arrow). The ends of the towel clamp have had their ends spread to better appose the tracheal ends. Stainless steel sutures (white arrows) are used to secure the anastomosis.

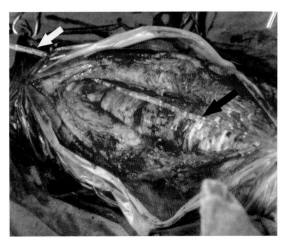

Figure 40.17   Completed tracheal anastomosis with a fenestrated drain in place (arrow) which exits through the skin ventral to the initial incision.

tied proximal to distal to be used as tension sutures. This is required if more than three tracheal rings have been removed. A continuous suction drain is placed next to the trachea and maintained for 3–4 days following surgery (Figure 40.17). The muscle bellies of the sternothyroideus and sternohyoideus are closed, followed by subcutaneous tissue and skin. The head is kept in the flexed orientation and the martingale apparatus is refitted for recovery. The horse will need to wear it for 3 weeks post surgery and receive broad-spectrum antimicrobials

for 5–7 days. The surgical wound is monitored for signs of infection and seroma formation once the drain is removed. The anastomosis is monitored by endoscopy and/or lateral radiographs for disruption and tracheal narrowing. Using endoscopy, it is often possible to visualize small buds of granulation tissue as they form along the anastomosis site. These tend to appear 10–14 days post surgery and generally remain small and insignificant. The horse should be stall rested and hand walked for an additional 3 weeks. With a successful anastomosis and re-establishment of a stable airway diameter, the horse can resume normal exercise after 60 days.

References

Aleman M, Nieto JE, Benak J, Johnson LR. 2008. Tracheal collapse in American Miniature Horses: 13 cases (1985–2007). *Journal of the American Veterinary Medical Association* 233(8):1302–1306.

Bienert-Zeit A, Roetting A, Reichert C, Ohnesorge B. 2013. Laryngeal fistula formation after laryngoplasty in two Warmblood mares. *Equine Veterinary Education* 26(2):88–92.

Busschers E, Epstein KL, Holt DE, Parente EJ. 2010. Extraluminal C shaped polyethylene prostheses in two ponies with tracheal collapse. *Veterinary Surgery* 39(6):776–783.

Carstens A, Kirberger RM, Grimbeek RJ, Donnellan CM, Saulez MN. 2009. Radiographic quantification of tracheal dimensions of the normal Thoroughbred horse. *Veterinary Radiology and Ultrasound* 50(5):492–501.

Collins NM, Barakzai SZ, Dixon PM. 2005. Tracheal obstruction by an eosinophilic polyp in a horse. *Equine Veterinary Education* 17(3):128–131.

Couetil LL, Gallatin LL, Blevins W, Khandra I. 2004. Treatment of tracheal collapse with an intraluminal stent in a miniature horse. *Journal of the American Veterinary Medical Association* 225:1727–1732.

Epstein K. 2008. Clinical commentary: Tracheal collapse: Are there other options for treatment? *Equine Veterinary Education* 20(2)91–92.

Freeman DE. 2005. Surgery for obstruction of the equine oesophagus and trachea. *Equine Veterinary Education* 17(3):135–141.

Graham SB, Schilpp D, Bradley WM, Cook G, Gayle J. 2010. Treatment of traumatic tracheal collapse with extraluminal titanium mesh screens. *Equine Veterinary Education* 22(11):557–563.

Kirker-Head CA, Jakob TP. 1990. Surgical repair of ruptured trachea in a horse. *Journal of the American Veterinary Medical Association* 196(10):1635–1638.

Lankveld DPK. 2001. Tracheal obstruction by an eosino-philic granuloma in a horse: Surgical and Nd:YAG laser treatment. *Equine Veterinary Education* 13(6):309–312.

Mair TS, Lane JG. 2005. Diseases of the equine trachea. *Equine Veterinary Education* 17(3):146–149.

Robertson JT, Spurlock GH. 1986. Tracheal reconstruction in a foal. *Journal of the American Veterinary Medical Association* 259:313–314.

Saulez MN, Gummow B. 2009. Prevalence of pharyngeal, laryngeal and tracheal disorders in thoroughbred race-horses, and effect on performance. *Veterinary Record* 165:431–435.

Spanton JA, Henderson ISF, Krudewig C, Mair TS. 2008. Tracheal rupture in a native pony mare associated with

a condition resembling tracheobronchopathia ostech-ondroplastica. *Equine Veterinary Education* 20(11):582–586.

Tate LP Jr, Koch DB, Sembrat RF, Boles CL. 1981. Tracheal reconstruction by resection and end-to-end anastomo-sis in the horse. *Journal of the American Veterinary Medical Association* 178(3):253–258.

Tetens J, Hubert JD, Eddy AL, Moore RM. 2000. Dynamic tracheal collapse as a cause of exercise intolerance in a Thoroughbred. *Journal of the American Veterinary Medical Association* 216(5):722–724.

Wong DM, Sponseller BA, Riedesel EA, Couetil LL, Kersh K. 2008. The use of intraluminal stents for tracheal col-lapse in two horses: Case management and long-term treatment. *Equine Veterinary Education* 20(2):80–90.

41 Permanent Tracheostomy in the Horse

Peter C. Rakestraw

Indications

Disorders such as recurrent laryngeal neuropathy, arytenoid chondritis, subepiglottic cysts, epiglottic entrapment, and dorsal displacement of soft palate are commonly encountered in horses that have upper airway disease. In all of these conditions the cross-sectional area of a portion of the airway, usually pharynx or larynx, is compromised resulting in decreased airflow. Often the abnormality becomes clinically significant only at exercise. In the majority of these cases, surgical correction specifically addresses the area of compromise and attempts to correct that abnormality. There are certain conditions, however, in which the lesion causes such severe stenosis of the upper airway that surgical correction of that lesion is met with guarded or poor long-term prognosis. For horses with those types of problems, permanent tracheostomy should be considered (Chesen and Rakestraw 2008; McClure et al. 1995; Rakestraw 2003; Rakestraw et al. 2000; Shappell et al. 1988).

The most common upper airway abnormalities requiring permanent tracheostomy are related to the nasopharyngeal cicatrix syndrome (Chesen and Rakestraw 2008; McClure et al. 1995; Rakestraw 2003; Rakestraw et al. 2000; Shappell et al. 1988). Horses with this syndrome often have scar tissue that forms primarily in the pharynx and larynx. The developing scar tissue is first seen on the lateral aspect of the pharynx as thin, elevated strips of white tissue that extend ventral to the pharyngeal openings of the guttural pouch and across the soft plate underneath where the tip of the epiglottis rests on the soft palate. In more severe cases the scar tissue extends over the dorsal pharynx resulting in a complete circular web of tissue. Arytenoid chondritis is commonly associated with the generalized inflammatory process involved in the development of this syndrome. In some cases the arytenoid chondritis is the predominant abnormality seen on endoscopic examination, with little pharyngeal scarring observed (Chesen and Rakestraw 2008; Rakestraw 2003; Rakestraw et al. 2000). While early stages of the disease can be treated medically, more advanced stages require a permanent tracheotomy. Surgical resection of the diseased cartilage or laser resection of the scar tissue have met with limited success due to continuation of inflammatory process as the horse is put back into the same environment with continued pharyngeal and laryngeal swelling, scar tissue formation, and subsequent airway compromise (Dean and Cohen 1990; Schumacher and Hanselka 1987). Permanent tracheotomy effectively bypasses the nasopharynx providing an alternative route for airflow. Other indications for permanent tracheotomy are neoplasia, persistent dorsal displacement of the soft palate, bilateral arytenoid chondritis not associated with cicatrix, fourth branchial arch defects, and severe deformity of the nasal passage or any condition of the upper airway that significantly restricts airflow and is not amenable to medical treatment or other types of surgical correction.

Tracheotomy technique

The surgery can be performed on the standing horse or with the horse anesthetized and positioned in dorsal recumbency (Chesen and Rakestraw 2008; McClure et al. 1995; Shappell et al. 1988). In most cases the standing position is preferred, as this eliminates the cost and potential complications associated with general anesthesia. There is also less distortion of the tissue planes relative to one another when the procedure is done in the standing horse compared to the anesthetized horse. A greater degree of head extension in either the standing sedated horse or the anesthetized horse will cause greater displacement of the trachea relative to the skin. If the stoma is made with this distortion there will be increased tension on the surgical site when the horse assumes its normal head position after the surgery, increasing the risk of dehiscence. In some horses a temporary tracheotomy is required to allow the horse an adequate airway before and during the surgery. The temporary tracheotomy sites should be far enough down the neck that it does not overlap the area where the permanent tracheostomy site is made. If the temporary tracheotomy site has already been placed too high to prevent overlap, the temporary tracheostomy site can be incorporated into the ventral aspect of the permanent tracheostomy site (Chesen and Rakestraw 2008).

Procaine penicillin G (20 000 IU/kg, IM), gentamicin sulfate (6.6 mg/kg IV), and flunixin meglumine (1.1 mg/kg, IV) are administered prior to surgery. The horse is placed in stocks and sedated with detomidine (0.02 mg/kg, half dose given IV

and the other half IM). Butorphanol tartrate (0.01–0.02 mg/kg, IV) is sometimes used but may cause twitching in some horses. Once the horse appears sedate, a dental halter is placed on the head and the horse is positioned forward in the stocks with the head and neck extended in front of the side poles of the stocks. Maintenance of this position is facilitated by attaching cross ties from the two side bars to the dental halter as well as suspending the head from a bar (if available) extending forward from the top of the stocks. The portion of the halter in contact with the mandible should have appropriate padding to prevent facial nerve paralysis. This positioning allows a surgeon seated in front of the stocks access to the surgical area.

The surgical area is clipped and aseptically prepared. The surgical site is centered over tracheal rings two through six. Local anesthesia is infiltrated subcutaneously in an inverted-U pattern dorsal and lateral to the surgical site. The underlying muscle is also infiltrated with local anesthesia. Starting approximately 3 cm distal to the cricoid and centered over midline, a 4-cm wide × 7-cm long elliptical segment of skin and subcutaneous tissue are removed. The underlying paired sternothyrohyoideus muscles are separated on the midline, dissected laterally from the surrounding tissue, and isolated for the length of the incision. It is often necessary to inject additional local anesthetic into these deeper muscles before transecting them. The muscle bellies are isolated and clamped (Ferguson Angiotribe Forceps; Miltex, Lake Success, NY) at their proximal and distal exposure in the incision. The forceps are left in place for several minutes to crush the vessels and allow for clot formation once the vessel has been crushed. The forceps are then removed and the muscle is transected. A 3-cm wide segment on the medial aspect of each omohyoideus muscle is next dissected from the parent muscle along the length of the incision and removed in a similar manner. Removal of these muscles decreases the amount of soft tissue around the border of the stoma which helps prevent future collapse of the stoma during exercise (Chesen and Rakestraw 2008; Rakestraw et al. 2000).

Dissection of the tracheal rings from the tracheal submucosa/mucosa can be challenging. Careful excision of the facial tissue that overlies the cartilaginous rings allows the rings to be more easily elevated off and dissected from the underlying tracheal submucosa/mucosa. Taking care not to

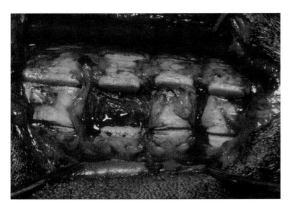

Figure 41.1   Division of four tracheal rings into segments. The segments are then carefully dissected from the tracheal mucosa using a combination of sharp and blunt dissection.

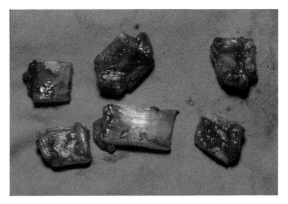

Figure 41.2   Dissected segments of tracheal cartilage removed in preparation for permanent tracheostomy.

penetrate through the tracheal mucosa, the most proximal tracheal ring is cut at its midline along its entire width using a No. 15 blade. It helps to squeeze the sides of the tracheal ring together to force the ventral aspect (the midline) to protrude out and away from the underlying submucosa/mucosa. Once the cut is complete and the two sides are separate, tissue forceps or small penetrating towel clamps are used to grasp and elevate one side of the cut border of the tracheal ring. With careful dissection, staying close to the underside of the tracheal ring, the cartilage ring is dissected off the submucosa/mucosa for approximately 1.5 cm abaxial to the midline cut (Figure 41.1). This segment of cartilage is transected by cutting from the inside to outside of the elevated cartilage. This process is repeated on the other side of the incised ring. This leaves a gap in the cartilage at the most ventral aspect of the ring approximately 3 cm wide. Approximately one-third of the ring is removed. The same surgical excision of cartilage is continued for the remaining four rings.

A variation of the above technique is to make the three parallel incisions in each tracheal ring before each segment of cartilage is removed (Figure 41.2) (Chesen and Rakestraw 2008; McClure et al. 1995; Shappell et al. 1988). In the author's opinion, this increases the risk of penetration of the mucosa at the abaxial borders of the incisions. In general the author removes five rings but this may range from four to seven rings. The tracheal rings may vary in width and in the proximity of spacing which influences how many rings are

removed in order to get an adequate stoma. The tracheal mucosa can be desensitized by injecting 30 mL of 2% lidocaine hydrochloride into the tracheal lumen at the most proximal part of the surgical area and let it flow ventrally over the mucosa, although in most cases this is not necessary. In some cases, before making the incision into the mucosa, the dead space can be reduced by suturing tracheal fascia abaxial to the removed tracheal cartilage to the subcutaneous tissue using a simple interrupted pattern with absorbable sutures. This step is not felt to improve the outcome significantly and consequently often not performed. The tracheal mucosa is then incised longitudinally as a simple linear incision or with a double "Y" incision (Figure 41.3). For the double "Y" incision the central midline incision ends approximately one tracheal ring width before the rostral and caudal ends

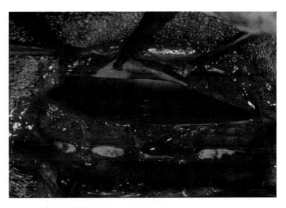

Figure 41.3   Retraction of tracheal mucosa prior to suturing of the tracheal mucosa to the skin.

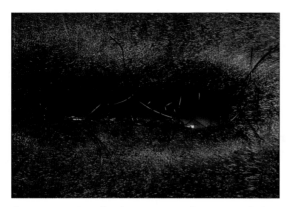

Figure 41.4   Completed permanent tracheostomy with the horse positioned in dorsal recumbency.

of the exposed tracheal mucosa. The midline incision is extended as a "V" with each leg connecting to the corners of one end of the exposed rectangular section of tracheal mucosa. The tracheal mucosa is then sutured to the skin using simple interrupted sutures of 0 polydioxanone or 0 or 2-0 polyglactin 910 (Figure 41.4). It is best to reconstruct the proximal and distal ends of the stoma first in order to have minimal tension on the tracheal mucosa/submucosa during this part of the procedure.

Aftercare

Horses are maintained on procaine penicillin (22 000 IU/kg, BID, IM) and flunixin meglumine (1.1 mg/kg, IV) for 5 days after surgery. Once flunixin meglumine is discontinued, they are often placed on phenylbutazone (2.2 mg/kg, BID, PO) for 3–5 days depending on the amount of swelling. The discharge around the stoma should be cleaned twice daily with a clean moist paper towel taking care not to disturb the sutures. The discharge will decrease significantly over a 3–4 week period and then more slowly over the next several months. After several weeks the stoma will only need to be cleaned once a day and eventually only periodically as needed. Postoperatively we recommend stall confinement for 3 weeks. The sutures should be removed in 2 weeks.

It is important to make sure the horse is kept in a stall that does not have any object protruding that would allow the horse to get its neck over and rub the incision. Until the incision is healed, the horse should be fed at a level where it does not have to extend its neck down or up to eat. They can be walked during the recovery period but should not be allowed to graze until the incision is healed. Once the incision is healed the only restriction on management is not turning them out in an area where they might swim!

Complications

Short term: The most common short-term postoperative complications are partial dehiscence (10% before discharge; 5% after discharge), transient fever (12%), and excessive swelling (16%) (Chesen and Rakestraw 2008; McClure et al. 1995). There is likely to be a cause and effect relationship between the excessive swelling and partial dehiscence. It is the author's opinion that the excessive swelling is either due to poor hemostasis during the surgical technique or from a postoperative infection. In order to decrease the occurrence of a hematoma forming around the incision, the surgeon should attend to any intraoperative bleeding. Adequate clamping of the resected muscles and ligation of any bleeders in the muscle or in the fascia removed around the tracheal rings will normally prevent hematoma formation. In order to decrease the risk of postoperative infection, we have changed our use of antibiotics from prophylactic to therapeutic for this procedure. The author does not like inserting drains at the time of the surgery as this can introduce contamination into the area. If sutures are pulled out of the repair due to excessive tension, replacement of some of these sutures with larger sutures or mattress sutures, particularly at the edge of the area dehiscing in order to reinforce it, will often allow the wound to heal without further problems. Since dehiscence may occur up to 10–14 days postoperatively, it is important to monitor horses closely in the short term in order to address the dehiscence and attempt to minimize it. If significant infection occurs, the stoma can be modified once the infection clears. In a few cases we have left a large tracheostomy tube in place until second intention healing has occurred.

Long term: The most common long-term complications are inversion of the skin edges around the stoma (3%) or stenosis of the stoma (1%) (Chesen and Rakestraw 2008; McClure et al. 1995; Rakestraw et al. 2000; Shappell et al. 1988). Inversion of the skin edge may occur because not enough muscle (sternohyoideus, sternothyroideus, or omohyoideus) was removed or the section of tracheal cartilage resected was either too much or not enough. Removal of a section of the omohyoideus muscle and a wedge-shaped section of skin lateral to each side of the stoma seems to correct most of the cases with collapsing or inverting skin edges. For stenosis of the stoma and occasionally for inversion of the skin edges the lateral borders of stoma can be opened and the cartilage exposed. Removal of additional cartilage will widen the incision. In some cases, if only one side of the stoma is opened and the rings shortened, it allows the stomal edges to be at different levels. When this occurs the edges are further apart and less likely to invert or collapse during inspiration. Other reported long-term complications are low-grade cough at exercise (17%), respiratory noise at exercise (11%), and intermittent episodes of respiratory distress (6%) (Chesen and Rakestraw 2008). We have not recognized an increased risk of pneumonia secondary to decreased filtration and humidification of inspired air. Since most of the reported cases have been performed in horses living in a relatively warm environment, it is possible that horses living in a cold environment may have more trouble.

Prognosis

The prognosis for long-term survival is excellent. Most horses can return to normal use following a permanent tracheotomy. Although many of the horses in the retrospective studies have been used as broodmares, many others have been used for pleasure riding and various Western performance activities. A small number of performance horses will have a mild cough at the beginning of exercise, but this does not appear to affect their performance. In the majority of cases (89–98%) owner satisfaction with permanent tracheostomy is high. It should be remembered that it is illegal in the United States to race a horse with a permanent tracheostomy.

References

Chesen AB, Rakestraw PC. 2008. Indications for and short- and long-term outcome of permanent tracheostomy performed in standing horses: 82 cases (1995–2005). *Journal of the American Veterinary Medical Association* 232:1–5.

Dean PW, Cohen ND. 1990. Arytenoidectomy for advanced unilateral chondropathy with accompanying lesions. *Veterinary Surgery* 19:364–370.

McClure SR, Taylor TS, Honnas CM, Schumacher J, Chaffin MK, Hoffman AG. 1995. Permanent tracheostomy in standing horses: Technique and results. *Veterinary Surgery* 24:231–234.

Rakestraw PC. 2003. Equine nasopharyngeal cicatrix syndrome. *Proceedings of the Texas A&M University Annual Equine Conference* 40–43.

Rakestraw PC, Eastman TG, Taylor TS, Schumacher J, Wright L. 2000. Long-term outcome of horses undergoing permanent tracheostomy: 42 cases. *Proceedings of the American Association of Equine Practitioners* 46:111–112.

Schumacher J, Hanselka DV. 1987. Nasopharyngeal cicatrices in horses: 47 cases (1972–1985). *Journal of the American Veterinary Medical Association* 191:239–242.

Shappell KK, Stick JA, Derksen FJ, Scott EA. 1988. Permanent tracheostomy in equidae: 47 cases (1981–1988). *Veterinary Surgery* 192:939–942.

Index

Advances in Equine Upper Respiratory Surgery, First Edition. Edited by Jan Hawkins.
© 2015 ACVS Foundation. Published 2015 by John Wiley & Sons, Inc.